DATE DUE	
MAR 0 2 2006	
GAYLORD	PRINTED IN U.S.A.

Nutrition in the community
The art of delivering services

Nutrition in the community
The art of delivering services

REVA T. FRANKLE, M.S., Ed.D., R.D.

Director of Nutrition, Weight Watchers International, Inc., Manhasset, New York;
formerly Coordinator, Nutrition Division, Department of Community Medicine,
Mount Sinai School of Medicine of the City University of New York;
Instructor and Field Supervisor, Program in Nutrition, Columbia University Teachers College;
Public Health Nutritionist, Bureau of Nutrition,
New York City Department of Health

ANITA YANOCHIK OWEN, M.A., R.D.

Nutrition Consultant, Office of Nutrition,
Michigan Department of Public Health, Lansing;
Lecturer in Nutrition, Human Nutrition Program,
University of Michigan School of Public Health, Ann Arbor, Michigan;
formerly Assistant Director for Community Health Services and Chief,
Bureau of Nutrition, Arizona Department of Health Services,
Phoenix, Arizona

with 49 illustrations

The C. V. Mosby Company

Saint Louis   1978

The C. V. Mosby Company
11830 Westline Industrial Drive, St. Louis, Missouri 63141

Library of Congress Cataloging in Publication Data

Frankle, Reva T.
    Nutrition in the community.

    Bibliography: p.
    Includes index.
    1. Nutrition policy. I. Owen, Anita
Yanochik, 1937-   joint author. II. Title.
[DNLM: 1. Nutrition. 2. Community health
services—United States. QU145.3 F83In]
TX359.F7   362.5   78-9144
ISBN 0-8016-1666-2

GW/CB/B 9 8 7 6 5 4 3 2 1

Foreword

Community nutrition has many health and social benefits to offer contemporary society. Its potential is staggering. Malnutrition as a public health problem can be virtually eliminated through modalities such as multimedia nutrition education efforts, economic aid and food programs for low-income groups, well-designed preschool and school lunch programs, special efforts for groups at high risk of malnutrition such as adolescents and the elderly, and continuing concern to progressively lower the unemployment rate. The developmental and behavioral defects that may result from fetal and infant malnutrition can be tragedies of the past if all children are given the opportunity to fulfill their God-given genetic potential through optimal nutritional status coupled with social and academic environments that favor psychological and intellectual growth and development.

What is equally as urgent and dramatic are the nutritional determinants of chronic diseases that have now been identified. And as the American diet progresses in its evolution, nutrition will continue to play an important role in blunting the epidemics of coronary heart disease, stroke, diabetes, and perhaps certain cancers. Newer knowledge derived from the basic and clinical nutrition sciences that relate to optimal levels of calories, proteins, various lipids, simple and complex carbohydrates, fiber, trace minerals, vitamins, and the metabolic aspects of alcohol and drugs as they interact with nutrients will provide the data base, opening new therapeutic avenues for the control of obesity, nutritional anemias, the hyperlipidemias, and the malnutrition associated with the public health nutritional problems posed by alcohol and drug abuse.

Provocative issues immediately surface: should the public health nutritionist have a solid foundation in clinical nutrition and the behavioral sciences before embarking on a career in community nutrition? New issues face today's community nutritionist. Can "hospital malnutrition" be solved among the elderly living in long-term care facilities? Can nutritional regimens be designed to meet the specific requirements of persons receiving chemotherapy for cancer? What new dietary recommendations may emerge from the Multiple Risk Factor Intervention Trial (MRFIT)?

But new nutritional regimens to meet the needs of preventive and therapeutic medicine require the knowledge and skills provided by the behavioral sciences. Cultural anthropology, psychology, and sociology are examples of disciplines in which the community nutritionist must be trained. How to effect behavioral changes that reverse nutritional risk factors of chronic disease indeed remains a basic problem of preventive health care.

However, the problems of community health are also its fascinations. Commitment and patience for the people to be served, the ability to communicate with colleagues of other disciplines who comprise the contemporary health care unit, adeptness in attracting political and administrative support for community nutrition programs, the ability to project energy and faith in long-term goals that often appear blocked by seemingly impregnable short-term barriers—these are

vii

just some of the special virtues required of the community nutritionist.

Reva T. Frankle and Anita Yanochik Owen have the contemporary experience, judgment, and enthusiastic realism to discuss community nutrition. They are fully cognizant of new currents in community nutrition and bravely depart from some of the stale precepts of yesterday's public health and community medicine methodologies and objectives. They summarize and interpret the major public health, political, legislative, administrative, and academic advances of the past decade and show how current knowledge can inject fresh goals and methods for the design of nutrition programs of the present and future. The authors also provide guidelines for approaching the community nutritional problems of special groups such as migrant workers and drug addicts and also include nutritional status assessments criteria and methodologies that can be used by all categories of health workers. The importance of budgeting, lobbying skills, and grantsmanship—almost never or weakly mentioned in previous texts—is given the recognition it deserves.

Here indeed is new, heady community nutrition "wine" in a sturdy new "bottle." It is capable of preparing the health worker—from municipal medical officer to community aide—in utilizing available nutrition knowledge to sharply reduce illness, disability, and death from both malnutrition of deficiency and excess.

GEORGE CHRISTAKIS, M.D., M.P.H.
Nutrition Division,
Department of Epidemiology and Public Health,
University of Miami School of Medicine

Preface

Several years ago when I became involved in the teaching of community nutrition to graduate nutrition students, as well as first- and second-year medical students, I was surprised to learn that there was no text available. There were journal articles and occasional chapters in books but not a single text to guide the teacher and student alike in pulling together the subject of community nutrition. As a member of the Department of Community Medicine of a new medical school, I saw my colleagues also struggling without a text for the teaching of community medicine. However, in addition to the classroom, we did have the laboratory field setting —the community.

We were concerned with the community —its diagnoses, health needs, on-going programs, need for new programs, priorities, and program planning, implementation, and evaluation. Students were placed in a field setting for a two-month period of block time during which they actually *did* plan, implement, and evaluate a program. Much enthusiasm was engendered by those placed in the Arizona State Department of Health for their two-month experience. For this reason I called on Anita Yanochik Owen, nutritionist and at that time assistant director, Community Health Services, Arizona State Department of Health, a former classmate and friend, to be the coauthor of a text that would meet the needs of students, teachers, and practitioners alike—a reference book that the student could use years later when assigned the task of designing and working in community nutrition programs. In her position she worked closely with community health services that were related to nutrition, nursing, and dental programs. As president of the Association of State and Territorial Public Health Nutritionists, she was aware of nutrition in public health programing across the country. She knew the concerns of the practicing nutritionist. As chairwoman of the National WIC-LIT Committee she sparked legislative action across the country.

From my attendance at meetings held by the Association of Faculties for Graduate Training in Public Health Nutrition and the Association of State and Territorial Public Health Nutrition Directors, I realized that no single formula had been developed for teaching community nutrition or for practicing community and public health nutrition. Some departments of graduate nutrition education have established programs wherein the student visits and perhaps works in a variety of settings that already have several types of community nutrition programs in operation. Another alternative is the placement of students in a specific community for the express purpose of studying the community as one would study a patient. Here students are encouraged to view the community as an ecological system with multiple subsystems but, while doing so, to adapt basic approaches to the cultural group with which they are working.

Since the mid-1960s, programs involving nutrition services have originated: Project Head Start; Maternal and Infant Care; Women, Infants, and Children Supplementary Feeding Programs; and, in addition, Food Commodities and Food Stamp Programs. New legislation such as The Child Nutrition

Act and Comprehensive Health Planning Acts with the involvement of health maintenance organizations further spurred nutrition services at the community level. Individual rights to health care and services for minority groups became law.

Simultaneously, new problems blighted the community; with the apparently less restrictive "hippie" scene came increased drug abuse and alcoholism. It was apparent that major medical problems of heart disease, obesity, alcoholism, hypertension, drug abuse, emotional disorders, and many chronic medical complaints rampant in communities could no longer be served effectively by the individual approach. Tools of community nutrition—epidemiology and biostatistics—helped to identify problems of population groups.

Prevention and life-style became keywords. Improvement of the health of populations required changing the way people lived —persuading them to modify their habits became the goal of health care. The skills needed to teach or change these habits had to be included in the educational programs for health personnel.

The community approach is by no means limited to activities of nutritionists and dietitians. Community nursing, community pharmacy, community pediatrics, community mental health, and community medicine are terms which illustrate the fact that the community was rediscovered simultaneously by other disciplines within the medical team. Some professionals have maintained that community health is not a discipline or even an area of interest but rather a social movement that also will pass. Others, in contrast, regard it as a discipline that matches other health specialties in scientific rigor. Although the Expert Committee of the World Health Organization emphasized the relevance of the study of the community to the medical student, their findings can apply as well to the nutrition student:

The education of every physician should . . . enable him . . . to understand how factors affecting health can be examined and measured and to discern the practical steps that can be taken to counteract hazards; he should know enough about the economics and priorities of public health programs, at both the local and national levels, to recognize when the local community must make important decisions and when the national cost of health services must be balanced against those of other community services. He should understand how health services operate and are related to one another, the principles governing the delivery of medical care, what parts are played by auxiliaries and other health workers, and the effects of culture on the demands for services and of the use made of them when they are provided. (The use of health service facilities in medical education, World Health Organization Technical Report Series, 1967, p. 355.)

Regardless of the method used in teaching this subject in classroom and community, it is essential to know the community and its demographic data, people, health problems, resources, and current programs. It is essential to know the art of program planning, implementation, and evaluation.

We humbly believe that our backgrounds and experiences, particularly ideas and services generated as a result of our many years in government and higher education administration, as well as teaching the public and student populations, place us in a position where we may be able to make a contribution toward solving the dilemma of the college student and the practitioner.

A work of this kind necessarily involves the assistance and expertise of many people —far too many, in fact, to make it possible for us to express our thanks individually to them in this volume. But we would be derelict, indeed, if we did not publicly acknowledge the help and encouragement of others, especially our contributing authors:

George M. Owen, M.D., Director, Human Nutrition Program, University of Michigan School of Public Health; Professor of Pediatrics, University of Michigan School of Medicine, Ann Arbor, Michigan

James Rye, M.S., R.D., Training Coordinator, Bureau of Nutrition Services, Arizona State Department of Health Services, Phoenix, Arizona

Alan Stone, Legislative Assistant to Senator George McGovern; formerly Staff Director, U.S. Senate Select Committee on Nutrition and Human Needs, Washington, D.C.

Morissa White, M.P.H., R.D., Chief, Bureau of Nutrition Services, Arizona State Department of Health Services, Phoenix, Arizona

Many of the ideas that led to the development of the community nutrition delivery system, which this book covers, were a result of the hard work of its pioneers, Carol Eichleberger, Sheryl Lee, Alice Shoemaker, and Janet Mastin, who worked with Anita Y. Owen in developing the system from its initial stages. This system herein described is now an integral part of the Arizona health care system because of the dynamic leadership of Morissa White, Chief of the Bureau of Nutrition Services; James Rye, Training Coordinator; and Philip Abadie, WIC Coordinator.

A very special notation must be made to Gladys Werner and Harriett Fanning, whose combined efforts contributed to the final draft of this text; and to Lorna Harkus, who acted as a mediator between the two authors, blending our styles and ideas. Anita would like to pay a special tribute to her husband, George, for his guidance, keen mind, and patience. And I would like to pay a special tribute to my many students—both nutrition and medical students—especially Lorelei King Groll and Kati McCloy, Phil Luloff,

M.D., and Alan Engelberg, M.D.—whose inquiries sparked precious moments of truth and taught me to continue learning with them; they gave me the courage to dare to be innovative.

We are most fortunate to have a Foreword written by our distinguished colleague, George Christakis, M.D., who has designed many innovative community nutrition programs in which graduate students—of nutrition, medicine, social work, nursing, and health education—all learned together. It is he who taught me that community nutrition is not only a subject to be studied and debated but also a method for accomplishing social ends, a means by which rational action can take the place of rhetoric. Community nutrition is not merely the practice of nutrition in the community; it is a discipline that requires a precise definition of health problems and a specific commitment to examine them and treat them in light of the full scope of their implications. When it fails to do this, when it becomes a tool of public pacification, confusion and discouragement follow.

REVA T. FRANKLE

Contents

GENERAL CONCEPT

Adequate food and sound nutrition are essential to good health, crucial for human survival, key factors in prevention and recovery from illness, prerequisites for improving the quality of life, and fundamental needs for all members of society. It is the responsibility of government at all levels to take the initiative to create an appropriate nutritional atmosphere; it is the responsibility of the public to take personal concern in their own health.

OUTCOMES

The student should be able to do the following:
- Review the politics of nutrition in the United States.
- List the nutrition problems of the 1970s and the effect of individual life-styles.
- Discuss the escalating cost of health care in the past 25 years and the annual savings due to nutritional care.
- List the six dietary goals proposed by the United States Senate Select Committee on Nutrition and Human Needs and discuss the advantages, disadvantages, and the implications of each.

Nutrition: is a national nutrition policy needed?

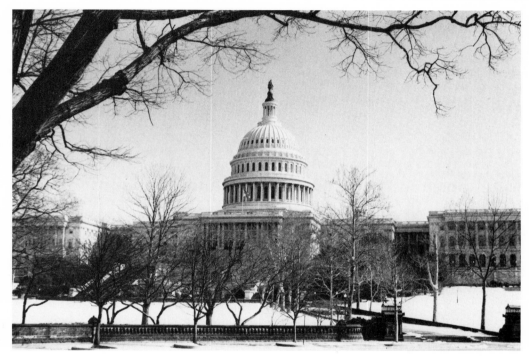

Nutrition as a public policy issue has become a major topic for discussion for an increasing number of individuals and agencies concerned with social, political, and economic development. The 1970s have brought an emerging awareness that resources are finite and that the United States will no longer be able to tolerate uncoordinated policies on food production, consumption, and trade. The immediate impetus for action may be a result of inflation, spot shortages, or the awareness that even in the United States abundance is not infinite. As more and more citizens, freed from the threat of the

nutritional diseases of poverty, fall prey to the nutritional diseases of abundance, a national nutrition policy is mandated.

Adequate food and sound nutrition are essential to good health. Not only are they crucial for human survival and key factors in the prevention and recovery from illness, but they are prerequisites for improving the quality of life of Americans and other peoples of the world. The element of nutrition can influence a broad spectrum of health concerns, from the quality and safety of the food supply and the maintenance of good health to the disorders of undernutrition and overnutrition and disease etiology and therapy. In effect, in all phases of the life cycle, from preconception to death, nutrition plays a vital role. Today there is growing concern at all levels of the government, the scientific community, and the public about the role of nutrition in human health and a greater recognition of the opportunities for enhancing the nation's health through improved nutrition.

By definition a sound nutrition policy and knowledge of the subject are in the public interest, since their application can make the members of society healthier, happier, and more productive. If nutritionists are to serve in the public interest, their philosophy must be concerned with the "public good."

EATING PATTERNS: A PUBLIC HEALTH CONCERN

. . . the eating patterns of this century represent as critical a public health concern as any now before us.

We must acknowledge and recognize that the public is confused about what to eat to maximize health. If we as a Government want to reduce health costs and maximize the quality of life for all Americans, we have an obligation to provide practical guides to the individual consumer as well as set national dietary goals for the country as a whole.

Such an effort is long overdue. . . .

Senator George McGovern. Chairman, United States Select Committee on Nutrition and Human Needs, United States Senate, January 14, 1977.

Interest in nutrition in the United States has fluctuated greatly. In the 1920s and 1930s there was interest in the nutrition deficiency diseases, and many American scientists contributed significantly to knowledge of the vitamins, including elucidation of their structure and metabolic functions. The economic depression of the late 1930s and the entry into World War II brought forth the discovery that large numbers of men were unfit for military service because of nutritionally related problems. Thus a Conference on Nutrition and National Defense was held that led to a wide-scale nutrition education program.

The 1950s became the era of biomedical research. In the mid-1960s there was again a surge of interest in nutrition, partly due to recognition of the prevalence of malnutrition among developing countries and the challenge to solve the increasingly apparent world food problem.

The 1960s produced important legislation, including the Maternal and Child Health Amendments in 1963 and Social Security Amendments in 1965, which created Medicare and Medicaid. These have and will continue to have a tremendous impact on the role, function, and identification of the nutritional care of the people in communities across the United States.

In 1966, President Johnson appointed a committee to study the world food supply that investigated many aspects of the food situation throughout the world. The findings, published in 1967, indicated that the scale, severity, and duration of the world food problem was so great that a massive, long-range, innovative effort unprecedented in human history, would be required to master it.[1]

The latter part of the 1960s and the 1970s were years of national and international concern about food supply, food consumption patterns, mass media advertising, and the role of government and industry in food and nutrition policies. There was the 1968 U.S. Senate Select Committee on Nutrition and Human Needs, the 1969 White House Conference on Food, Nutrition and Health, and a 1971 Follow-up Conference. These will be discussed at greater length later on in this chapter, since they too were concerned with the politics and problems of nutrition of the 1970s.

The greatest drop in world food production since World War II occurred in 1972. This crisis led to hunger and famine in many countries and large price increases on the world markets. The world stock of basic food commodities declined to a new low level and has not increased since. At the 1974 World Food Conference held in Rome, it was agreed that a solution of the world's food problems must take place within the framework of general development and international economic cooperation.

The World Food Conference adopted a declaration on the elimination of hunger and malnutrition and passed twenty-two resolutions relating to the following three main elements of a global food policy:

1. Increased food production in all countries
2. Improved nutrition through a better distribution of food and improved consumption patterns
3. Establishment of a system of global food security

To assure a coordinated follow-up of the resolutions of the World Food Conference, it was recommended to the General Assembly of the United Nations that a World Food Council be created as the central body for food questions and agricultural development. The World Food Conference accorded the World Food Council responsibility for an overall coordination and follow-up of matters concerning food production, nutrition, food security, food trade, and food aid in all United Nations bodies. The first session of the new council was held in Rome in June, 1975, and the results were comparatively limited. However, in the debate on food questions during the 59th session of the United Nations Economic and Social Council, all members expressed support for the further work of the World Food Congress Council.[2]

POLITICS OF NUTRITION

It was only in the 1960s that malnutrition became a national issue. The state of hunger and poverty in the United States was brought to the attention of the American people, not by nutritionists, but by the Southern Christian Leadership Conference and its guiding spirit, Dr. Martin Luther King. He and his followers created a new climate of concern about many urban problems and poverty in the United States.

In spring, 1967, many people in the United States were shocked to learn of the existence of hunger and malnutrition in their country. Senators Robert Kennedy and Joseph Clark, members of a Senate Poverty Committee, took an unscheduled field trip to Mississippi and discovered the appalling conditions of poverty and hunger in the Delta area. They also learned that the federal food stamp program was inadequate in alleviating the problem. Visits to the area by physicians sponsored by the Field Foundation stimulated the establishment of a Citizens' Board of Inquiry and led to the publication of a report entitled "Hunger U.S.A."[3]* This was followed by a Columbia Broadcasting System documentary on the subject that provoked citizenry across the country to ask questions.

As a result of such publicity, in June, 1967, the Senate passed a law directing the U.S. Department of Health, Education, and Welfare to make a comprehensive survey of the incidence and location of serious hunger and malnutrition and other health problems and to report their findings to the Congress within 6 months. This task was delegated to Arnold Schaefer, a nutrition scientist in charge of the Interdepartmental Committee on Nutrition and National Defense (ICNND), who had conducted many surveys in developing countries and had long been seeking authorization to conduct surveys in the United States.

In a preliminary report to the Senate Select Committee on Nutrition and Human Needs, chaired by Senator George McGovern, Schaefer[4] reported significant amounts of low vitamin levels in blood serum, growth failure in children, anemia, and obesity.

United States Senate Select Committee on Nutrition and Human Needs, 1968

The U.S. Select Committee on Nutrition and Human Needs was appointed by the Senate, and hearings began in December, 1968. As a result, much testimony has been gathered regarding the importance of nutrition in health and the nutritional problems that are present in the United States. These hearings have been published and are avail-

---

*The reader is referred to Katz, N.: Let them eat promises: the politics of hunger in America, Englewood Cliffs, N.J., 1969, Prentice-Hall, Inc.; and Simon, P., and Simon, A.: The politics of world hunger; grass-root politics & world poverty, New York, 1973, Harper's Magazine Press.

able from the U.S. Government Printing Office.

UNITED STATES SENATE ESTABLISHED SENATE SELECT COMMITTEE ON NUTRITION AND HUMAN NEEDS

Following the Congressional legislative mandate to investigate malnutrition in the U.S.A., the United States Senate authorized and established a Select Committee on Nutrition and Human Needs in 1968. This has provided an opportunity for scientists, legislators, government employees, the poor and industry to testify and assist in structuring legislative support for improvement of nutrition, health, housing and education needs of the less fortunate of our country.

This congressional interest and the Ten-State Nutrition Survey stimulated the assembly of the First White House Conference on Food, Nutrition and Human Needs. Even though the bureaucracy stymied many of the recommendations for action, much good was accomplished. For example, the Department of Agriculture, with Congressional urging, truly revamped an unimaginative, ineffective food donation program. The Food and Drug Administration has introduced a new system of nutrition labelling directed towards an updated consumer education program. The Department of Agriculture took action in requiring the fortification of dried skim milk with vitamins A and D and an improved cereal enrichment with iron, lysine, thiamine, riboflavin, niacin, and vitamin A was evaluated in selected test areas in the United States.

Arnold E. Schaefer: Nutrition in the United States of America. In McLaren, D. S.: Nutrition in the community, New York, 1976, John Wiley & Sons, Inc., p. 381.

A Ten State Nutrition Survey was carried out between 1968 and 1970, including a survey of New York City, with attention directed primarily to the lower income segment of the population. Findings which were reported in 1972 indicated that a significant proportion of the population surveyed was malnourished or at high risk of developing nutritional problems and that the types of malnutrition differed in prevalence and severity among various segments of the population. Obesity was prevalent particularly among adult women. A high prevalence of low hemoglobin and hematocrit values was found in all segments of the population. Low serum albumin levels found in pregnant and lactating women suggested marginal protein

nutrition. Low levels of vitamin A were common, and riboflavin status was poor in certain population groups.[5]

White House Conference, 1969

On May 6, 1969, President Nixon sent a message to Congress on the subject of hunger and malnutrition in the United States. He requested the Secretary of Health, Education, and Welfare "to work with state agencies to combat nutrient deficiencies, to expand the national nutrition survey, and to initiate detailed research into the relationship between malnutrition-related diseases." In June, 1969, President Nixon appointed Jean Mayer as a special consultant to organize a White House Conference on Food, Nutrition and Health. The conference was intended to "focus national attention and national resources on the country's remaining —and changing—nutritional problems."[6]

In December, 1969, some 3,500 participants assembled, including nutrition scientists, nutrition educators, dietitians, physicians, public health workers, clergymen, and agricultural workers, and representatives from the food industry, civil rights organizations, the Office of Economic Opportunity, consumer organizations, ethnic minorities, welfare administrators, and the poor.

The conference pointed out that there was no single agency coordinating food, nutrition, and health programs, and it recommended the appointment of a special assistant to the President, specializing in nutrition problems. Other recommendations were that the Secretary of Health, Education, and Welfare be responsible for coordinating government policy regarding food and nutrition activity as they relate to health; that the food stamp and distribution programs be transferred from the Department of Agriculture to the Department of Health, Education, and Welfare; and that an Office of Nutrition be established as a part of the Department of Health, Education, and Welfare. This Office of Nutrition would develop a program and priorities that would survey and monitor state, county, and local nutrition and health systems and would plan appropriate programs for the Department of Health, Education, and Welfare and other federal agencies.

The conference also recommended that health and nutrition delivery programs be provided for needy areas and that centers for research, diagnosis, and training also be established. It said that the need for manpower in the areas of nutrition had been overlooked, and in addition to training professionals, consumer education should be encouraged through federal funds. Joint programs in medicine and nutrition among schools of public health medicine, allied health, dentistry, nursing, and home economics should also be implemented.

White House Conference follow-up, 1971

A follow-up in 1971 to the 1970 conference noted some achievements that resulted from the conference. These included the expansion of the food stamp and school lunch programs; training of nutrition aides by the Department of Agriculture (EFNEP, or Expanded Food and Nutrition Education Program); enlargement of the nutrition program; and research by the Food and Drug Administration into additives, food-borne diseases, and environmental contamination. Voluntary efforts by citizen groups and the food industry have also increased.[7]

A nutrition program was established by the Center for Disease Control in Atlanta after the completion of a Ten State Nutrition Survey. On the basis of the data collected, the center initiated an applied nutrition program to determine means of solving certain of the problems that were revealed. An objective of this program was to evaluate the nutrition status of the whole United States, as well as trying to improve specific problems in various areas.

NUTRITION PROBLEMS OF THE 1970s

At the present time, six of the ten leading causes of death in the United States have been related to diet: heart disease, stroke and hypertension, cancer, diabetes, arteriosclerosis, and cirrhosis of the liver. These diseases are caused largely by factors that do not lend themselves to direct medical solu-

tions. The American diet and life-style are implicated in each of these "killer diseases." The urgency and seriousness of these diseases mandate that the population understand and practice the basic principles of good nutrition.

NUTRITION? HEALTH VS. DISEASE

National food and health policies, however effective, can help only those who help themselves. Increasingly, research findings tell us that we are in large measure responsible for our state of health. It is becoming common knowledge much cardiovascular disease, most cirrhosis of the liver, obesity and its consequences, and many gastrointestinal problems are self-induced by overeating, smoking, over-drinking, and eating the wrong foods. Changes in bad eating and drinking habits, therefore, can make dramatic improvements in the health of the population. Such improvements, however, depend to a great extent on the will and capability of the people to take personal responsibility for their own health.

Senator Charles H. Percy, United States Select Commitee on Nutrition and Human Needs, United States Senate, July, 1976.

The reasons for nutritional problems are many and complex. Inadequate income is a major determinant of nutritional status. Other factors have an effect, such as lack of knowledge; lack of interest; lack of skill; complications of disease; sedentary life-styles; mental and emotional factors; social isolation; lack of means for food purchasing, preparation, and storage facilities; consumer confusion and misinformation; overabundance of foods of low nutritive value and high cost; faddism; and geographic location.

Data from national nutrition studies

To define nutrition problems and their effect on health, three major nutrition studies have been sponsored by the Department of Health, Education, and Welfare during the past decade: the Ten State Nutrition Survey of almost 30,000 families, chiefly low income,[8] the Health and Nutrition Examination Survey (HANES), which studied a national sample of 10,126 persons representative of the United States civilian, noninstitutionalized population,[9] and the Preschool Nutrition Survey of a national probability sample of approximately 3,000 children.[10] In addition, there have been smaller studies of special population groups.[11-13] The studies indicate that in spite of advances in nutrition knowledge, food technology, medicine, and sanitation which have helped to reduce the prevalence of nutritional deficiency diseases in the United States, many Americans continue to suffer from poor nutrition or are at nutritional risk. There is mounting evidence that those who fail to attain a diet optimal for health can be found at every socioeconomic level. The studies show the widespread prevalence of nutritional problems such as obesity, retarded growth and development, iron-deficiency anemia, and dental caries.

Iron-deficiency anemia was a common finding in all of the national studies. The Ten State Nutrition Survey found low hemoglobin or hematocrit values in 25% of the persons below the poverty level and in 12% of those above the poverty level. In the Preschool Nutrition Survey, iron-deficiency anemia was a common finding among children who were 1 to 5 years of age, regardless of their socioeconomic status.

In the Ten State Nutrition Survey and HANES, the prevalence of obesity was high, particularly among adult women, of whom nearly one third were found to be obese. Men, children, and adolescents also had a high prevalence of obesity. In the pilot Center for Disease Control Nutrition Surveillance System in five states,[13] the number of children enrolled in health care programs such as Title V/Maternal and Child Health, Head Start, and Early Periodic Screening, Diagnosis, and Treatment falling below the 5th percentile of height for age ranged from nearly 10% to 15%. Data also indicated that a considerable portion of the population under surveillance was relatively overweight, with the number falling in the 95th percentile of weight for height ranging from 8% to 13%. There was a high percentage of overweight in the very young—about 16% of the 1-year-old infants were above the 95th percentile,

whereas 9% of 13- to 17-year-old girls were above the 95th percentile. Not only is obesity associated with a high incidence of degenerative diseases but it is also associated with disorders in cardiopulmonary and metabolic function, which often create problems in physical mobility.

These investigations have demonstrated that Americans who fail to attain a diet optimal for health can be found at every socioeconomic level. The reasons are many and complex, but it is clear that many people in various situations are affected by improper diet. For instance, there is the increased risk involved in the pregnancies of poorly nourished women; the chance that these infants may be of low birth weight with accompanying risk of retarded physical and mental development; the high prevalence of overweight and underweight in school children and in adults; the debilitation of the elderly population because of malnourishment; widespread dental diseases in the total population; and the high prevalence of chronic illnesses, many of which are nutrition related and require dietary treatment, monitoring, and follow-up.[14] These facts would surely seem to answer the question: "Is a national nutrition policy needed?" Nutrition is recognized as a vital part of health and, as stated in the constitution of the World Health Organization ". . . the enjoyment of the highest attainable standard of health is one of the fundamental rights of every human being without distinction of race, religion, political beliefs, economic or social condition."[15]

In attempting to answer the foregoing question, in addition to the diseases resulting from poor nutrition, there are three basic issues to be considered. The first is the escalating cost of health care, the second is the monetary and economic savings that nutrition services and education could make possible, and the third, which necessarily follows, is that prevention encompassing an awareness of the effects of life-styles must be the theme for health program planning. All three of these issues are pertinent when considering, "Is a national nutrition policy needed?"

COST OF HEALTH CARE

American families can ill afford to spend unnecessarily for medical care. Large and persistent increases in health costs, which continue to outpace inflation in the rest of the economy, boosted national health expenditures in the fiscal year 1975 to an unprecedented $118.5 billion, or 8.3% of the gross national product as shown in Table 1-1. Americans now spend on the average of 10% of their total income on health care alone. Table 1-2 shows sources of payments for personal health care services in the United States. If nothing else, the pocketbook incentive should encourage each individual to test the thesis that good nutrition and living habits can go a long way in preventing disease and maintaining good health.

Burger[16] has maintained that the phrase "crisis in health," which became a household term during the late 1960s and the first two years of this decade, emerged from a crisis in health services—especially in the *costs* of health services and their *availability* and *accessibility*.

The past three decades of intensive bio-

Table 1-1. Health care expenditures in the United States and their relation to the gross national product, 1950, 1965, and 1975*

	Expenditures					
	In billions of dollars			In percentage of gross national product		
	1950	1965	1975	1950	1965	1975
Gross national product	$263.4	$655.6	$1424.0			
Total health care expenditures	12.0	38.9	118.5	4.6	5.9	8.3
Hospitals	3.7	13.2	46.6	1.4	2.0	3.3
Physicians	2.7	8.4	22.1	1.0	1.3	1.6
Drugs	1.6	4.6	10.6	0.6	0.7	0.7
Dentists	0.9	2.7	7.5	0.3	0.4	0.5
Nursing homes	0.2	1.3	9.0	0.1	0.2	0.6
Other†	2.9	8.7	22.8	1.1	1.3	1.6
Funded by government	3.1	9.5	49.9	1.2	1.4	3.5
Funded by private insurance‡	1.3	9.6	31.7	0.5	1.5	2.2

*From Kristein, M. M., Arnold, C. B., and Wynder, E. L.: Health economics and preventive care, Science **195:**457, 1977. Copyright 1977 by the American Association for the Advancement of Science.
†Includes public health and research.
‡Benefit payments made by all private insurance organizations, including Blue Cross and Blue Shield.

Table 1-2. Sources of payments for personal health care services in the United States, 1950, 1965, and 1974*

	Payments					
	In billions of dollars			In percentage of total personal health care expenditures		
	1950	1965	1974	1950	1965	1974
Government	2.1	7.0	34.0	20.2	20.9	37.7
Private insurance	1.2	9.0	24.4	11.5	26.9	27.0
Consumers	7.1	17.6	32.0	68.3	52.5	35.4

*From Kristein, M. M., Arnold, C. B., and Wynder, E. L.: Health economics and preventive care, Science **195:**457, 1977. Copyright 1977 by the American Association for the Advancement of Science.

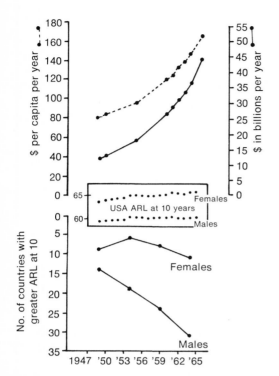

Fig. 1-1. Health expenditures, average remaining lifetime (ARL) and rank among other countries, 1949-1964. Two upper curves show the annual expenditures on health in the United States from 1949 through 1966 (1966 estimated). The dotted curve and left-hand scale give the per capita expenditures adjusted for the fall in the purchasing power of the dollar. The solid line and right-hand scale give the actual amounts in billions of dollars. The central insert gives the average remaining lifetime at 10 years of age for males (dots) and females (circles) from 1949 through 1964. The lower curves give, at five-year intervals, the number of countries with a greater average remaining lifetime at 10 years of age than the United States from 1949 through 1964 (dots for males and circles for females). By the inversion of the ordinate scale, the falling position of the United States is indicated by a falling line. The average remaining lifetime in the United States has remained nearly constant, but its rank among the nations has fallen sharply for males and slightly for females. (Reprinted by permission from Forbes, W. H.: N. Engl. J. Med. **227:**74, 1967.)

medical research have resulted in clinical intervention in certain diseases, and disease patterns have changed also. But how does one account for the startling fact that there has been little or no improvement in life expectancy for adults since the 1920s? And how does one account for the rising costs of health care, which led William Forbes to conclude that in the United States there is no longer any significant relation between money spent and results achieved?

Forbes[17] in 1967 was among the first to explore analytically the relation between national expenditures for health and health itself. His analysis was prompted by the promises implied by the then new Regional Medical Program. What characterized this program was the proposition that investment of money for the early location, therapy, and prevention of heart disease, cancer, and stroke would buy increased health. However, as seen in Fig. 1-1, Forbes[17] concluded that there was not necessarily any correlation, at least in the United States.

Six years later, Glazer[18] shared this finding when he suggested that little should be expected in the way of correlation between health conditions on the one hand and health expenditures, use of health care facilities, or the system of health care on the other.

Cornely[19] has said there is more to health than just paying bills, and he argues that prevention is the most significant single deterrent to present-day spiraling medical costs, and one that is frequently overlooked by health legislators.

Although a total of $94 billion was spent last year, 1973, and this figure continues to rise annually by 10 to 15 percent, it has not improved the health of our citizens and has, in some instances, jeopardized it. Most of the money has been spent for hospitals, drugs, medical hardware, and intensive care units, with the major emphasis on *cure*. Yet our infant mortality rate continues to be high: coronary care units have not measurably affected deaths from coronary heart disease; patients who enter hospitals are dying from prescribed drug interactions or infections which they contracted while in the hospital; and the life expectancy at age 20 has changed very little during the last quarter of a century.

As demonstrated in Fig. 1-2, in 1975 annual national health expenditures reached a total of $118.5 billion. In the decade from 1965 to 1975, per capita expenditures rose from $198 to $547—an average annual increase of 10.7%. As a proportion of the gross national product, health care outlays rose significantly from 5.9% in 1965 to reach 8.3% in 1975. Factors affecting increases in personal health care expenditures are shown in Fig. 1-3.

General share of health care financing has

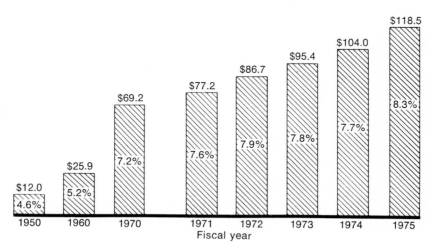

Fig. 1-2. National health expenditures and percent of gross national product, selected fiscal years 1950-1975 (in billions of dollars). (From U.S. Department of Health, Education, and Welfare: Forward Plan for Health FY 1978-82, Aug., 1976; source: Social Security Administration Office of Research and Statistics.)

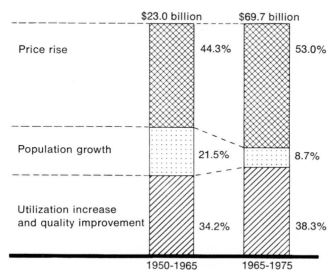

Fig. 1-3. Factors affecting increases in personal health care expenditures, fiscal years 1950-1965 and 1965-1975. (From U.S. Department of Health, Education, and Welfare: Forward plan for health FY 1978-82, Aug., 1976.)

Table 1-3. Magnitude of benefits from nutrition research *

Health problem	Magnitude of loss	Potential savings from improved diet
	Part A. Nutrition-related health problems	
Heart and vasculatory	Over 1 million deaths in 1967	
	Over 5 million people with definite or suspect heart disease in 1960-1962	25% reduction
	$31.6 billion in 1962	20% reduction
Respiratory and infectious	82,000 deaths per year	
	246 million incidents in 1967	20% fewer incidents
	141 million work-days lost in 1955-66	15%-20% fewer days lost
	166 million school days lost	15%-20% fewer days lost
	$5 million in medical and hospital costs	$1 million
	$1 billion in cold remedies and tissues	$20 million
Mental health	2.5% of population or 5.2 million people are severely or totally disabled; 25 million people have manifest disability	10% fewer disabilities
Infant mortality and reproduction	Infant deaths in 1967—79,000	50% fewer deaths
	Infant death rate 22.4 per 1,000	50% fewer deaths
	Fetal death rate 15.6 per 1,000	50% fewer deaths
	Maternal death rate 28.0 per 100,000 live births	50% fewer deaths
	Child death rate (1-4 years) 96.1 per 100,000 in 1964	Reduce rate to 10 per 100,000
	15 million with congenital birth defects	3 million fewer children with birth defects
Early aging and lifespan	49.1% of population, about 102 million people have one or more chronic impairments	10 million people without impairments
	People surviving to age 65 years %	
	White males 66	1% improvement per year to
	Negro males 50	90% surviving
	White females 81	
	Negro females 64	
	Life expectancy in years	
	White males 67.8	Bring Negro expectancy up to
	Negro males 61.1	White
	White females 75.1	
	Negro females 68.2	
Arthritis	16 million people afflicted	8 million people without afflictions
	27 million work days lost	13.5 million workdays
	500,000 people unemployed	125,000 people employed
	Annual cost $3.6 billion	$900 million per year
Dental health	44 million with gingivitis; 23 million with advanced periodontal disease; $6.5 billion public and private expenditures on dentists' services in 1967; 22 million endentulous persons (1 in 8) in 1957; ½ of all people over 55 years have no teeth	50% reduction in incidence, severity, and expenditures
Diabetes and carbohydrate disorders	3.9 million overt diabetic; 35,000 deaths in 1967; 79% of people over 55 years with impaired glucose tolerance	50% of cases avoided or improved
Osteoporosis	4 million severe cases, 25% of women over 40	75% reduction

*From benefits of human nutrition research. Appendix A, Nutrition and health II, Select Committee on Nutrition and Human Needs, U.S. Senate, July, 1976, Government Printing Office, p. 77.

Table 1-3. Magnitude of benefits from nutrition research—cont'd

Health problem	Magnitude of loss	Potential savings from improved diet
Obesity	3 million adolescents; 30%-40% of adults; 60%-70% over 40 years	80% reduction in incidence
Anemia and other nutrient deficiencies	See improved work efficiency, growth and development, and learning ability	
Alcoholism	5 million alcoholics; one half are addicted	33%
	About 24,500 deaths in 1967 caused by alcohol	33%
	Annual loss over $2 billion from absenteeism, lowered production and accidents	33%
Eyesight	48.1% (86 million people) over 3 years wore corrective lenses in 1966; 81,000 become blind every year; $103 million in welfare	20% fewer people blind or with corrective lenses
Cosmetic	10% of women age 9 years or more with vitamin intakes below recommended daily allowances	
Allergies	32 million people (9%) are allergic 16 million with hayfever asthma	20% people relieved
	7-15 million people (3%-6%) allergic to milk	90% people relieved
	Over 693,000 persons (1 in 3,000) allergic to gluten	90% people relieved
Digestive	8,495,000 workdays lost; 5,013,000 school days lost; About 20 million incidents of acute condition annually	25% fewer acute conditions
	$4.2 billion annual cost; 14 million persons with duodenal ulcers; $5 million annual cost; 4,000 new cases each day	Over $1 billion in costs
Kidney and urinary	55,000 deaths from renal failure; 200,000 with kidney stones	20% reduction in deaths and acute conditions
Muscular disorders	200,000 cases	10% reduction in cases
Cancer	600,000 persons developed cancer in 1968; 320,000 persons died of cancer in 1968	20% reduction in incidence and deaths
Part B. Individual satisfactions increased		
Improved work efficiency		5% increase in on-the-job productivity
Improved growth and development	113,000 deaths from accident; 324.5 million workdays lost; 51.8 million people needing medical attention and/or restricted activity	25% fewer deaths and workdays lost
Improved learning ability	Over 6.5 million mentally retarded persons with I.Q. below 70; 12% of school-age children need special education	Raise I.Q. by 10 points for persons with I.Q. 70 to 80
Part C. Increased efficiency in food services		
Improved efficiency in food preparation and menu planning		Not estimated
Reduced losses of nutrients in food storage, handling, and preparation		Not estimated
Improved efficiency in food selection		Not estimated
Improved efficiency in food programs		Not estimated

increased by a proportion comparable to the decrease of private funds. From 1966 to 1975 the proportion of federal outlays for health more than doubled—to 11.2%. By fiscal year 1978 the *increases* in federal Medicare and Medicaid equaled the total Public Health Service budget.

Until costs can be contained, federal policy making in health will be dominated by these basic economic considerations. Proposed solutions must address the total health care system, not merely a major component or program in that system. Comprehensive national health insurance is such a total system approach, but rises in health care cost as well as economic and social policy make the timing and phasing of a national program uncertain and difficult to implement at optimum efficiency.[20]

ANNUAL SAVINGS DUE TO NUTRITION CARE

The statistics on poor nutrition are overwhelming, even when considered in terms of dollars rather than in terms of lives. Testimony given by George M. Briggs, Professor of Nutrition at the University of California at Berkeley, before the U.S. Senate Select Committee on Nutrition and Human Needs in 1972, revealed that poor dietary habits cost this nation about $30 billion in health care each year. This is a tremendous bill to continue paying. At that time this was about one third of the nation's health costs. By 1974, the Department of Health, Education, and Welfare reported total health care costs to be $104 billion. Briggs' estimate was based on a report issued in 1971 by the Department of Agriculture, as shown in Table 1-3.

Another rather staggering statistic came from John W. Farquhar, of the Stanford University Medical Center, who told the National Nutrition Policy hearings that the elimination of obesity in the United States could cut in half the $24 billion being spent on treatment of premature cardiovascular disease.[21] In a paper prepared for the Select Committee in 1969, "Economic Benefits from the Elimination of Hunger in America,"[22] Barry M. Popkin, of the Institute of

Research on Poverty at the University of Wisconsin, made estimates of the economic benefits that might result from eliminating malnutrition. Popkin[22] stressed that there are both direct and indirect costs to society from continued neglect of nutritional care services in the total health care systems and has estimated annual savings due to nutritional care services in the following areas:

Education—Improved nutrition improves learning mental development and increases the ability to concentrate and work ($6.4-19.2 billion).

Physical performance—Improved nutrition increases the capacity for prolonged physical work and raises the productivity of workers and increases the motivation to work ($6.4-25.8 billion).

Morbidity—Improved nutrition results in higher resistance to disease and lowers the severity of disease ($201-502 million).

Mortality—Improved nutrition decreases fetal, infant, child, and certain types of maternal mortality ($68-157 million).

Intergenerational effects—Improved nutrition makes healthy mothers who have healthy children. Also, better educated parents lead to better educated children ($1.3-4.5 billion).

PREVENTION
Medical cure versus health care

In the past, consideration of proper nutrition care has been linked to the clinical management of disease states with modified diets. However, nutrition no longer can be considered only in terms of the diagnosis and treatment of nutritional deficiency diseases and the prescription of standard dietary regimens for the management of certain metabolic diseases, such as diabetes, obesity, and coronary heart disease, for which a special diet is required. Butterworth[23] corroborated the present antiprogressive status of nutrition education in medicine in the following statement:

Under-graduate teaching of nutrition often is centered around nutritional deficiency disease. *This is too limited a focus* for present-day problems. . . . I suggest that, as physicians, we have been guilty of misdirected effort and possibly even misappropriation of funds. To cite one example, we continue to treat a virtual epidemic of ischemic heart disease after it has occurred, often at an advanced stage, with only token efforts to find primary causes and long-range preventive measures. We have developed elegant techniques to measure coronary artery blood-flow, and to perform at great expense coronary artery bypass grafts. Elaborate, expensive coronary care units exist in areas where large segments of the population, such as migrant farm laborers, do not have access to basic health care, running water, sewage disposal, and an adequate diet. We have allowed these things to happen, because we have not properly educated ourselves, our colleagues, and our legislators.

Our health delivery system is suffering from the lack of primary care, or rather, primary prevention. Simply defined, primary prevention alters some factor in individuals or in the environment so that the disease never develops. The basic concept that health service is a privilege or even a luxury must be changed to the concept that it is both a necessity and a right.

Millis[24] explores the world of health services and refers to its two subworlds, that of medical cure and that of health care. He explains that the words "care" and "cure" are *not* synonymous, even though they are used as such by both laypersons and physicians. The words have different roots and have undergone different histories, but most importantly, they carry very different concepts. "Care" is a process and thus is continuous. "Cure" is an event and thus is episodic.

For most individuals the mental image created by the expression "health care" has to do with illness or disability and with the persons, institutions, and technology needed to cure that illness or alleviate that disability. Similarly, when most physicians speak of "health care," they are expressing the same mental image. It is disease oriented, situated in the specific environment of hospital, clinic, or doctor's office, and it involves the several medical arts—the application of which hopefully will result in a cure. In the concept of both the provider and the recipient, the necessary precedent is illness, not health. Thus, both many laymen and many professionals mean "medical cure" when they say "health care."

The Millis report[24] cites the need for improved comprehensive and continuing health care. He points out that there is little "well-adult care."

The great sources of morbidity and mortality for adults are automobile accidents, obesity, alcoholism, drug and cigarette-induced lung cancer, organic and mental disease frequently related to tension and an unself-disciplined life style . . . The physician is regarded by himself and by his patients as a healer and rarely as a teacher. We are still concerned with mortality and not with morbidity.

Life-style

In two neighboring states, Nevada and Utah, there are startling differences in morbidity and mortality statistics. How can this be accounted for? Fuchs[25] presents the situations of these two states that enjoy the same levels of income and medical care and are alike in many other respects but whose levels of health differ enormously. In his challenging and important book, *Who Shall Live? Health, Economics and Social Change*, Fuchs, one of the nation's leading authorities in the field of health economics, surveys every aspect of the nation's health care system in relation to what the latest data reveal about the nation's health needs. His startling but fully documented conclusion once again demonstrates that in the United States, health has less to do with what people spend on medical care than with their heredity, environment, and personal life-styles which could effect prevention. As Fuchs[25] draws his comparison between Nevada and Utah, he explains:

The answer almost surely lies in the different life-styles of the residents of the two states. Utah is inhabited primarily by Mormons, whose influence is strong throughout the state. Devout Mormons do not use tobacco or alcohol and in general lead stable, quiet lives. Nevada, on the other hand, is a state with high rates of cigarette and alcohol consumption and very high indexes of marital and geographical instability. The contrast with Utah in these respects is extraordinary.*

---

*From Fuchs, V. R.: Who shall live? health, economics, and social choice, p. 53, © 1974 by Basic Books, Inc., Publishers, New York.

Consider also the following 1973 statistics wherein hundreds of thousands of Americans died prematurely from causes primarily related to their individual life-styles—life-styles that could have included preventive care but most likely did not to any discernible extent: 755,864 deaths from heart disease; 115,040 from accidents; 33,360 from cirrhosis of the liver; 24,440 from suicide; 19,700 from homicide; and 8,010 from hypertension.[26] In the same year, death rates for men were 1,070 per 100,000; for women, 820 per 100,000.[26] The difference here can be traced primarily to life-style, as can the following statistics. In 1972, 13,208 children under 14 years of age died from accidents or homicide.[27] When both parents smoke, children are twice as likely to get pneumonia or bronchitis in their first year of life as when neither parent smokes.[28] An estimated 9 million Americans are alcoholics.[29] Nearly 4 million Americans have histories of heart attack or angina pectoris.[30]

This relationship between death rates, health status, and life-style is becoming increasingly clear, and documentation is accumulating at a rapid rate. Yet individual behavior changes in response to this information have been extremely slow. Smoking, overeating, excessive drinking, and unfastened seat belts are still common facts of American life.

With the rise in the cost of health care in the United States, it seems understandable for the government and people to become concerned about spending 8% or more of the gross national product on health services, and more so, because this is at a time when questions are being asked about the relation of value to money: the formulas for balancing the exchange of energy and resources for benefits. Since there is a finite amount of the gross national product that the American people wish to use for health care, choices have to be made.

The type of question to consider is which resources will produce the greatest benefit for society, for example, those applied to infant nutrition and prenatal care or those applied to a chronic renal dialysis program? Judging both from statistics and economics,

it seems that there is little choice—prevention must become the underlying concept of health programs and of health education programs. Are health providers not best advised to broaden their approach from treating symptoms of a disease that has already appeared and devote more of their efforts to identifying problems that have major impact on the quality of people's lives and on the nature of their life-styles?

The ultimate goal of a prevention strategy is to enable each person to live long and free from disability by reducing the occurrence of disease or injury. Prevention is often described as consisting of three stages: primary, secondary, and tertiary prevention. Primary prevention includes actions or interventions designed to prevent etiologic agents from causing disease or injury in humans. Secondary prevention is concerned with the early detection and treatment of disease to cure or control its course. Tertiary prevention includes those activities directed at ameliorating the seriousness of disease by reducing the disability and dependence resulting from it.

Behavior change

For planning purposes it is more productive to focus on the underlying conditions or antecedent causes of preventable diseases than to concentrate on the diseases themselves. With this suggestion that higher priority be given to the development of primary prevention programs directed at the underlying causes of disease, it goes without saying that in some instances this calls for fundamental changes in the behavior of people and in the traditional practices of social and economic institutions.

Almost all patient and consumer health education assumes, explicitly or implicitly, that if people know what is most healthful, they will do it. However, as Milio[31] points out, it is a paradox that health professionals, in their efforts to improve people's health-related practices, seem to expect more of the ordinary consumer than they do of themselves:

Perhaps the most obvious test of this assumption is to look at the health professionals themselves. If *knowing* what is health-generating were directly related to *doing*, then surely we in the health field would be among the most robust in the nation, slim, agile, nonsmoking, temperate eaters of complementary protein, low fat and cholesterol, low-sucrose, and nonrefined carbohydrate foods, avoiders of drugging levels of alcohol and other artificial mood-changers, evenly paced in our daily patterns . . . Most will recognize that it is not much more likely for a physician earning $85,000 a year to change his life pattern than for a $6,000 a year hospital aide to do so. However, the *potential* for lifestyle change, the array of options available to these two individuals, may differ considerably.

Speaking in the most general terms, Dr. Lester Breslow, Dean, School of Public Health, University of California at Los Angeles, has noted that the life expectancy of a 45-year-old man has increased only about four years since 1900. He estimates that an additional eleven years could be added to such life expectancy (and seven years to adult female life expectancy) if people were to exercise regularly, maintain moderate weight, eat breakfast, not snack between meals, avoid smoking, limit liquor consumption, and sleep at least 7 hours a night. Thus, according to Breslow, a 45-year-old man who followed three or less of these health habits on the average could expect to live another 21.6 years, or until 66.6 years of age; whereas if he followed six or seven of them, on the average he could add 33.3 years, or live until he was 78.1 years of age.[32]

The solution of health problems demands a comprehensive approach that not only looks to the individual to accept primary responsibility for maintaining his health but to the industrial society to moderate those practices that are potentially hazardous to humans. For this reason prevention programs should be organized on at least two levels: they should be directed at educating the general public and at specific individuals and groups most susceptible to disease.

COMPREHENSIVE HEALTH SERVICES

Preventive health care in American society is only one part of comprehensive health services. The goals of comprehensive care are closely linked with the goals of optimum health in the World Health Organization sense: that is, comprehensive care is directed toward helping people achieve and maintain optimum health status, which is perceived not merely as the absence of disease but as the realization of an individual's full potential for satisfactory social function. Thus it is dependent on the collaborative efforts of a variety of professional and nonprofessional personnel, institutions, and services and is not the exclusive domain of any single profession or institutional entity.

Beloff[33] offers a definition of comprehensive health services that indicates its broad base, including preventive care, acute care, rehabilitation, and management of chronic illness. It also involves consideration of the social, emotional, and biologic causes and effects of health and disease.

He includes the roles of the specialist, the health care team, and the family in his definition of health care management.[33] Many definitions can be found in the literature, but despite the multiplicity of definitions, health care always implies the synergistic use of psychodynamic and sociologic knowledge along with biologic skills.[34]

The importance of comprehensive health care, for example, the availability of preventive, diagnostic, therapeutic, and rehabilitative ambulatory service under the same umbrella, is being recognized in recent legislation. The concept of continuity of patient care, which means that a patient has the opportunity for ongoing contact with a single health professional or with the same team of health professionals, is also being incorporated into federal and state legislation and regulations.[35]

In addition to government recognition, many issues concerning comprehensive health care are finding contemporary expression in the priorities of medicine and medical education. The renaissance of family practice and the primary care model may be viewed as an offshoot of this trend. This was slow in coming and is slow in taking hold.

In the past, and generally, the teaching hospital was concerned only about specific types of illness. Little or no attention has been given to the great bulk of illness that exists and medical care that is provided outside of the hospital. In a classic paper prepared by White and co-workers,[36] data were presented from the United States and Great Britain which suggest that, in a population of 1,000 adults, in an average month 750 will experience an episode of illness, 250 of these will consult a physician, 9 will be hospitalized, 5 will be referred to another physician, and 1 will be referred to a university medical center. Based on these estimates, programs limited to hospital services will cover 3% of sick adults and 1% of the adult patients in a community. As White[36] has said, a sick person's "entry into the system should not be a blind alley or the portal to a labyrinth; it should lead to a medical and social evaluation of the patient's needs," including a nutritional assessment.

There are at present little baseline data about the general state of health. Vital statistics provide mortality and morbidity data but lack health data. There are no reliable estimates on the distribution of health problems in populations. There are no reliable estimates on the symptoms and complaints brought to physicians at the time of their initial contact with patients, and only limited estimates are available on medical reasons for using hospitals or long-term care facilities.

In the absence of such data, it is virtually impossible to define the overall objectives of health care today. It is known what the needs of society and the present health care system are. It is also known that the two are incompatible today. The health professional is now beginning to deal with patients in a community—a population group. What is the health professional's new role? Is it enough to tell the patient that he has a chronic heart disease and prescribe a suitable regimen, or should he and his family be taught to manage the problem so that he can live a satisfying life? And what is the responsibility to the community? Should the health professional educate the community so that its members can better cope with current epidemics—alcoholism, drug addiction, inadequate parenting, the plight of the aging, loneliness,

occupational boredom, and suicide? The answer here clearly should be yes, but implementation is still a large problem to tackle. The National Consumer Health Information–Health Promotion Act of 1976 provides authority for new federal actions in prevention, but it appears too diffuse in its objectives to be effective on the individual level. Furthermore, it appears much too underfunded to be effective in the fiscal year 1978.

It becomes apparent that life-style determines nutrition and health. It becomes apparent that a national nutrition policy is needed.

NATIONAL NUTRITION POLICY
National Nutrition Consortium's guidelines

In the mid-1970s a concise statement of a national nutrition policy became timely and desirable. In preparation for the Senate hearings on a national nutrition policy in 1974, the National Nutrition Consortium designed a five-part document that discussed (1) the need for a national nutrition policy, (2) the goals of a national nutrition policy, (3) measures for attaining the goals of a national nutrition policy, (4) the programs needed to meet these objectives, and (5) requirements for the establishment of a national nutrition policy.

TOWARD A NATIONAL NUTRITION POLICY

The past year may represent a turning point in history. Numerous developments including the energy crisis, inflation, rising food costs and depletion of our food reserves have convinced many knowledgeable people that we are now entering an era which will be characterized by a shortage of resources including food. The high energy cost of producing food makes it clear that food and the energy supply are inextricably linked. For the first time, the capacity of the United States to feed itself and meet its world food commitments is being seriously questioned. A world food crisis exists at this time, and this will have serious repercussions in this country. . . .

D. Mark Hegsted: Special report: guidelines for a national nutrition policy, The National Nutrition Consortium, Inc., April, 1974.

1974 National Nutrition Policy Study Hearings

On February 24, 1974, the opening session of the National Nutrition Policy Study Hearings on Nutrition and Health was held and many experts testified. The point was made that there is much greater recognition today of the fact that the kinds and amounts of food and alcohol consumed by the public and the style of living of a sedentary society are major contributing factors to the development of chronic illnesses. Evidence was presented concerning the role of nutritional factors in coronary heart disease, diabetes mellitus, hypertension, liver disease, moderate alcohol drinkers, alcoholism, cholesterol, gallstone formation, oral health, anemia, reproduction and family planning, the health of infants and children, aging, and cancer.

The experts testify
Jean Mayer

Jean Mayer, acting as General Coordinator of the National Nutrition Policy Study Hearings, spoke of the rapidly increasing growth in world population, adverse changes in the world weather pattern, poor agricultural productivity in lesser developed countries, a possible worldwide shortage of chemical fertilizers, and the increasing intake in developed countries of animal products, especially of beef, with its concomitant inefficient conversion of grain into meat calories and protein. Mayer hoped that within the framework of these hearings there was the power to create, on the international as well as the national scene, a pattern of "distributive justice" to cope with the problems of supply, distribution, education, and disease and mortality prevention.

Mayer had established six panels of nutrition and food experts to research information that would lead to the formation of a national nutrition policy. The panel of Nutrition and Health had strong implications regarding the diseases of overabundance. The relative abundance of food in the United States, the panel reported, has led to a whole new spectrum of diseases in which nutritional factors either play the prime etiologic role or are highly contributory. The panel[37] states specifically:

These are: *Coronary Heart Disease*—dietary cholesterol, saturated fats, and excessive calories; *Hypertension*—dietary salt and excessive calories with associated obesity; *Diabetes Mellitus*—excessive calories, high dietary cholesterol and saturated fat intakes leading to obesity and vascular complications; *Obesity*—excessive calories and lack of physical activity; *Dental Caries*—high sugar intake; *Liver Disease*—excessive use of alcohol. . .

The Sub-panel on Health Care Systems recommended that the role of nutrition be clearly spelled out in future health legislation, and provision made for adequate funding and training of personnel.*

William E. Connor

A common theme ran through almost all of the reports emanating from this panel on Nutrition and Health. It was that the vast majority of Americans suffer from an overabundance of food—a problem of overconsumption. Connor[38] stressed the relationship between diet and heart disease. His testimony presented a statement from the Inter-Society Commission for Heart Disease Resources (1970), and three other studies by Kannel, Keys, and Connor. These provided the background material for Connor's[38] strong statement about nutrition and cardiovascular disease being interrelated.

The Commission recommends that a strategy of primary prevention of premature atherosclerotic disease be adopted as long-term national policy for the United States and to implement this strategy that adequate resources or money and manpower be committed to accomplish: changes in diet to prevent or control hyperlipidemia, obesity, hypertension and diabetes. [Connor refers to Report of the Inter-Society Commission for Heart Disease Resources: Primary prevention of atherosclerotic disease. Atherosclerosis and Epidemiology Study Groups, Inter-Society Commission for Heart Diseases, Circulation **42**:A-55, 1970.]

Kannel had said: . . . only with a strategy of primary prevention can this nation hope to curb

---

*Reproduced with permission of *Nutrition Today* magazine, 101 Ridgely Ave., Annapolis, Md. 21404 © July/August, 1974.

the continuing epidemic of atherosclerotic cardio-vascular disease. There is every indication that this epidemic has evolved from our way of life and the remedy would appear to entail restoration of the ecology to one more favorable to cardiovascular health. [Connor refers to Kannel, W. B.: The disease of living, Nutr. Today **6**(2), 1972.]

Keys was more specific: Nutritional factors have the most crucial role in the causation of atherosclerosis and coronary heart disease. The link between dietary lipids (cholesterol and fat) and the obstructive lesions of atherosclerosis is the level of cholesterol in the blood. Atherosclerotic coronary heart disease does not occur as a major disease entity when the blood cholesterol remains low, below 180 mg%, over the lifetime of the individual. [Connor refers to Keys, A., editor: Coronary heart disease in seven countries, Circulation **41**(suppl.):1-211, 1970.]

And W. E. and S. L. Connor were most concise: For the most part, in both man and animals, dietary cholesterol and fat are the sine qua non factors necessary to cause elevation of the blood cholesterol levels. [Connor refers to Connor, W. E., and Connor, S. L.: The key role of nutritional factors in the prevention of coronary heart disease, Prev. Med. **1**(49), 1972.]

Senator Richard S. Schweiker

Senator Richard S. Schweiker[39] made the following remarks, indicating the role of nutrition in diabetes:

Diabetes is a national problem, not just one of diabetics, their families and relatives. Americans are nearing the point where diabetes will affect nearly one in every five of us . . . Experts estimate that by 1980 diabetes will be the leading cause of blindness in the United States. In addition, diabetes can lead to the failure of a vital body organ, such as the kidney or heart. And diabetes can cause vascular and capillary degenerations, forcing the amputation of body extremities. It is a complicated, systemic disease of which, unfortunately, we know very little . . . The question I want to ask is this one: "Are we Americans bringing a diabetes crisis unknowingly upon ourselves? Are we eating our way into a diabetic epidemic?"

George F. Cahill

George F. Cahill,[40] Professor of Medicine, Harvard Medical School, Director, Joslin Research Laboratories, Boston, Massachusetts,

was another of the witnesses to speak on the relationship between the American diet and diabetes:

. . . how does nutrition fit into the above simplified description of the metabolic abnormalities in diabetes? It has been known for centuries that overnutrition leads to diabetes. This is primarily due to the fact that overweight people need much more insulin for it to do its job. Therefore, an individual predisposed to diabetes develops the overt disease when overfed, and proper nutrition is thus crucial . . . Nutritional education is necessary to combat the cultural concentration we have in America on the dinner table and all the advertising made to prompt our already overfed population to ingest even more calories. . . .

Nutrition and diabetes are culturally and scientifically intertwined and for the prolonged well-being of the population, appropriate and enlightened nutrition programs are mandatory.

Senator Edward M. Kennedy

On June 21, 1974, Senator Edward M. Kennedy,[41] at the start of 3 days of deliberation on the National Nutrition Policy Study Hearings, delivered a similar message. He indicated that a panel of experts would provide testimony and thoughtful recommendations. Before calling upon the impressive group of authorities, he delivered an opening statement:

Nutritional adequacy is a prerequisite for good health. No matter what conditions the body may be forced to suffer, the provision of adequate nutrition is the most fundamental requirement for survival. No internist can substitute for proteins. No surgeon can excise iron deficiencies, and no pediatrician can replace the nutrients lost in premature birth due to poor prenatal care . . . The delivery of good nutritional care is, in the long run, the most important "medicine" that each of us can and must administer to ourselves. . .

So much of the suffering and debilitation endured by Americans today could be avoided if we ate properly. Because we eat nearly 3,000 calories per day, it is easy to assume we are a healthy people . . . as a nation we are too fat. Obesity is America's number one health defect . . .

Special stress should be placed on nutrition education in medical schools, and special attention also should be directed toward those physicians who deal with high risk nutrition patients.

While the poor have traditionally belonged to this group, it is now apparent that malnutrition can and does affect all economic classes.

Directors, Society for Nutrition Education

The Panel on Consumer Programs and Public Education representing the Society for Nutrition Education[42] made a statement on the needs for nutrition education:

Nutrition education should be viewed as the means to develop each individual's nutritional knowledge in such a way that he will be motivated to choose a nutritionally adequate diet. It is the right of every individual to be able to easily obtain sufficient knowledge to choose an adequate diet. This right is basic and has been too long neglected. . .

Nutrition education as a part of health education and preventive medicine and dentistry should be greatly increased in federal and state programs. It is the areas of health and disease where the tremendous waste of national income exists. For example, it is possible that up to 50 percent of the money spent on dental care could be saved by nutrition programs. Effective nutrition education could reduce the incidence of obesity by as much as 80 percent.

Nutritionists: Collins, Forbes, Kocher, Yanochik

As a subgroup of the panel on Nutrition and Health, four nutritionists presented a position statement on the implementation and delivery care services in health care systems. They recommended that a nutritional care plan, determined by a dietitian/nutritionist should utilize an appropriate combination of nutrition services through all the following phases of health care: (1) primary care, (2) preventive services, (3) diagnostic services, (4) acute inpatient care, (5) chronic inpatient and extended care, (6) ambulatory care, and (7) rehabilitation.[43] The suggested patterns of nutrition care are shown in Chapter 2.

U.S. DEPARTMENT OF HEALTH, EDUCATION, AND WELFARE (DHEW), NUTRITION POLICY STATEMENT

Such testimonies as the preceding gave impetus to a policy statement issued by the Department of Health, Education, and Welfare. The policy statement describes the department's major program objectives with respect to the health aspects of nutrition. The statement also serves as a framework around which DHEW agencies can shape program initiatives, increase or redirect resources, and establish more collaborative relationships among themselves with other departments and with nonfederal agencies.

The goal of the DHEW nutrition policy[44] is to improve the quality of life by enabling all Americans to reap the health benefits of good nutrition. It has the following three main points:

1. A high priority is to ensure that every American has access to an adequate supply of wholesome food which provides all nutrients known to be essential to maintain or improve health and vitality.

Government agencies (DHEW, Social Security Administration and the Social and Rehabilitative Services) should work together to develop a Departmental nutrition policy with special attention directed at the relationship between sound nutrition, the availability and cost of food, and the policies of the United States Department of Agriculture.

2. Nutrition concerns shall permeate all health-related activities. Nutrition shall become a mandatory component of these programs of public education, primary care and comprehensive health care funded or supported by the Department, and should be included in the planning, organization and implementation of health care systems and direct health especially should be extended to those populations with special risk of malnutrition and special nutrition requirements: infants, young children, pregnant and lactating women, and the aged.

Especial attention too should be given to health problems which are initiated or aggravated by inappropriate or poor diets—e.g., dental caries, diabetes mellitus, hypertension, obesity, iron deficiency, anemia, and certain forms of arteriosclerosis and cardiovascular disease, and also diseases that require special diets, e.g., peptic ulcer, gout, heart failure, food allergy, phenylketonuria and other inborn errors of metabolism.

Nutrition concerns should also be part of the training of all health-related personnel.

3. Monitoring activities shall be needed to establish the nutritional status of the nation. This

shall be accomplished through general surveillance activities at the national level, and through local surveys of high-risk populations. It should also include monitoring trends of the eating habits of the American people, as well as determining the long-range effects of chronic ingestion of various nutrients. Studies should explore the immediate and long-term linkages between dietary habit, nutrition, and health. The results of surveillance and monitoring shall be linked programmatically to activities of the Department to promote and enhance the health and well-being of the population.

To ensure the consumption of safe and wholesome food and nutrients, it is required that there be determined the nutrient composition of foods and the presence of potentially hazardous substances—additives, artificial coloring and fortifiers—as well as inadvertent contaminants, infectious agents, toxins, or other dangerous materials as might naturally occur in foods. This also recognizes potential problems associated with changing agricultural practices, preparation, processing, packaging, transportation, and storage. Such measures require monitoring of food safety. Finally, in order that the public may make safe and intelligent selection of foods, full and accurate labeling must be assured.

1977 DIETARY GOALS OF THE UNITED STATES[44a]

On January 14, 1977, Senator George McGovern, alarmed by the diet patterns of Americans, called a press conference at which he released the first comprehensive statement by any branch of the federal government on risk factors in the American diet.

ACTION IS NEEDED NOW

Without Government and industry commitment to good nutrition, the American people will continue to eat themselves to poor health . . . Action is needed to determine how changes can be made regarding the content of nutritional information provided to the public; the kinds of food produced, how foods are processed and advertised; and the selection of foods offered by eating establishments. Our national health depends on how well and how quickly Government and industry respond.

Senator Charles H. Percy, United States Select Committee on Nutrition and Human Needs, United States Senate, January 14, 1977.

The simple fact is that individuals' diets have changed radically within the last fifty years, with great and often very harmful effects on health. Too much fat and too much sugar or salt can be and are linked directly to heart disease, cancer, obesity, and stroke, among other killer diseases.

Senator McGovern[45] announced that those within the government had an obligation to acknowledge this drastic change in the composition of the average diet in the United States. He stated that the public wanted some guidance, wanted to know the truth, and "hopefully today we can lay the cornerstone for the building of better health for all Americans, through better nutrition." He presented the following statistics:

Last year every man, woman and child in the United States consumed 125 pounds of fat, and 100 pounds of sugar.

The consumption of soft drinks has more than doubled since 1960—displacing milk as the second most consumed beverage. In 1975 there was a per capita intake on the average of 295 twelve ounce cans of soda.

In the early 1900's, almost 40 percent of caloric intake came from fruits, vegetables and grain products. Today, only a little more than 20 percent of the calories come from these sources.[45]

To illustrate a plan of action to meet the urgency of this situation, six basic goals were set for changing the national diet:

UNITED STATES DIETARY GOALS

1. Increase carbohydrate consumption to account for 55 to 60 percent of the energy (caloric) intake.
2. Reduce overall fat consumption from approximately 40 to 30 percent of energy intake.
3. Reduce saturated fat consumption to account for about 10 percent of total energy intake; and balance with polyunsaturated and monounsaturated fats, which should account for about 10 percent of energy intake each.
4. Reduce cholesterol consumption to about 300 mg. a day.
5. Reduce sugar consumption by almost 40 percent to account for about 15 percent of total energy intake.
6. Reduce salt consumption by about 50 to 85 percent to approximately 3 grams a day.[45]

The goals are expressed graphically in Fig. 1-4.

To meet these goals, the following changes in food selection and preparation by consumers were recommended:

1. Increase consumption of fruits and vegetables and whole grains.
2. Decrease consumption of meat and increase consumption of poultry and fish.
3. Decrease consumption of foods high in fat and partially substitute polyunsaturated fat for saturated fat.
4. Substitute non-fat milk for whole milk.
5. Decrease consumption of butterfat, eggs and other high cholesterol sources.
6. Decrease consumption of sugar and foods high in sugar content.
7. Decrease consumption of salt and foods high in salt content.[45]

There were also four very specific recommendations for government to encourage the achievement of the foregoing dietary goals:

1. That Congress provide money for a public education program in nutrition based on the foregoing or similar goals. The initial minimum period for the promotion of these dietary goals should be five years.

   Such a campaign should utilize and coordinate efforts emphasizing the following five functional areas:
   a. Health and nutrition education in the classroom and cafeterias of our schools
   b. Nutrition and health education for school food service workers
   c. Nutrition education in the federally-funded food assistance programs
   d. Nutrition education conducted by the Extension Service of the Department of Agriculture
   e. Extensive use of television to educate the

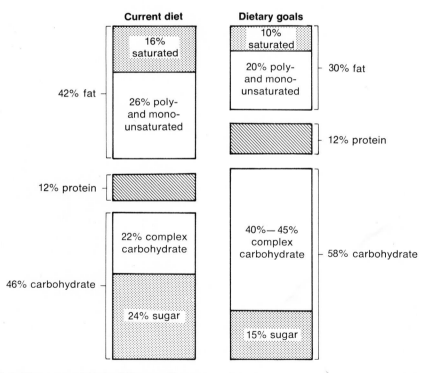

Fig. 1-4. The current United States diet versus the dietary goals. Proportions of saturated versus unsaturated fats based on unpublished Agricultural Research Service data. (From Friend, B.: Sources for current diet: changes in nutrients in the U.S. diet caused by alterations in food intake patterns, Washington, D.C., 1974, Agricultural Research Service, U.S. Department of Agriculture.)

A REQUIEM: NOVEMBER 16, 1977
Requiem for the Hunger Committee

It has had hairbreadth rescues before, but this time, barring some parliamentary miracle, a young institution of uncommon compassion and extraordinary impact seems certain to die. The least that can be done now is to mourn it well.

Its formal title is the Senate Select Committee on Nutrition and Human Needs, but for nine years it has been known throughout Washington simply as the Hunger Committee, a body that has ceaselessly prodded a disbelieving country on behalf of millions of people too poor, often, to eat.

Now the committee, chaired by Senator McGovern, is itself a victim, of the simplification of Senate committees and of enmity in the Senate Rules Committee. The Hunger Committee's work is far from finished; just last month it won passage of an act, welcome in a junk food era, to fund nutrition education in the public schools. But now the committee is scheduled to expire on Dec. 31, to be succeeded by a small subcommittee of the Senate Agriculture Committee.

The Hunger Committee will be survived by, and remembered for, an array of accomplishment. In 1968, when it began, the Federal Government was spending $228 million to help feed 2.2 million people through food stamps. This year, spending has increased 25-fold, to nearly $6 billion, benefiting 17 million people. In 1968, there was no Federally supported school lunch program. Now, 11 million children from low-income families receive subsidized lunches—and 2 million receive subsidized breakfasts.

Once the nation came to recognize how many Americans went hungry each day, the idea of helping to feed them had many friends. But it also had enemies, or at least enemies of increased Federal anti-hunger spending. The Hunger Committee was instrumental in fighting off the budget axes. Some innovations came wholly from the committee—like the W-I-C program (for women, infants and young children) designed to combat the lifelong problems caused by malnutrition during infancy. This program, instituted in 1972, now serves a million people a year.

One of them is Katherine Combs, a young mother from Appalachia, who testified before the committee last year. In talking about her sick baby and W-I-C, she uttered words that provide a fitting eulogy for the Hunger Committee: "When a man's family is starving to death and dying and turned down the help they need because of a lack of money or because the Government doesn't think they need it bad enough, just what are they supposed to do, lay down and die? . . . What I'm really trying to say is, W-I-C is great. It helped my son when nobody else would."

---

public in the potential benefits of following certain dietary goals

2. That Congress require food labelling for all foods, containing the following information to enable the consumer to make informed comparisons between foods:
   a. Percent and type of fats
   b. Percent sugar
   c. Milligrams of cholesterol
   d. Milligrams of salt
   e. Caloric content
   f. A complete listing of food additives for all foods, including those now covered by standards of identity
   g. Nutrition labelling which is currently voluntary
3. That Congress provide money to the Departments of Agriculture and Health, Education and Welfare to jointly conduct studies and pilot projects that would develop new techniques in food processing and institutional and home meal preparation aimed at reducing risk factors in the diet.
4. That Congress increase funding for human nutrition research in the Department of Agriculture in accordance with the plan of the Agricultural Research Service, and that Congress establish a committee for the coordination of human nutrition research undertaken by the Departments of Agriculture and Health, Education and Welfare.[45]

These dietary goals ignited much discussion. The comments ranged from Goodwin's "Let's get on with the dietary goals, one of the most significant contributions to the public's health in recent years,"[46] to the opposition of the American Medical Association, the meat industry, and the sugar lobby.

The American Medical Association[47] indicated that "While the goals set forth would appear to be laudable in many respects, the AMA believes that at this time it would not be appropriate to adopt such dietary goals . . . carry with them the underlying potential for prohibiting the sale or for discouraging the agricultural production of certain food products which may not in the view of the government be supportive of the dietary goals."

In addition, the meat industry actively sought to discredit the dietary goals report because of the recommended increased substitution of poultry and fish for red meat in an effort to reduce fat and cholesterol consumption.[47]

The evaluation of the role of cholesterol in foods and its relation to serum cholesterol levels continues. Alfin-Slater[48] reported that "Although there is a segment of the population who are genetically disposed to hypercholesterolemia and atherosclerosis and who therefore should not limit their dietary cholesterol intake, this should not apply to the population as a whole. Obviously much more research is needed in this area."

Dietary Goals for the United States, second edition[48a]

Since the release of the first edition of *Dietary Goals*, eight more hearings have been held in the series, "Diet Related to Killer Diseases."[49] They are *Diet and Cardiovascular Disease*,[50] *Obesity*,[51] *Dietary Goals for the U.S.—Re Meat*,[52] *Dietary Fiber and Health*,[53] *Nutrition: Mental Health and Mental Development*,[54] *Dietary Goals for the U.S.—Re: Eggs*,[55] *Nutrition: Aging and the Elderly*,[56] and *Nutrition at HEW: Policy, Research, and Regulation*.[57]

These hearings, which have included dozens of independent researchers and numerous governmental health officials, have

brought to light more evidence from epidemiologic studies and basic clinical research and have highlighted further the areas of controversy. Their responses and others solicited by the Select Committee were immediately sought, and those received are printed in their entirety in *Dietary Goals for the United States—Supplemental Views*.[58] There continued to be concern about the shift in per capita civilian consumption of food energy, protein, fat, and carbohydrate as shown in Fig. 1-5. Since 1910 there has been a decrease in carbohydrate and an increase in fat as energy sources in the United States diet.

The intense discussion and debate that prompted the issuance of this second edition are good signs. The sense of immediacy has not lessened, nor has the concern among those charged with developing the nation's health policy.

New goal added. Of all the comments received on *Dietary Goals*, perhaps the one heard most often was that there should be a goal addressing total energy (caloric) consumption. The second edition includes such a new goal: To avoid overweight, consume only as much energy (calories) as is expended; if overweight, decrease energy intake and increase energy expenditure.

The alarming prevalence of obesity in the

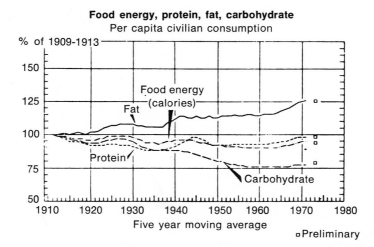

Fig. 1-5. 1910 to 1980 per capita consumption of protein, carbohydrates, fat, and calories. (From Friend, B.: Changes in nutrients in the U.S. diet caused by alterations in food intake patterns, Washington, D.C., Agricultural Research Service, U.S. Department of Agriculture.)

United States is attributable partly to the fact that the energy requirements of Americans have decreased steadily over recent decades. This decline in energy expenditure has not been paralleled by a decline in energy intake. The physical activity of people in the United States is generally considered to be light to sedentary rather than heavy as was true earlier in the century.

Obesity resulting from the overconsumption of calories is a major risk factor in many killer diseases. Therefore it is extremely important either to maintain an optimal weight or to alter one's weight to reach an optimal level. Altering one's calorie consumption is not the only way to control weight and thus lessen the risk factors associated with obesity. Exercise can and should play an important and integral role as well. Even if dietary patterns remain the same, the influence of an increasingly sedentary life-style may turn what was previously a diet adequate in calories into one with too many calories.

Revised goals of the second edition follow:

UNITED STATES DIETARY GOALS

1. To avoid overweight, consume only as much energy (calories) as is expended; if over-

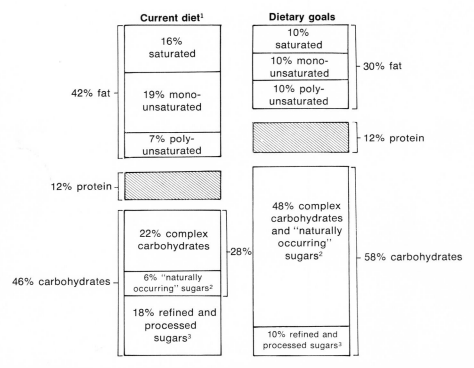

Fig. 1-6. The current United States diet versus the dietary goals. [1]These percentages are based on calories from food and nonalcoholic beverages. Alcohol adds approximately 210 calories a day to the average diet of drinking-age Americans. [2]"Naturally occurring" sugars that are indigenous to a food as opposed to refined (cane and beet) and processed (corn sugar syrups, molasses, and honey) sugars that may be added to a food product. [3]In many ways alcoholic beverages affect the diet in the same way as refined and other processed sugars. Both add calories (energy) to the total diet but contribute little or no vitamins or minerals. (Sources for current diet from Friend, B.: Changes in nutrients in the U.S. diet caused by alterations in food intake patterns, 1974, Agricultural Research Service, U.S. Department of Agriculture. Proportions of saturated versus unsaturated fats based on unpublished Agricultural Research Service data.)

weight, decrease energy intake and increase energy expenditure.

2. Increase the consumption of complex carbohydrates and "naturally occurring" sugars from about 28 percent of energy intake to about 48 percent of energy intake.
3. Reduce the consumption of refined and processed sugars by about 45 percent to account for about 10 percent of total energy intake.
4. Reduce overall fat consumption from approximately 40 percent to about 30 percent of energy intake.
5. Reduce saturated fat consumption to account for about 10 percent of total energy intake; and balance that with poly-unsaturated and mono-unsaturated fats, which should account for about 10 percent of energy intake each.
6. Reduce cholesterol consumption to about 300 mg. a day.
7. Limit the intake of sodium by reducing the intake of salt to about 5 grams a day.[48a]

The goals suggest the following changes in food selection and preparation:

1. Increase consumption of fruits and vegetables and whole grains.
2. Decrease consumption of refined and other processed sugars and foods high in such sugars.
3. Decrease consumption of foods high in total fat, and partially replace saturated fats, whether obtained from animal or vegetable sources, with poly-unsaturated fats.
4. Decrease consumption of animal fat, and choose meats, poultry and fish which will reduce saturated fat intake.
5. Except for young children, substitute low-fat and non-fat milk for whole milk, and low-fat dairy products for high fat dairy products.
6. Decrease consumption of butterfat, eggs and other high cholesterol sources. Some consideration should be given to easing the cholesterol goal for pre-menopausal women, young children and the elderly in order to obtain the nutritional benefits of eggs in the diet.
7. Decrease consumption of salt and foods high in salt content.[48a]

Although the dietary goals are stated in terms of specific levels, each specific level should be considered as the center of a range. A revised graphic representation is expressed in Fig. 1-6.

NORWEGIAN NUTRITION POLICY

A comprehensive nutrition policy was proposed by the Ministry of Agriculture of Norway in December, 1975.[59] It is comprehensive in that it was developed as a cooperative effort between experts in agriculture and public health and it is promising in that it is the culmination of a long development of policy in the health and agricultural sectors.

Winikoff[60] has presented a comparison of the approaches of Norway and the United States to the subject of a national nutrition policy. Whereas Ringen noted that the Norwegian nutrition and food policy is "somewhat of a milestone," Winikoff offers the following three reasons why the Norwegian document is even more remarkable in relation to the United States' efforts in the same area:

1. The goals of the proposed nutrition and food policy are based on scientific understandings of nutrition/health interrelationships. Real numbers, based on nutritional knowledge, are the foundation of the proposal. This is a document which does not rely only on humanitarianism, morality, or pious hopes for the future.
2. The stated goals themselves are the desired end points against which policy must be measured. These goals take primacy over the institutional or functional arrangements of government structures designed to deal with nutrition.
3. The national government takes itself seriously as an institution responsible for setting overall policy directions. The government's responsibility is first to the well-being of its own citizens, and as far as possible, in congruence with the aspirations and needs of other citizens of the world.

Do we need a national nutrition policy? Do we need dietary goals?

SUMMARY

The 1970s brought an emerging awareness that food resources are finite, and while much of the world is suffering from nutritional disease of poverty, a large proportion of the population of the United States is suffering from diseases related to overabundance and over-consumption of food. Gradually, through the 1930s, 1940s, 1950s, and 1960s, there has been increased legislation regarding public health care, including some mention of nutrition, but it was not until the early 1970s that there was a specific White House Conference on Food, Nutrition and Health. This conference recommended coordination of nutrition and health programs among the various agencies of government and delivery of health and nutrition services to needy areas, and it generally stimulated recognition and discussion of prevalent nutrition-related diseases.

Among the most serious diseases related to diet in the United States are heart disease, stroke and hypertension, cancer, diabetes, arteriosclerosis, and cirrhosis of the liver. In addition to improper diet, these diseases are aggravated by contemporary life-styles, which include lack of physical exercise and a large amount of mental stress and emotional tension.

At the National Nutrition Policy Study Hearings held in the early 1970s, the extraordinarily high costs of medicine and the huge amount of the gross national product spent on health bills were pointed out. These costs are incurred by treatment of diseases, rather than by a health delivery system that offers primary care, or rather, primary prevention. It is in the area of primary prevention programs that priorities should be established and thus, ultimately, reduce excessive expenditures. Many experts have noted that whereas medical expenditures have increased enormously, life expectancy in the United States has remained the same over the past twenty-five years.

To combat this state of affairs, the National Nutrition Consortium issued guidelines for a national nutrition policy. It stressed the need

for such a policy, its goals, the programs necessary to meet objectives, and the requirements for a national nutrition policy. In 1974 further U.S. Senate hearings at which experts presented evidence and findings were held. They reiterated the need for a national nutrition policy.

An urgency was expressed when Senator McGovern called a press conference in January 14, 1977, at which he called attention to the radical change in the average American diet during this century. He linked this change in dietary patterns to the high toll of killer diseases. To reverse the trend and to combat these diseases, the dietary goals of the United States and changes in food selections necessary to meet these goals were outlined. Later in 1977, as a result of a series of hearings, a second edition of the Dietary Goals were released. A new goal addressed to the problem of obesity appeared in this edition. To implement these important recommendations, carefully designed programs and program implementation are needed. To whom should this task be delegated? The need for manpower trained specifically in the areas of nutrition and preventive health care cannot be overestimated. The nutritionist is the health professional whose training is based solely and specifically in the knowledge, skills and art required in translating the findings of nutritional science into action so that programs can be designed to meet the public's need. Thus Chapter 2 is concerned with the public health nutritionist. Who is she, who is he, and how do they function, in what agencies and settings?

REFERENCES

1. The World Food Problem, Report of the President's Science Advisory Committee, Washington, D.C., May, 1967, Government Printing Office, vol. I.
2. Royal Norwegian Ministry of Agriculture: Report to the Stortling, no. 32 (1975-1976) on Norwegian nutrition and food policy, Oslo, 1975.
3. Hunger U.S.A., Report of the Citizens' Board of Inquiry into Hunger and Malnutrition in the United States, Boston, 1968, Beacon Press, Inc.
4. Statement by Arnold E. Schaefer, Chief Nutrition Program, Division of Chronic Disease Programs, Regional Medical Programs Service, U.S. Department of Health, Education, and Welfare, before U.S. Senate Select Committee on Nutrition and Related Human Needs, Jan., 22, 1969.
5. Center for Disease Control, U.S. Department of Health, Education, and Welfare: Ten-state nutrition survey, Publication no. 72-8134, Atlanta, 1972, vol. 1.
6. White House Conference on Food, Nutrition and Health, Final Report, Washington, D.C., 1970, Government Printing Office.
7. White House Conference on Food, Nutrition and Health. Report on Follow-Up Conference, Williamsburg, Va., Feb. 5, 1971.
8. U.S. Department of Health, Education, and Welfare; Ten-state nutrition survey, 1968-1970, Washington, D.C., 1972, Publication no. (HSM) 72-8130-8134, Government Printing Office.
9. U.S. Department of Health, Education, and Welfare: Preliminary findings of the first health and nutrition examination survey, U.S., 1971-72, Washington, D.C., 1973, Publication no. (HRA) 74-1219-1, Government Printing Office.
10. Owen, G., et al.: A study of nutritional status of preschool children in the United States, 1968-1970, Pediatrics 53(suppl.):597, 1974.
11. Kaufman, M., et al.: Families of the fields—their food and their health, Division of Health State of Florida Monograph Series, No. 13, 1973.
12. Larson, L., et al.: Nutritional status of children of Mexican-American migrant families, J. Am. Diet. Assoc. 64:29, 1974.
13. Center for Disease Control, U.S. Department of Health, Education, and Welfare: Nutrition surveillance, Washington, D.C., 1975, Publication no. (CDC) 75-8295, Government Printing Office.
14. The nutritional components of health care delivery systems, J. Am. Diet. Assoc. 58:537, 1971.
15. Constitution of the World Health Organization, Geneva, 1948.
16. Burger, E. J., Jr.: Health and health services in the United States—a perspective and a discussion of some issues, Ann. Intern. Med. 80:645, 1974.
17. Forbes, W. H.: Longevity and medical costs, N. Engl. J. Med. 287:77, 1967.
18. Glazer, N.: Perspectives on health care, Public Interest 31:110, Spring, 1973.
19. Cornely, P. B., There is more to health than just paying bills (editorial), Am. J. Public Health 64:9, Sept., 1974.
20. U.S. Department of Health, Education and Welfare: Forward plan for health FY 1978-82, Washington, D.C., 1976, Government Printing Office, p. 1.
21. Farquhar, J. W.: Prepared statement to U.S. Senate Select Committee on Nutrition and Human Needs. Part 5. Washington, D.C., June 21, 1974, Government Printing Office, p. 2630.
22. Popkin, B. M.: Economic benefits from the elimination of hunger in America, Institute for Research on Poverty Discussion Paper No. 102-71, Madison, Wis., 1971, University of Wisconsin Press.
23. Butterworth, C. E., Jr.: The present status of nutrition education in medicine. In White, P. L., Mahan, K., and Moore, M. F., editors: Conference on guidelines for nutritional education in medical schools and post-doctoral training, Williamsburg, Va., June 25-27, 1972, Chicago, 1972, Council on Foods and Nutrition, American Medical Association, p. 16.
24. Millis, J. S.: A rational public policy for medical education and its financing, New York, 1971, The National Fund for Medical Education, p. 23.
25. Fuchs, V. F.: Who shall live? Health, economics and social change, New York, 1974, Basic Books, Inc.
26. U.S. Department of Health, Education, and Welfare, National Center for Health Statistics: Monthly vital statistics report—annual summary for the United States, 1973, Washington, D.C., June 27, 1974, Government Printing Office.
27. U.S. Department of Health, Education, and Welfare, National Center for Health Statistics; Monthly vital statistics report—summary report, final mor-

tality statistics, 1972, Nov. 6, 1974, Table 1, p. 3.

28. The New York Times, citing an article in The Lancet by scientists at St. Thomas Hospital and the London School of Hygiene and Tropical Medicine, Nov. 12, 1974, p. 35.

29. National Institute on Alcohol Abuse and Alcoholism, U.S. Department of Health, Education, and Welfare: Personal communication, Rockville, Md., Jan., 1975.

30. Heart facts reference sheet, New York, 1975, American Heart Association.

31. Milio, N.: A framework for prevention: changing health-damaging to health generating life patterns, Am. J. Public Health **65**:435, 1976.

32. Belloc, N., and Breslow, L.: Relationship of physical health status and health practices, Prev. Med. **1**: 409, 1972.

33. Beloff, J. S.: The teaching of comprehensive patient care (editorial), Am. J. Public Health **60**:430, 1970.

34. Steiger, W. A., Hoffman, F. H., Hansen, A. V., et. al.: A definition of comprehensive medicine, J. Health Human Behav. **1**:83, 1960.

35. Kresky, B.: Ambulatory care: impact on changes and concepts on planning for facilities, N.Y. State J. Med. **74**:562, 1974.

36. White, K., Williams F., and Greenberg, B. G.: The ecology of medical care, N. Engl. J. Med. **265**: 887, 1961.

37. Hearing of the McGovern Committee on Nutrition and Human Needs, Nutr. Today **9**:25, July/Aug., 1974.

38. Connor, W. E., and Connor, S. L.: The role of nutritional factors in coronary heart disease, Panel paper for the Senate Committee on Nutrition and Health, Subpanel on Nutrition and Health, Iowa City, 1974, Department of Internal Medicine and Clinical Research Center, University of Iowa (mimeographed).

39. Schweiker, R. S.: Nutrition and diseases: diabetes and the daily diet, U.S. Senate Select Committee Hearing on Nutrition and Human Needs, Feb. 26, 1974, Washington, D.C., 1974, Government Printing Office, p. 405.

40. Cahill, G. F., Jr.: Prepared statement for Hearings before the U.S. Senate Select Committee on Nutrition and Human Needs. Part 4. Diabetes and the daily diet, Washington, D.C., Feb. 26, 1974, Government Printing Office, p. 408.

41. Kennedy, E. M.: Opening statement, National Nutrition Policy Study Hearings on Nutrition and Health, June 21, 1974.

42. Board of Directors, Society for Nutrition Education: National nutrition policy: nutrition and the consumer II. Working Paper for the U.S. Senate Select Committee on Nutrition and Human Needs, June, 1974.

43. Collins, M. E., Forbes, C., Kocher, R., and Yanochik, A.: Position statement of implementation and delivery of nutritional care services in the health care system, Subpanel of Health Care Systems of the Panel on Nutrition and Health, U.S. Senate Select Committee on Nutrition and Human Needs. Part 6. Washington, D.C., June 21, 1974, Government Printing Office, p. 2626.

44. U.S. Department of Health, Education, and Welfare, Public Health Service, Bureau of Community Health Services: Preliminary guide for developing nutrition services in health care programs, Washington, D.C., 1976, Government Printing Office.

44a. Select Committee on Nutrition and Human Needs: Dietary goals for the United States, Washington, D.C., Jan., 1977, Government Printing Office.

45. McGovern Press Release, Jan. 17, 1977 (mimeographed).

46. Goodwin, M. Y.: Let's get on with the dietary goals, Community Nutrition Institute Weekly Report **7**:4, Aug., 4, 1977.

47. CNI Weekly Report: AMA opposes dietary goals, June 23, 1977. AMA opposes dietary goals, Community Nutrition Institute Weekly Report **7**:8, June 23, 1977.

48. Alfin-Slater, R. B.: Nutrition—styled to protect against heart disease: the moderately styled approach (abstracts), 60th Annual Meeting, Oct. 10-14, 1977, Los Angeles, The American Dietetic Association.

48a. Select Committee on Nutrition and Human Needs: Dietary goals for the United States, ed. 2, Washington, D.C., Dec., 1977, Government Printing Office.

49. Diet related to killer diseases, July 27 and 28, 1976, Washington, D.C., U.S. Government Printing Office.

50. Diet related to killer diseases, Vol. II, Part I, Diet and cardiovascular disease, Feb. 1, 1977, Washington, D.C., U.S. Government Printing Office.

51. Diet related to killer diseases, Vol. II, Part 2, Obesity, Feb. 2, 1977, Washington, D.C., U.S. Government Printing Office.

52. Diet related to killer diseases, Vol. III, Response to dietary goals for the U.S.—re meat, March 24, 1977, Washington, D.C., U.S. Government Printing Office.

53. Diet related to killer diseases, Vol. IV, Dietary fiber and health, March 31, 1977, Washington, D.C., U.S. Government Printing Office.

54. Diet related to killer diseases, Vol. V, Nutrition: mental health and mental development, June 22, 1977, Washington, D.C., U.S. Government Printing Office.

55. Diet related to killer diseases, Vol. VI, Response to dietary goals for the U.S.—re eggs, July 26, 1977, Washington, D.C., U.S. Government Printing Office.

56. Diet related to killer diseases, Vol. VII, Nutrition: aging and the elderly, Sept. 23, 1977, Washington, D.C., 1977, U.S. Government Printing Office.

57. Diet related to killer diseases, Vol. VIII, Nutrition at HEW: policy, research and regulation, Oct. 17, 1977, Washington, D.C., 1977, U.S. Government Printing Office.

58. Dietary goals for the United States—supplemental views, Nov., 1977, Washington, D.C., U.S. Government Printing Office.

59. Ringen, K.: The Norwegian food and nutrition policy, Am. J. Public Health **67:**550, 1977.

60. Winikoff, B.: Nutrition and food policy: the approaches of Norway and the United States, Am. J. Public Health **67:**552, 1977.

GENERAL CONCEPT

The public health nutritionist is the health professional who must assume leadership required to promote, elevate, and maintain the nutritional status of all members of society, especially as the role of nutrition in health maintenance and disease prevention is becoming better recognized.

OUTCOMES

The student should be able to do the following:
- Define the role and functions of the nutritionist.
- Indicate how and at what levels the nutritionist operates.
- Differentiate the types of care and teams in the health delivery system.
- Define the procedures for quality assurance.

Role of the public health nutritionist: who? where? how? how well?

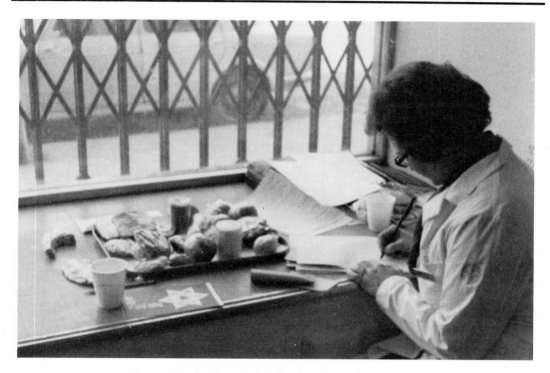

Exodus House Drug Rehabilitation Center Storefront, New York, New York.

WHY THE NUTRITIONIST?

Public health programing that contains a strong nutrition component is a definite public need, since nutrition has been identified and proved to be a vital environmental factor affecting human development, health, productivity, and longevity. National nutrition surveys have shown the existence of major nutritional problems that result in growth deficits, iron-deficiency anemia, obesity, elevated blood lipids, and dental caries. In 1977 the U.S. Senate Select Committee on Nutri-

tion and Human Needs pointed out that six of the ten leading causes of death in the United States are related to diet—heart disease, stroke and hypertension, cancer, diabetes, arteriosclerosis, and cirrhosis of the liver. Such findings document the need for nutrition programs.

Radical changes for the worse in the diet habits of Americans during this century have been linked to these disease-inducing nutritional problems. To reverse this trend, carefully designed programs must be planned,

A PHILOSOPHY OF PUBLIC HEALTH NUTRITION

It involves the point of view that nutrition is not only a science, but also a social means to help meet the health needs of the people. People are not to be viewed as passive consumers of food and nutrients who are simply to be fed or told what to eat. They are human beings with rights and potential, whose well-being is the goal of all nutritional endeavors. Food, as a prime tool for meeting nutritional needs, must be viewed as intimately tied to a total way of life—socially, politically, and economically. Nutrition must be seen in perspective as but one important part of the total health picture.

Ruth L. Huenemann and *Mary M. Murai:* Philosophy and status of an educational program for public health nutritionist-dietitians, J. Am. Diet. Assoc. **61:**669, 1972. Reprinted by permission. Copyright The American Dietetic Association.

implemented, and evaluated. This necessitates a willingness on the part of the nutritionist in public health to assume the leadership required to promote, elevate, and maintain a nutritional status that is consistent with recognized health norms for all members of society. Once such a goal is established, the questions may be asked: Who is the nutritionist? What is inherent in the education and training of the nutritionist that qualifies him or her for this task?

WHO IS THE NUTRITIONIST?

The nutritionist, as a member of the health planning team, is the professional whose specialized education, training, and experience is based solely and specifically on the science and art of nutrition. The nutritionist translates the findings of biomedical science into action so that they can reach the people. The nutritionist interprets these findings into specific food plans to meet the requirements for health and to alleviate disease throughout the life cycle. In addition, the nutritionist has a working or practical knowledge of dietetics, food practices, food economics and budgeting, the psychological and social significance of eating behavior, and educational methodology. The nutritionist is aware of the pa-tient as part of the institutional setting, the home environment, and the community. The nutritionist is familiar with the resources at the community, city, state, and federal level.

In the past the public health nutritionist had little or no training and education in administration and advocacy and therefore neither accepted nor was given administrative and legislative responsibilities. Fortunately, the attitudes toward preventive measures in health care and the best means to implement and administer them are becoming increasingly more sophisticated.[1]

Educational background, qualifications, and responsibilities

The nutritionist, whether trained to work primarily with individuals or groups, is concerned foremost with maintaining a desirable nutritional status and is responsible as planner, promoter, initiator, and evaluator for the nutrition component of health services. This task requires specific qualifications and training. At the college undergraduate level, education is designed to prepare the student to enter the profession at the staff level, usually to function in a direct service setting such as a hospital outpatient clinic, a neighborhood health center, or a health maintenance organization under the supervision of the public health nutritionist who has had graduate education and training.

Graduate education at the master's level includes advanced study in the science of nutrition, in special aspects of public health, in the behavioral and psychological sciences, in sociologic sciences, and in education theory and practice. The public health courses introduce program planning, health care administration and evaluation. The behavioral science and educational courses are directed toward understanding behavioral change. This further study, plus field practice, instructs the nutritionist how to operate at the supervisory program planning and administrative level. Doctoral level training prepares one for teaching, service, and research in public health practice, whether it be under the auspices of medical center, government, or industry.

Each level—baccalaureate (undergraduate), master's, and doctoral—demands continuing education in the expanding science and art of nutrition. This is usually done through workshops, seminars, and refresher courses, as well as attendance at professional meetings at the local, national, and international levels. Additional depth and understanding can be gained by prearranged visits to other nutrition agencies and programs. Specific guidelines for the education and training of public health nutritionists at each level are described in detail by an American Dietetic Association publication, *Personnel in Public Health Nutrition.*[2]

The various titles, qualifications, and responsibilities of personnel in public health nutrition have been carefully outlined in this American Dietetic Association publication by an expert committee of nutritionists and physicians. The titles that may be assigned are those of the public health nutritionist; the community dietitian; the public health nutritionist in a specialized area—administration, maternal and child health, adult health, geriatrics, chronic diseases, and rehabilitation; clinical dietetics; group food service (consultant dietitian and dietitian); the college and university teacher of public health nutrition; the medical public health nutritionist; the research public health nutritionist; and the community health nutrition aide.

The titles "nutritionist" and "dietitian" as used in this American Dietetic Report refer to the specialists in human nutrition who direct their knowledge and competence toward the maintenance and improvement of human health. This publication further delineates the titles, responsibilities, and qualifications of persons to be employed by both official and voluntary public health agencies and those in educational institutions that are preparing personnel for such agencies.

Such a professional, who is a member of the health team that assesses community nutrition needs and also plans, implements, and evaluates the nutrition component of health services, is the kind of nutritionist being addressed in this text. The specific responsibilities of the public health nutritionist have

THE HOSPITAL DIETITIAN: EXPANDED HORIZONS

The major part of professional nutrition care provided in this country is to hospitalized patients. As a hospital nutritionist, I am aware that this severely limits our ability to influence nutritional practices by the population at large. However, in order to permit the expansion of hospital nutrition services to people in the community, third-party payor reimbursement must become reality . . .

The involvement of health care in the average American's life can be illustrated by the person who has a heart attack at age fifty. For almost forty-five years of his life, he does well, experiencing few health problems beyond colds and minor aches and seldom relating to the medical care system. At forty-five, obvious signs of atherosclerosis may appear—elevated blood pressure, poor circulation, and perhaps angina. At age fifty, the crisis strikes. Last year, approximately one million Americans went through this particular crisis—myocardial infarction. For two or three weeks of hospitalization, he is treated with the intensive care intervention of a modern hospital with a resulting bill, usually over $3,500. After that, he requires less intensive, but still costly, medical care providing rehabilitation and support. Nutritional care often enters this scenario only at the point of crisis intervention . . .

Agencies in Washington and most states will not pay for rehabilitative or preventive health care, and because of this, our clinic may be forced to limit or eliminate welfare patients. Third-party payors, such as medical insurance companies, have been hesitant to pay for nutritional counseling for out-patients. In fact, some patients have been hospitalized for little more than nutritional counseling and general health teaching. That is, at best, a costly answer to this problem . . .

A belief is prevalent outside the health care area that anyone can teach nutrition by means of the "Basic 4" food groups. However, nutrition is a much broader subject than this comment would indicate. Nutritional services should be provided by professionals adequately educated in nutrition and in the physical and social sciences.

The dietitian and dietetic technicians working as a team can effectively provide both education and care. We have a rapidly growing group of well trained individuals who could help American people adjust to a permanent change in eating habits, leading to a healthier, more vigorous life. What is needed now is financial commitment to make this expertise available to the public in time to prevent a medical crisis.

Joan M. Karkeck: Dietary counseling in ambulatory care—viewpoint of the hospital dietitian, J. Am. Diet. Assoc. **68:**249, 1976. Reprinted by permission. Copyright The American Dietetic Association.

been outlined by a special committee of the American Dietetic Association[2, p.5] as follows:

1. To identify nutritional needs: plan, organize, direct, coordinate, and evaluate the nutrition component of health services, programs, and projects.
2. To participate in assessing the nutritive quality of food eaten by people in the community and identify the probable relationship of food intake to the number and kind of health problems reported.
3. To provide consultation with physicians, nurses, social workers, therapists, teachers, and other professional workers on current nutrition research findings and the practical application to personal and community health.
4. To plan, direct, and/or carry out in-service education and orientation programs for workers in nutrition and allied professions.
5. To plan and supervise public health field experience for students in public health nutrition, dietetics, and allied health professions.
6. To advise administrators of health care facilities and food service personnel in group care facilities (hospitals, nursing homes, extended care facilities, child care centers, and institutions) on appropriate nutrition and management standards; determine need for employment of qualified dietitians; recruit and consult with dietitians as necessary.
7. To plan and evaluate dietary studies and participate in nutritional status studies and epidemiological studies with a nutrition aspect.
8. To coordinate the public health nutrition services with related programs and so bring about appropriate action.
9. To select, plan, prepare, and evaluate teaching aids and materials that will disseminate nutrition and diet information to professional and nonprofessional audiences through various media.
10. To keep records of work performed: evaluate programs in terms of objectives, and develop plans for the future.
11. To interpret food labeling and food legislation for other professionals and the consumer.
12. To provide assistance in establishing food assistance programs or feeding programs such as congregate meals and "Meals on Wheels" for the elderly or child nutrition and school feeding programs as needed.

The job description is even further defined for the public health nutritionist in administration. The nutritionist administrator establishes policies, develops, organizes, and administers a coordinated program of nutrition services. The responsibilities for this job are as follows:

1. To plan policy and action related to changing health needs as influenced by nutrition practices and social and economic forces.

ECONOMICS, MANAGEMENT, AND PUBLIC HEALTH NUTRITION

In a study in which the efficiency of comprehensive health care delivery was examined . . . , the presence of a nutritional function area in a comprehensive health care project for children and youth had the net effect of reducing average annual registrant cost.

Thus, the inclusion of public health nutritionists is a cost-effective strategy in formulating a program of comprehensive health care for children and youth. However, once the nutritional functional area is included, the cost of delivering this care should be analyzed further.

In making the above inferences about nutritional care efficiency, the assumption could be made that nutritionists are equally qualified and competent across projects. In spite of carefully defined job descriptions and specifications for education and experience, it is, of course, unlikely that all nutritionists perform equally well in all projects. Consequently, the measurements of nutritional performance will reflect, at least in part, different personal productivities across nutritionists.

However, the economics of health indicates that the most effective and desirable strategies must involve the public in a much more active role. Not only must people take the major responsibility for their own health, they must be prepared to change their life style, placing a major prescriptive focus on the improvement and maintenance of personal health. Nutritionists should assume a leading role in developing this new direction in health policy and participate in what could yield the greatest return to investment in public health of any feasible and available healthy strategy. Research has demonstrated the promise of this approach. Professionals from all relevant disciplines are trained and available. It is time to act.

2. To determine program priorities through projection of anticipated benefits and expected costs.
3. To establish effective working relationships between state and local government and voluntary agencies in matters related to nutrition.
4. To evaluate the effectiveness of program services provided and report findings.
5. To recruit and direct a staff of multidisciplinary personnel.

WHERE IS THE NUTRITIONIST EMPLOYED?

The public health nutritionist may be employed at the international, federal, state, county, city, or neighborhood level. Depending on the program's organization, the nutritionist may be employed either as a generalist who develops all nutrition services or as a specialist who serves in a specific program or population group. For example, health programs designed to meet different population groups may be organized to meet specific needs: special high-risk periods of the life cycle, such as pregnancy, infancy, childhood, and old age; or populations with special needs for care because of socioeconomic status or life-style, such as the elderly living alone or in groups and migrant workers; or various health problems, such as dental health, chronic disease control, communicable disease control, starvation, and malnutrition.

International level

Nutrition at the international level was the theme of the International Conference on Nutrition, National Development, and Planning at Massachusetts Institute of Technology in 1971, which was attended by representatives from fifty-five countries. The paramount question of this conference was: Should the nutritionist logically have a major role in national development plans all over the world, especially in the lower income countries of the Third World, for economic as well as for humanitarian reasons, bearing in mind the other very great claims on limited resources of all types?

One of the conclusions of this highly im-

portant conference was that there was a need for change in the roles of the development planner and of the nutritionist. Reference was made to a growing need for the eco-nutritionist, or the nutritionally oriented government planner, who could be more instrumental than the classic nutritionist in improving nutrition around the world.

Nutritionists employed at the international level can be found in such international agencies as WHO, PAHO, FAO, and UNICEF. The contemporary nutritionist in such agencies must have a much wider scope and vision than in the past. Jelliffe[3] suggests that one of the roles of the international nutritionist is to inform the planner and to give technical advice. To do this adequately, he says,

There is a need, for example, in the training program to study political science, the techniques of decision-making and policy-making, modern managerial methods, and the like . . . The nutritionist has become much more aware of the financial burden of malnutrition to the community, especially through the drain on the health services, and of the need to consider cost-benefit implications of alternative programs.

National level

At the federal level most nutrition programs and services are within the U.S. Departments of Agriculture and Health, Education, and Welfare. The nutritionist at that level is a program planner. As the outline below indicates, there is wide variety in the kinds of programs that require the services of a nutritionist—from direct food programs such as the food stamp, child nutrition, and elderly need programs; to less direct activities such as surveys and basic research; to practical procedure operations such as administrative training programs, establishing of nutritional guidelines, enrichment procedures, and food labeling; to general health services programs.

FEDERAL NUTRITION PROGRAMS/SERVICES*

I. U.S. Department of Agriculture
   A. Food and Nutrition Service

---

*Anonymous, 1976.

1. "Food Stamp Program"
2. "Child Nutrition Programs"
   a. National School Lunch Program
   b. School Breakfast Program
   c. Nonfood Assistance Program
   d. Special Food Service Program for Children
   e. Special Milk Program
   f. Women, Infants, and Children (WIC)
3. "Food Distribution Program"
B. Agricultural Research Service
   1. Consumer and Food Economics Research Division
      a. Family Economics Branch—surveys food, housing and clothing expenses
      b. Food Consumption Branch—food consumption surveys—nutritional adequacy of diets
      c. Food and Diet Appraisal Branch—food composition data
      d. Daily food guides
   2. Human Nutrition Research Division
C. Cooperative State Research Service—grants of landgrant colleges for basic research
D. Extension Service—education agency of USDA, EFNEP among others
E. Economic Research Service—research and technical service for AID
II. U.S. Department of Health, Education, and Welfare
A. Public Health Service
   1. Food and Drug Administration
      a. Nutrition labeling
      b. Nutritional Guidelines
      c. Enrichment of Foods
      d. Food safety programs
   2. Health Resources Administration
      a. Training Programs
      b. Comprehensive health planning
   3. Health Services Administration
      a. Maternal and Child Health Service
         (1) Maternal and Infant Care Projects
         (2) Children and Youth Projects
         (3) Maternal and Child Health Programs
      b. Community Health Service
         (1) Neighborhood and Family Health Centers
      c. Migrant Health Programs
      d. Others

4. National Institutes of Health
   a. Heart and Lung Institute et al.—basic research
5. National Institute of Alcoholism, Drugs and Mental Health
B. Office of Human Resources
   1. Administration on Aging—elderly feeding programs
   2. Others
C. Office of Education
   1. School Health and Nutrition Services Project—demonstration projects to improve health and nutrition services in needy schools

State level

Prior to 1937 little existed in the way of nutrition services in state health departments, chiefly because neither the health officer nor the public related nutrition to the maintenance of health and the prevention of disease. However, from 1933 to 1935, during the depression years, hundreds of workers trained in nutrition were employed by state and local emergency relief administrations to give advisory service to directors concerned with their responsibility for preserving the health of unemployed families and individuals.[4]

Federal funding became available to state and local health services at about this time. The Social Security Act of 1935 provided some funds to extend nutrition services in maternal and child health programs and opened the way for the application of both preventive and curative measures as a basic part of child health care.

In 1935 there were 9 nutritionists in three state health departments; by September, 1937, fifteen state health departments employed 27 nutritionists. With the continued financial support of federal agencies and the impetus arising from the discovery of the poor nutritional status of World War II army recruits, the rapid expansion continued. By 1943 there were about 100 nutritionists and 150 vacancies in forty-four state and territorial health departments and an unknown number of city and county agencies. A 1946 estimate of all public health nutritionists was 400. By this time official state agencies employed the largest number, with the American Red Cross next. Others were employed by visiting nurses associations, health councils, and tuberculosis associations.[5]

The directors of nutrition in the state and territorial health departments organized in 1952 so that they would be able to communicate formally with the state and territorial health officers and exchange information about common problems. A few medical nutritionists entered public health and became directors of some nutrition programs, but the great majority of directors were nonmedical nutritionists.[6]

By way of comparison, Table 2-1, compiled by Nichaman and Collins,[7] shows the number of state and territorial nutrition positions

budgeted and filled as of May, 1973. The administrative location and the number of nutritionists reported to be employed is shown in Table 2-2.

At the state level, nutritionists spend a large proportion of their time providing consultation to others in the agency, to local health departments, and to nonagency personnel concerned with nutrition and health such as teachers, agricultural workers, and welfare employees. Depending on the individual state structure, considerable time also may be devoted to various group care facilities. In general, direct patient counseling is provided by local departments or by local clinic staff.[7]

A sample position description of a public

Table 2-1. Number of state and territorial nutrition positions budgeted and filled, May, 1973*†

Number of positions budgeted per state and territory	Number of states and territories reporting	Total number of positions budgeted	Positions vacant
None	2	—	—
1-3	14	27	4
4-6	17	83	10
7-9	6	47	4
10-20	12	160	21
Over 20	4	179	12
Total	55	496	51

*From Nichaman, M. Z., and Collins, G. E.: Nutrition programs in state health agencies, Nutr. Rev. **32:**65, 1974.
†Includes 32 part-time positions.

Table 2-2. Administrative location and number of nutritionists reported to be employed in state and territorial health agencies, May, 1973*†

Number of nutritional positions	Number of states and territories reporting	Total number of nutritionists in reporting states and territories	Number and location of nutritionists				
			Separate nutrition unit	Health care facilities	Chronic diseases	Maternal and child health	Other
None	3	—					
1-3	24	48	25	10	1	8	4
4-6	11	57	21	16	5	8	7
7-9	8	66	37	14	1	5	9
10-20	5	75	36	5	—	1	33
Over 20	4	167	54	8	1	32	72
Total	55	413	173	53	8	54	125

*From Nichaman, M. Z., and Collins, G. E.: Nutrition programs in state health agencies, Nutr. Rev. **32:**65, 1974.
†Excludes part-time nutritionists and vacancies.

health nutritionist's duties at the state level is presented below. As Nichaman and Collins suggest, there are four major areas of involvement within which optimum nutrition programs may evolve at the level of the state health agency: (1) nutritional surveillance, (2) nutritional standards, (3) nutritional consultation, and (4) applied nutrition research.

SAMPLE POSITION DESCRIPTION OF A PUBLIC HEALTH NUTRITIONIST AT THE STATE LEVEL*
Definition

Under the direction of the medical director, the nutritionist is responsible for the nutrition component of the health care program. He or she is expected to:

- Plan, develop, direct, and evaluate the nutrition component of the program; determine the nature and extent of nutrition needs and problems of the target population; and develop policies, standards, and services to meet needs.
- Provide nutrition consultation to professional staff as well as to other agencies.
- Recruit and provide technical and administrative direction to the nutrition staff, including training and supervision of community health aides assigned to nutrition.
- Coordinate nutrition services with other health services and with existing nutrition programs of other community agencies.
- Plan, prepare, and conduct in-service educational programs in nutrition for professional and auxiliary health personnel.
- Prepare, review, and select nutrition education materials.
- Supervise field experience in nutrition.
- Possibly plan for and provide nutrition and food service management and technical assistance to group feeding programs.
- Cooperate with or initiate plans with appropriate community agencies for provision of food assistance to families.
- Provide or arrange for diet counseling to patients; participate in case conferences, evaluation, and planning conferences which involve health care providers.
- Participate in health studies, possibly initiate

---

*Modified from guide class specifications in state and local public health programs, Rockville, Md., 1971, U.S. Department of Health, Education, and Welfare.

nutrition studies, and analyze nutrition services.
- Report and summarize progress and activities at regular intervals; prepare periodic and special reports.

Education and experience

A master's degree in nutrition, including or supplemented by public health courses, from an accredited college or university; an approved hospital dietetic internship or equivalent training and experience in a health care program which meets requirements for registered dietitian; two years of full-time progressively responsible experience in nutrition, one year of which must have been in a public health agency. Experience in health services for adults, mothers and children, and chronically ill patients would be desirable.

Nutritional surveillance. Although this facet of nutrition care seems basic to planning, implementing, and evaluating a program, thus far it generally has not received much attention. A surveillance program for a specific area is the best way to identify the nutritional needs unique to that area. Whereas national surveys give an indication of problem areas and high-risk population groups, a continuing planned surveillance will ensure the most efficient, well-founded program.

Surveillance implies a continuous process, whereas a survey occurs once at a particular time. A survey may highlight problems but is best followed with periodic monitoring of various indices that have been selected to measure nutritional problems. Such indices may include the nutritional status of selected population groups, dietary patterns, monitoring of the food supply, or availability of health and nutrition services, to cite a few (Chapter 7).

Nutritional standards. The setting of nutritional standards should be a foremost responsibility of the health agency. For example, these might include meal service standards for group facilities, professional standards for personnel, guidelines for nutrition education programs, and norms against which to measure the nutritional status that has to be discovered by either surveys or a surveillance system. Most recently, there has been added emphasis on congregate feeding for the elderly and also on generally providing nutritional services as a functional component of health maintenance organizations. With larger numbers of non-nutritionists being utilized to extend nutritional care, it is vital that standards be set and methods established to assure their implementation.

Nutritional consultation. Nutritional consultation is a third important area for a state program. Although, in general, direct patient counseling is performed at the local level, and often the same is true for consultation to institutions, the nutritionist at the state level should be able to help in identifying problems, to interpret these in terms of the program, and to assist in setting up an operational program at the local level. The state nutrition unit should also provide consultation to various state agencies and the state legislature with regard to long-range and immediate nutrition needs and program plans for the state.

Applied nutrition research. Finally, the state nutrition unit should conduct a research program for applied nutrition that is directed toward designing, implementing, and evaluating model programs. These, if successful, can be instituted at the local level.

For many, the foregoing ideas will not be new. However, using them as functional guidelines may require an in-depth review of existing programs and a realignment of manpower and objectives. Despite existing shortages of money and manpower, a new look at priorities and a willingness to abandon traditional approaches if they are no longer effective will move the nutritionist much closer to optimum nutrition for the population.

As already stated, funding for the state positions in many instances originated from maternal and child health (MCH) monies. Legislative provisions for health services for mothers and children, first initiated in Title V of the Social Security Act of 1935, provided formula grants to states for maternal and child health programs. In 1974 the Social Security Act required that each state develop a state plan providing five projects, including maternal and infant care, intensive infant care, health services for children and youth,

dental health of children, and family planning services.

These programs, administered either directly or through contracts from the state maternal and child health unit, provide comprehensive health care, continuity in supervision of care, and health management to low-income and high-risk population groups. The approach is multidisciplinary, offering services in the areas of medicine, dentistry, nutrition, nursing, and social work. A discussion of the multidisciplinary team effort follows. The MCH nutrition consultant at the state level concentrates on the agency's planning, organization and administration of services to accomplish the desired change in the health status of specific population groups.*[8]

Local level

At the local and community level the nutritionist usually acts as a specialist in a specific program serving a particular population group. There are a variety of needs. The nutritionist may work in a maternity and infant care project, a children and youth program, a day care center, a school setting, an adolescent clinic, a drug rehabilitation center, or a geriatric center, among others. In this role the nutritionist often is involved in direct services. Coincident with this, the community nutritionist must also plan, implement, and evaluate a specific program (Chapter 5).

Nutrition services at the local and community level should be supported by existing specialized programs and services. These include programs for particular populations such as health services for mothers and children, the elderly, and other special groups such as migrant agricultural workers and low-income families; family planning programs;

---

*For more details see Federal Register **40:**225, HEW Maternal and Child Health and Crippled Children's Services, Thursday, Nov. 20, 1975. Guidelines for the Nutrition Component of Comprehensive Health Care Services for Mothers and Children, HEW, Health Services and Mental Health Association, Jan., 1971. Interim Guidelines for Maternal and Child Health Services Program of Projects under Title V, Social Security Act, HEW, Health Services Administration, Bureau of Community Health Services, April, 1975.

chronic disease control services; home health services, rehabilitation services for drug and alcohol addicts; and group care services in facilities such as hospitals, nursing homes, extended care facilities, day care centers, and residential institutions; and detention centers, detoxification centers, and prisons.

UNDERSTANDING THE CLIENT REQUIRES KNOWLEDGE OF HIS HOME AND COMMUNITY

Where do clients in health care facilities come from? To what conditions do they return? What life styles, food habits, fears, beliefs, knowledge do they bring with them to the hospital or health care facility? What community services and resources hasten the client's return to his home and support him there to contribute to his comfort, recovery, and potential for independence? For most people, a hospital stay is a short episode set in a longer life in the home and community. Understanding the client requires knowledge of his home and community.

Mildred Kaufman and *Frances Hoffman:* Dietetic trainees learn about their community, J. Am. Diet. Assoc. **71:**5, 1977. Reprinted by permission. Copyright The American Dietetic Association.

WHAT DOES THE NUTRITIONIST DO? WHAT IS THE OVERALL GOAL?

As the public health nutritionist functions with the planning and policy-making level of international, federal, regional, state, and local comprehensive health planning bodies, he or she is in a position to ensure that an appropriate nutritional care component is incorporated into all comprehensive health care planning.

The American Dietetic Association has issued a position paper on the importance of nutrition as a component of health care for all health and health-related programs so that the total population is reached. Priority is given to nutritionally vulnerable groups such as infants, children, and youth in the growing years, women in the childbearing years, and the older age population.[9]

The American Dietetic Association's position is that the inclusion of nutrition as a component of health care will significantly reduce the number of people requiring sick care service and therefore will contribute directly to (1) a relief of strain on the nation's health care delivery system; (2) a decrease in the escalating rate of health care costs; and (3) an increase in the physical, mental, and social well-being of people so that they may achieve and maintain productive and independent lives.

Nutritional care is the application of nutrition science to the health care of people. In its broadest sense, nutritional care is provided to the general population through studies on food consumption and nutritional health, mass education, and food assistance programs. As applied to patient care and service delivery at the local level, it has the same components (assessment of food practices and nutritional status, nutrition education, and food assistance) plus dietary counseling and the service of appropriate food. These nutritional care services must be combined and coordinated to meet individual needs.

A suggested model of nutritional goals and activities in a health maintenance organization is shown in Table 2-3. It is a synthesis of preventive, diagnostic, curative, and restorative health services. Any contemplated health services delivery system should include a nutrition component in its preventive as well as remedial services if the maximum benefits to health are to be achieved.

Comprehensive health care plans include appropriate administrative placement of the nutrition care component, staffing patterns and qualifications for personnel, identification of the nature and extent of nutrition problems, standards of nutritional care, methods to be used for delivery of nutrition services, and evaluation.

What services are needed?

Specific nutrition services in health care programs should include screening for nutritional problems and the assessment of the nutritional status of individuals. This would involve a review of food availability and dietary practices reflecting cultural socioeconomic factors, biochemical measurements of nutrients in body fluids and tissues, and, to

Table 2-3. Suggested pattern of nutritional care*

Phase of delivery	Nutritional care goal	Nutritional care activities†
Health appraisal and referral	To identify potential problems and plan for continuing surveillance or appropriate care	Assessment of food practices and nutritional status Referral for corroboration Data input into patient information systems
Environmental protection and disease prevention; health maintenance	To prepare patients and their families to assume responsibility for their own care and manage early symptoms to prevent complications	*In addition to the activities described above:* Individual counseling Group teaching Recording of progress in record Development and/or evaluation of nutrition methods and materials Training, continuing education and technical consultation to medical, dental and other professional staff Training and continuing education for dietetic supportive personnel Referral to, and liaison with, food assistance and other nutrition-related community programs Leadership in seeking solutions to community-wide nutrition problems Consultation to group care facilities
Acute and intensive care	To develop and implement immediate and long-range individualized nutrional care plans for in and outpatients	*In addition to the activities described above:* On-going participation in health-team planning, direct nutritional assessment and counseling and evaluation Planning and/or supervision of appropriate group food service Health team staff conferences Initial and follow-up counseling for normal and therapeutic nutritional needs Input into clinical records
Restoration and extended care	To assist patients and their families with long-term health problems to attain and maintain adequate diets	*In addition to the activities described above:* Assistance in adjusting home environment to maximize independent functioning in activities in and outside the home Liaison with non-contract services or programs helpful in carrying out the nutritional care plan

*From Collins, M. E., Forbes, C., Kocher, R., and Yanochik, A.: Position paper on the implementation and delivery of nutritional care services in health care systems, U.S. Senate Select Committee on Nutrition and Human Needs. Part 6. Washington, D.C., June 21, 1975. Modified from American Dietetic Association: Position paper on nutrition services in health maintenance organizations, J. Am. Diet. Assoc. **60:**4, 1972.

†Nutritional care activities as listed are not intended to be sequential. They may clearly overlap and are seldom restricted to a single phase of delivery.

be most thorough, clinical examinations including an assessment of growth.

In the planning and development of a health delivery system, the nutrition component should be integrated with medical and multidisciplinary support. The following services should be among the key considerations:

• Analyzing the food and nutrition needs of the target population
• Establishing criteria for identification of the "nutritionally vulnerable"—those who are most likely to need nutrition services
• Establishing measurable objectives and determining priorities in nutrition
• Planning for the most efficient and effective use of nutrition resources, including nutrition professionals and other health personnel, and identifying and establishing referral systems with available nutrition resources

SO YOU'RE A NUTRITIONIST! WHAT DO YOU DO?*

When I joined the nutrition staff of the Department of Health of the City of New York in 1943, I was assigned to serve as consultant to the personnel in the four district health centers in the borough of Queens (population approximately 1,200,000). At the first professional meeting I attended in the community, which included representatives of all the disciplines in the various health and welfare agencies, I was bombarded with questions such as these: "So you're a nutritionist. Now just what do you do?"

Typical tasks of nutritionists—New York City Department of Health

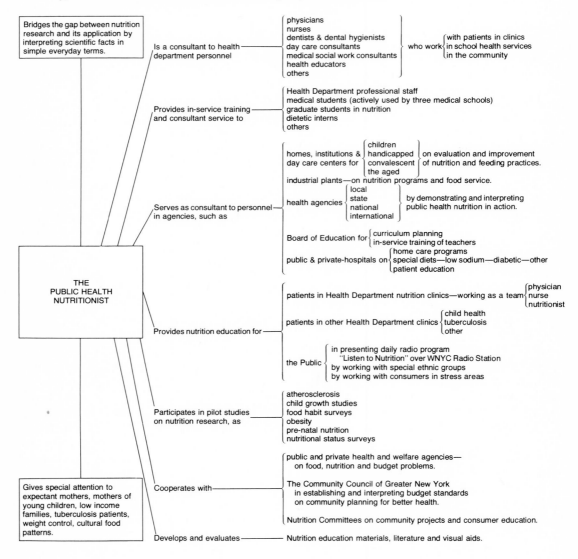

*From *Bennett, I.*: So you're a nutritionist! Tell me—just what do you do? Am. J. Home Economics **53**:93, Feb., 1961.

- Integrating nutrition services into the total pattern of health services
- Evaluating the efficiency and effectiveness of the nutrition component of the health care services

Special services having to do with planning and implementation of care for individuals with nutrition and diet problems should include individual and group counseling to meet normal and therapeutic dietary needs, which to be most effective, would include nutrition education that is responsive to consumer beliefs, attitudes, environmental influences, and understanding about food. The service should also provide specific referrals to community food assistance resources— home-delivered meals, community meals for the elderly, supplemental food programs for high-risk groups such as pregnant women and infants, food stamps, and child nutrition services such as school lunch and breakfast programs and child day care feeding.

WHEN AND HOW SHOULD NUTRITION SERVICES BE PROVIDED?

Sometimes nutrition services are categorized as *primary, secondary,* and *tertiary* levels of care, whether they be provided in hospitals, outpatient departments, family and neighborhood health centers, group practices, rehabilitation centers, or mental health centers. (See Glossary.)

At the primary level, which would include ambulatory care and health maintenance organizations, nutrition should be included in screening and diagnosis, health maintenance, and health supervision. This is true in a single provider situation or in a project involving a multidisciplinary health care team. Health promotion activities involving community-wide efforts such as the development of food assistance programs, water fluoridation, and nutrition education are also important aspects of this level.

At the other levels of care, which include the secondary or tertiary provider institutions that receive referrals from primary care, nutrition is a significant element in diagnosis, treatment, and rehabilitation. Expertise in specialized areas of nutrition may be required in medical centers that serve patients with complex nutritional problems.

In recent years the need for primary health services of far greater scope than can be provided by any one health professional alone has virtually mandated the use of multidisciplinary teams for maintaining health and treating illness. One reason has been that increasing pressure for greater efficiency and lower costs necessitates trials of new methods and careful monitoring of quality.

The multidisciplinary team

The primary care team model has become a highly organized multidisciplinary group of professionals and lay health workers. Disciplines represented vary in many instances, but the usual team consists of an internist, pediatrician, nurses, social worker, nutritionist, and paraprofessionals such as the family health worker.

The internist not only provides medical direction and participates in establishing standards, criteria, and policies for nutrition services but also has major responsibility for the assessment of nutritional status and making the diagnosis, followed by appropriate referral for dietary counseling. The internist also reinforces the need for the patient's attention to nutritional advice.

Nursing personnel can assist with nutritional assessment and provide education and counseling in normal nutrition. They also can assist in interpreting dietary prescriptions and in making appropriate referrals of more complicated problems to nutrition personnel.

Social workers can contribute to the mobilization of community resources and social services that are needed to support adequate nutritional care. They can assist in developing referral mechanisms and in counseling patients whose nutritional problems are complicated by social and emotional factors. They have experience in group diagnosis and counseling and skills involving crisis situations, interviewing techniques, and knowledge of family dynamics.

Other professionals such as physical therapists, occupational therapists, dentists, dental hygienists, and representatives of other health disciplines frequently aid in counseling individuals who have physical conditions that interfere with adequate nutrition. Health educators and behavioral scientists can assist in implementing educational programs in nutrition for patients and staff.

No health team member can cover the complete care of a patient. Neglect of the expertise of any members of the health care team will diminish the quality of service rendered to individuals. One person, however, should have overall responsibility for the management of an individual patient's care and that of his or her family.

The 1960s were marked by innovations in the use of medical manpower. The domains of the physician and the nurse, which had become more or less sacrosanct in the preceding decades, were invaded by a variety of physician assistants, nurse practitioners, clinical associates, patient-care expediters, family health workers, and community nutrition aides.

Yanochik[10] has reported that the "backbone" of the innovative nutrition delivery system in Arizona is one member of the team, the community nutrition worker, who combines a specific nutrition background with a general understanding of health care and training in simple laboratory procedures. The community nutrition worker also reflects the culture and life-style of the local residents. This person's sensitivity and concern for the community make him or her an effective change agent.

The whole team functions as a kind of transitory social system, a number of persons working together for a defined and mutually accepted goal and according to a mutually accepted program in which each member understands his contribution to the goal. In the health care system the team's goal is the satisfaction of specific needs of an individual patient, a family, or a whole community. (See Suggested readings.)

The purpose of a group or team approach is to optimize the special skills and knowledge of each team member so that the individual or community needs can be met more competently, effectively, and considerately than would be possible by independent and individual action. Without question the patient himself is a member of the team and, in a democratic society, can be expected increasingly to exert his prerogative to participate in decisions that affect his well-being.

Because it is a transitory system, each team has an existence only as long as the needs it is designed to meet exist. Its composition is determined by those needs, and its leadership may be expected to vary with the nature of the needs and which of them is preponderant at any particular time.

Teams may be classified according to a variety of organizing principles. In the health delivery system there are three possibilities: the patient care team, the medical care team, and the health care team.

The *patient care team* comprises any group of professionals, semiprofessionals, and nonprofessionals who jointly provide needed services that bring them into direct personal and physical contact with the patient according to his individualized program of management. The smallest team of this type consists of the physician and the nurse. Others enter it in different settings: social workers, dietitians, physical therapists, and so on. All these are the people who deal directly with the patient, have the most sustained contact with him as a whole person rather than as a representation of certain symptoms and characterizations. They must experience with him the joy of cure or the burden of failure and death. Some patient care teams have a well-established composition, for example, the operating team, the coronary care team, the mental health team. All patient care teams introduce others transiently for the benefit of the patient, and all need the support of the next level of team organization.

The second team, the *medical care team*, provides essential backup services for the patient care teams. It is not in close continual contact with the patient, and although some of its members may deal on a personal basis with the patient, it is usually for a short period. Others do not work with the patient personally at all. They deal with a part of the patient—his sputum, urine, x-ray examinations, medications, and so forth. Members of these teams are, for example, laboratory technicians, pathologists, radiologists, x-ray technicians, and pharmacists.

The members of the medical care teams may, in turn, be members of more permanent teams organized along functional lines, such as the entire pharmacy team or laboratory team. They move into and out of the sphere of influence of the patient care teams as the needs of the patient require, but they do not participate in the day-by-day management of the personal and psychosocial requirements of the patient's illness.

The third team category, in this method of classification, is the *health care team*. Its members are the most distantly related to the individual patient and usually have as their concern the entire community. This team is the one most likely to have the public health nutritionist as a member. Such teams concentrate on the health of the aggregate population, the delivery of all services, their availability and accessibility, the costs of care, the distribution of resources in facilities and personnel, the regulation of quality, and the production of manpower adequate in number and kind to meet society's needs. The members of the health care team are varied and may include a broad spectrum of disciplines and professions—public health officers, hospital administrators, epidemiologists, medical economists and sociologists, a community medicine specialist, public health nutritionists, engineers, insurance carriers, and others. In this broad category almost every profession may play a role, depending on the problems that the community faces in planning and implementing a regional or national health policy.

Cruickshank[11] states: "Position in the interdisciplinary structure is of little import; each discipline uses its skills of the moment in the best possible way to seek solutions to the problem before it. The leadership role is not defined by historical prerogatives, regulation, or law . . . but by pertinence of the discipline to the agenda before the team and by the capacity of the individual representing that discipline to weld the other members . . ."

Achieving a stage of true collaboration between the disciplines cannot be forced. There should be a feeling of need for a discipline in the solution of existing problems. On the other hand, to be ready for interdisciplinary collaboration, the disciplines involved must have arrived at a certain degree of sophistication. Immaturity or insecurity may force a member to retreat into his own discipline. The development of an effective method of communication or a "neutral terminology," instead of using the special jargon of each particular discipline, may help to weld the disciplines together.

Therefore it is clear that the characteristics most emphatically desired in interdisciplinary workers are personal and professional security, emotional maturity, flexibility, humility, and open-mindedness. It is desirable that staff should be discovery minded and program oriented rather than status minded and reward oriented.[12]

The outcomes of the influence of the health care team are not yet apparent. Since the uses of medical manpower in the 1970s and the 1980s will certainly be affected by these innovations, the results of these experiments should be referred to in program planning of the future and assessed carefully.

As indicated earlier, communication among team members is essential. In addition to conferences at which dialogue and discussion between team members occur, the written record is a vital link as well.

Recording data

The accurate and careful recording of data obtained through interview and observation and objective data, such as laboratory findings and anthropometric measurements including heights and weights, is an essential part of the health care plan. A record permits monitoring the patient's progress and communicating information about the patient to other members of the health care team. Specific guidelines drafted by the American Hospital Association indicate that concise information about dietary intake, food habits, nutritional status, recommendations, adherence, and follow-up should be recorded chronologically in the patient's medical record.[13]

Although the method of recording should

be keyed to the clinic system, there is one method, the problem-oriented medical record (POMR) that has gained prominence in recent years and is having a profound impact. The POMR, developed and pioneered by Lawrence L. Weed, is not only a different way of writing charts but it represents an entire philosophy that stresses the long overdue alignment of the health care team with the patient and his needs. The problem-oriented philosophy requires the discipline of maintaining an awareness of each of the patient's problems precisely and of all of the patient's problems at the same time.

The physician's admission note, instead of containing the usual impressions and plans, appears as a list of the patient's problems precisely stated. There is also a plan for each problem that uses a three-pronged attack— diagnosis, treatment, and patient education. Then, even more importantly, there is a day-by-day work plan. The problem list on the front cover of the record is updated hour by hour or day by day as new information accumulates and as problems are added, dropped, or changed.

There are four essential elements in problem formulation that are summed up by the acronym SOAP:

S *Subjective data.* What information is available from talking to the patient. What statements are made by the patient when the history is being taken. How does the patient feel, his concerns, his description of his status that would include dietary intake and food habits.

O *Objective data.* New facts. A summary of physical observations, findings, and laboratory data, for example, height, weight, skinfolds.

A *Assessment.* What is the impact of the information on understanding the problem as defined. This includes two elements: (1) diagnosis and (2) severity or degree.

P *Plan.* New diagnostic, therapeutic and patient education ventures, counseling, anticipatory guidance, referrals, and future appointments for follow-up.

In the POMR the SOAP note is always problem specific in that it refers to a specific problem on the problem list which is identified by a common number, and it only contains data relevant to that single problem. This is in contrast to the traditional medical record, the "source-oriented record" (SOR), which groups data for several different problems together. The progress notes begin with the patient's complaints, then they present relevant historic data, results of physical examination, a diagnostic impression, and the therapy. Regardless of format, the patient's records should contain sufficient data to be used in a peer review and to assess standards of care. The records should also contain data on selected indices of nutritional status to be used in nutrition surveillance of the population served. These data will highlight problems, identify gaps in service for individuals or populations being served, help set priorities for service, and show manpower needs. (See Suggested readings.)

Quality assurance

Health professionals are becoming increasingly aware of the need to engage in self-assessment to assure quality in the delivery of nutritional care. The assessment of quality care becomes somewhat complex when it is likely to be or has been mandated. Many of the federal legislative proposals relating to health care are focusing on peer review as a means of assuring high standards of health care. (See Suggested readings.)

Professional Standards Review Organizations (PSROs) have been established to evaluate the quality of health care services rendered under the various maternal and child health programs of the Social Security Act and Medicaid and Medicare (Public Law 92-603, Sec. 249F, U.S. Statutes at Large, 92nd Congress, 2nd Session, 1972). The review process seeks to ensure that health services are (1) medically necessary and (2) consistent with professionally recognized health care standards.[*]

Although professional standards review was originally directed toward the physician

---

[*]See Guidelines for evaluating dietetic practices, Chicago, 1976, American Dietetic Association.

and hospital administrator because of increased health care costs, the implications for other allied health professions have been made clear. Each health professional involved with quality care is part of this quality assurance program, which, in turn, implies peer review. Winterfeldt[14] indicated that one of the functions of PSRO is to provide evidence over time that nonphysician health care practitioners have become involved in the development of norms, criteria, and standards for their areas of practice, as well as in the development of peer review mechanisms for their respective discipline.

The Department of Health, Education, and Welfare has come forth with certain basic principles and concepts used in assessment that can be applied to nutrition services. Quality of services can be considered in each of three categories: structure, process, and outcome.

Structure relates to environmental and personnel factors in the service delivery, for example, the adequacy of the facility and necessary equipment, the availability and training of skilled personnel (nutritionist), the scheduling of patient visits, and the storage and availability of patient records.

Process of care relates to the interaction between providers and patients, the data collected, the diagnostic assessments made, the therapeutic plans and how they are carried out, and the follow-up of problems over time. The main focus for process of care is the medical record.

Outcomes of care are measures of the success or failure of the structure and process of the care provided. In the context of nutritional services, it is sometimes possible to define what are sometimes termed *proximate* outcome measures—which are believed *probably* to influence long-term measures such as death or morbidity but which are relatively easy to measure over a reasonably short period of time.

In other clinical areas, where nutrition services play a role together with other services, determining proximate outcomes is more difficult, for example, in the care of diabetics, it may be difficult to separate out the effectiveness of the diet as opposed to medication in the control of blood glucose levels. In prenatal care it is well known that maternal nutrition is a major determinant of the normal development of the fetus. Nonetheless, it is not always possible to assess the contribution of nutrition to a problem situation, such as premature birth or a child who is ultimately found to be retarded or to have minimal brain dysfunction.[15]

There is another distinction in quality assessment that the DHEW guide for developing health services points out is useful to make: external as opposed to internal assessment. *External assessment* involves bringing in "experts" from outside to interview, observe, and examine medical records and then make judgments about the effectiveness of patient services. Whether or not certain identified deficiencies are corrected is another question.

Internal assessment refers to the criteria and standards developed by those actually responsible for providing care. These same individuals assess the actual care provided by one another, generally using the medical record as a basis. Limited evidence suggests that internal assessment is much more effective than external assessment in actually changing the way care is provided, since it is the direct responsibility of those providing care and should be integrated into the day-by-day operation of the program. The problem-oriented record is considered to be a precondition for effective internal assessment, or else it may be the quality of the record, rather than the care, that is at issue.

In situations where problems are nutritional, such as obesity, the process of care can be assessed by determining proximate outcomes (weight, skinfold thickness) over time. In other situations, such as diabetes, the data base is still readily defined, and the plan for management usually follows in a logical sequence. Assessing the proximate outcome in these instances, however, such as blood glucose levels, may involve an assessment of the efforts of several services.

At the national level, PSRO was created in October, 1972. Geographic areas by states were designated as PSROs in January, 1974, with the provision that the PSRO systems would function at a national, state, and local level. In April, 1974, the Coalition of Independent Health Professions (CIHP), of which the American Dietetic Association is a member organization, appointed a special task force to meet with the office of Professional Standards Review to discuss the means by which the CIHP might participate in the orderly development of PSROs.

The PSRO guidelines, which have been evolved by the American Dietetic Association, are aimed at those dietitians involved in the delivery of dietetic services to hospitalized patients. However, the guidelines may be expanded to cover the care provided in the ambulatory facilities as well. Dietitians

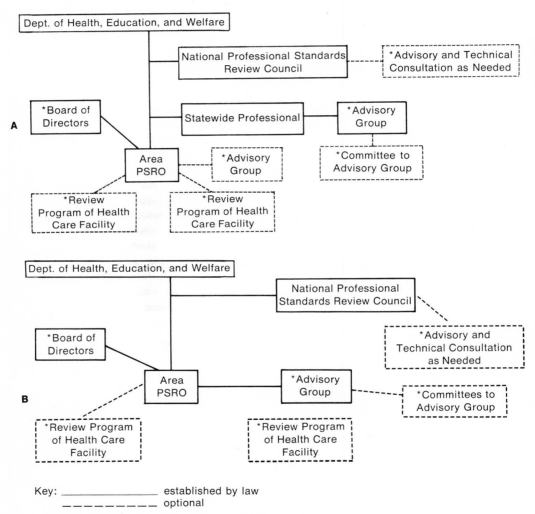

Key: _____ established by law
     _ _ _ _ _ _ _ _ optional

*Registered dieticians can seek the opportunity to serve on these groups.

Fig. 2-1. A, Diagram of PSRO structure for states with *three* or *more* PSROs showing areas of potential activity for registered dietitians. **B,** Diagram of PSRO structure for states with *less* than *three* PSROs showing areas of potential activity for registered dietitians. (From *Professional standard review procedure manual,* Chicago, 1976, American Dietetic Association.)

in the field of education are also affected by the PSROs, since they must utilize the findings of the peer review process to plan and modify educational programs for dietetic students and practicing dietitians. Dietitians need to understand their relationship between the hospital patient care audit committee and the local PSRO. The potential activity for registered dietitians and public health nutritionists in the PSRO structure is shown in Fig. 2-1.

The report of a workshop meeting conducted by the CIHP in April, 1975, published by the American Dietetic Association, indicates necessary specifics for a PSRO such as a descriptive background, objectives, functions, the role of the registered dietitian, and the patient care audit program. Because the patient care audit is the primary evaluation instrument for a PSRO, it seems pertinent to list the following important characteristics of a patient care audit:

1. An objective analysis of a specific aspect of the care for a particular patient from a defined population group
2. A form of quality assessment to determine the effectiveness of care for specific groups of patients with the implied obligation to effect a change where needed
3. The determination of the criteria establishing quality care by the peers of those delivering the care
4. An application of "Management By Objectives" principles for a health care setting including the establishment of "expected performance objectives," analysis of actual performance compared with the objectives, and improvement of performance when the actual is less than the desired
5. A means for determining needs for continuing education of the health care professional
6. The effective use of group dynamics in attaining commitment to the audit program with the concomitant requirements of time, effort, skill, and if possible, finances
7. A process that has the potential for

achieving organizational change in the health care setting and for resulting in a saving of professional time

The suggested procedure for patient care audit, consisting of nine steps, is shown in Fig. 2-2. The patient care audit, at times also referred to as "medical care evaluation," is oriented toward the best possible health care at the least cost, or in essence, cost effectiveness in health care. In addition, it must be borne in mind that the patient care audit does not imply any punitive action in the form of a peer review. It is vital in the multidisciplinary exercise of the patient care audit that confusion of responsibility, or what is known as cross criteria, among the separate professions be avoided whereas consultation, discussion, and cooperation are welcomed.[16]

In a study, two areas relevant to establishing guidelines for peer review of the clinical dietitian were explored: Parameters useful in assessing the nutritional status of individuals and written communication by a dietary staff for its possible role in a peer review process.

Findings show that biochemical and anthropometric indicators of nutritional status are available in the medical record but are not being utilized by the dietitian to the degree expected. Measurements recommended in the minimal appraisal of a patient's nutritional status are age, sex, race, height, weight, ideal weight, hemoglobin, and mean corpuscular hemoglobin concentration. Serum iron and iron-binding capacity can provide specific information about the patient's iron nutriture, but these measurements are not done routinely. Serum albumin, folic acid, and vitamin B_{12} determinations give a more definitive picture of nutritional status if interpreted in light of other diagnostic tests.

Better documentation is needed in the areas of dietary history recording, computation of ideal weights, utilization of laboratory data, and development of nutritional care plans.

Ideally, the clinical dietitian is responsible for the nutritional assessment and care of all patients, whether they are receiving regular

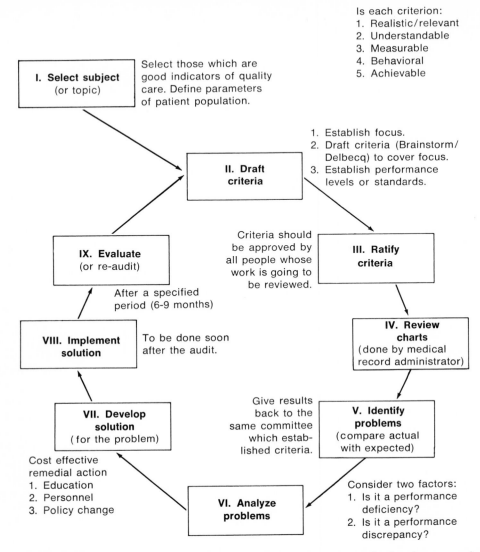

Fig. 2-2. Procedure for patient care audit. (From Professional standard review procedure manual, Chicago, 1976, American Dietetic Association.)

or modified diets. Implementation of the peer review process hopefully will be another means of improving performance and preserving the dietitian's unique role as a member of the health team.[17]

To have an effective review and screening process, *norms*, *standards*, and *criteria* should be developed by the health care practitioners who are providing the service at the local level.

1. Norms are defined as "numerical or statistical measures of usual, observed performance." For example, a norm may be the average number of hours needed to instruct effectively a diabetic patient about the prescribed diet.

2. Standards are professionally developed expressions of the range of acceptable variation from a norm or criterion. Using the above example, a standard would be the

range in number of hours needed to instruct effectively a patient with diabetes about the prescribed diet.

3. Criteria are predetermined elements or rules against which the quality of health care service may be measured; criteria are developed by professionals relying on their expertise and literature in the field. Registered dietitians may develop, for example, criteria of nutritional care for treatment or management of conditions such as diabetes mellitus, renal failure, and malnutrition.

If a local PSRO does not develop these norms, standards, and criteria, they may be established for that PSRO by the National Professional Standards Review Council.

Typically the establishment of a PSRO will occur in the following three steps:

1. The Planning Contract. This is established by a Planning Organization, a group that often needs short-term financial assistance to meet the necessary organizational and membership requirements. It develops a formal plan for the gradual assumption of PSRO duties and responsibilities, and may apply to the Department of Health, Education, and Welfare for a planning contract.

2. The Conditional Contract. Groups that have developed an acceptable formal plan may be awarded a conditional contract for a period of up to 2 years. During this time, the "Conditional PSRO" must develop and expand its review activities and capabilities. Groups may apply to become a Conditional PSRO without having been a Planning Organization.

3. If (at the end of the conditional period) the Conditional PSRO can demonstrate satisfactory performance, the Department of Health, Education, and Welfare will enter into an agreement with it for a period of one year, during which the Conditional PSRO will serve as the PSRO for its area. These contracts are renewable on an annual basis.

Contracts are available also for Statewide Support Centers, which are organizations designed to provide professional and administrative assistance to Planning Organizations and Conditional PSROs and, subsequently, to Operational PSROs and to State Professional Standards Review Councils. Support Centers are composed primarily of physicians who have continuing relationships with other health professional societies, agencies, and organizations.

PSRO is the first step in the application of the review procedures to all health services. Since it will undoubtedly apply to all health services supported by federal funds in the future, dietitians must accept it to be a feature of any national health insurance program that may be enacted. Because the concept and practice of PSROs are in the formative stage and because new updated guidelines will be appearing, it is the duty of dietitians and nutritionists actively to seek to update their knowledge of the new guidelines and their future modification. The American Dietetic Association[16] states: "To participate in shaping the course of the practice for the future is to become involved now."

SUMMARY

The nutritionist is a recognized professional whose responsibility it is to provide nutrition services by identifying problems and designing, implementing, and evaluating appropriate programs at the international, national, state, county, city, and local level. As the importance of preventive care is becoming more recognized, as well as the role of nutrition in disease, it is up to the nutritionist to assume more responsibility and leadership as a member of the health care team.

Public health problems indicate that the programs to be designed by the nutritionist will involve working with groups of people on the problems that they perceive as important. The public health team has developed into an interdisciplinary activity that encompasses practitioners and scientists from fields of medicine, epidemiology, nutrition, nursing, laboratory and sanitary science, health education, behavioral and social sciences, biostatisticians, and others. The nutritionist as a team member may direct planning to population groups living in communities. This will require a careful observation of community needs and a recognition of how people perceive their problems and their causes. They will also have to decide on the assignment of priorities and how to remove barriers standing in the way of getting what is necessary. What a community may need first is not new nutritional data but assistance in ordering the information it lacks and redefining goals. In this role the nutritionist must often subordinate nutritional expertise to the role as a community developer. The nutritionist must keep professional antennae ready to receive signals from the community for the best and most helpful intervention.

At the same time the professional must be prepared to maintain quality assurance, which is done on the state level through Professional Standards Review Organization (PSRO). To make a successful and effective assessment of the services of a multidisciplinary team, the necessity of keeping accurate records and data cannot be overemphasized. A problem-oriented medical record (POMR) is the best means for this.

If one defines public health nutrition as the practical discipline that deals with the identification and solution of health problems with nutrition implications for an individual within a community or human population group, the work of the nutritionist is spelled out. It is to efficiently identify nutrition problems and effectively develop and implement solutions to alleviate these nutrition problems.

This involves program planning, which is basic to the performance and evaluation of good, effective nutrition care and will be discussed in Chapter 3.

REFERENCES

1. Peck, E. B.: The development of a public health nutritionist, 1870-1969, University Microfilm, Ann Arbor, Mich., No. 71-9753, 1971.
2. American Dietetic Association: Personnel in public health nutrition, Chicago, 1976, The Association.
3. Jelliffe, D. B.: Summation. In Berg, A., Scrimshaw, N. S., and Call, D. L., editors: Nutrition, national development, and planning, Cambridge, Mass., 1973, M.I.T. Press, p. 379.
4. Heseltine, M. M.: The nutritionist in public health work, J. Am. Diet. Assoc. 14:241, 1938.
5. Stacey, H.: Public health nutrition: a summary, J. Am. Diet. Assoc. 19:281, 1943.
6. Directors of public health nutrition organize, J. Am. Diet. Assoc. 30:72, 1954.
7. Nichaman, M. Z., and Collins, G. E.: Nutrition programs in state health agencies, Nutr. Rev. 32:65, 1974.
8. Federal Register 40:225, HEW Maternal and Child Health and Crippled Children's Services, Nov. 20, 1975.
9. American Dietetic Association: Position paper on the nutrition component of health services delivery systems, J. Am. Diet. Assoc. 58:538, 1971.
10. Yanochik, A.: Community nutrition workers—their effectiveness in a nutrition delivery system, Public Health Curr. 13:5, Sept.-Oct., 1973.
11. Cruickshank, W. M.: An interdisciplinary model for manpower development for mental retardation. In Cohen, J. S., editor: Proceedings, First Annual Spring Conference of the Institute for the Study of Mental Retardation, May 15-16, 1970, Ann Arbor, 1971, University of Michigan Press.
12. Springer, N. C.: The nutritionist in the university-affiliated center, J. Am. Diet. Assoc. 59:494, 1971.
13. Recording nutritional information in medical records, Chicago, 1976, American Hospital Association.
14. Winterfeldt, E.: Professional Standards Review Organizations (PSRO's). I. Professional standards and peer review, J. Am. Diet. Assoc. 65:654, 1974.
15. Division of Clinical Services, U.S. Department of Health, Education, and Welfare: Preliminary guide for developing health services, Washington, D.C., 1976, Government Printing Office.
16. American Dietetic Association: Professional standard review procedure manual, Chicago, 1976, The Association.
17. Weed, J. E., and Molleson, A. L.: Establishing guidelines for peer review of the clinical dietitian, J. Am. Diet. Assoc. 70:157, 1977.

SUGGESTED READINGS
Team
Brunetto, E., and Birk, P.: The primary care nurse—the generalist in a structured health care team, Am. J. Public Health 62:6, 1972.

Frankle, R. T., and Christakis, G.: Community nutrition teams, Hospitals 47:56, Dec. 16, 1973.

Fry, R. E., and Lech, B. A.: An organizational development approach to improving the effectiveness of neighborhood health care teams, Master's thesis, Cambridge, Mass., 1971, Massachusetts Institute of Technology.

Torrey, E. F., Smith, D., and Wise, H.: The family health worker revisited: a five-year follow-up, Am. J. Public Health 63:1, 1973.

White, K. L.: Primary medical care for families—organization and evaluation, N. Engl. J. Med. 277:847, 1967.

POMR

Bjorn, J. C., and Cross, H. D.: Problem oriented practice, Chicago, 1971, Modern Hospital Press.

Hurst, J. W., and Walter, H. K., editors: The problem oriented system, New York, 1972, Medcom, Inc.

Hurst, J. W., and Walter, H. K., editors: Quality control in health care—application of a problem-oriented system, New York, 1972, Medcom, Inc.

Voytovich, A. E.: The dietitian/nutritionist and the problem-oriented medical record. I. A physician's viewpoint, J. Am. Diet. Assoc. 63:639, 1973.

Walters, F. M., and De Marco, M.: The dietitian/nutritionist and the problem oriented medical record. II. The role of the dietitian, J. Am. Diet. Assoc. 63:641, 1973.

Weed, L. L.: Medical records, medical education and patient care, Cleveland, 1970, The Press of Case Western Reserve University.

Weed, L. L.: Quality control and the medical record, Arch. Intern. Med. 127:101, 1971.

Quality assurance

Bistrian, B. R., Blackburn, G. L., Hallowell, E., and Heddle, R.: Protein status of general surgical patients, J. Am. Diet. Assoc. 230:858, 1974.

Bollet, A. J., and Owens, S.: Evaluation of nutritional status of selected hospital patients, Am. J. Clin. Nutr. 26:931, 1973.

Butterworth, C. E., Jr.: The skeleton in the hospital closet, Nutr. Today 9:4, March-April, 1974.

Hallahan, I. A.: The American Dietetic Association—pace-setter for the profession, J. Am. Diet. Assoc. 64:603, 1974.

Hansen, S. G.: Professional Standards Review Organizations (PSROs). 2. Developing professional standards review in dietetics, J. Am. Diet. Assoc. 65:656, 1974.

Leevy, C. M., Cardi, L., Frank, O., Gellene, R., and Baker, H.: Incidence and significance of hypovitaminemia in a randomly selected municipal hospital population, Am. J. Clin. Nutr. 17:259, 1965.

Sanstead, H. H., and Pearson, W. N.: Clinical evaluation of nutrition status. In Goodhart, R. S., and Shils, M., editors: Modern nutrition in health and disease, Philadelphia, 1973, Lea & Febiger.

Sauberlich, H. E., Skala, J. H., and Dowdy, R. P.: Laboratory tests for assessment of nutritional status, Cleveland, 1974, CRC Press.

Schiller, M. R., Sr., and Vivian, V. M.: Role of the clinical dietitian. I. Ideal role perceived by dietitians and physicians, J. Am. Diet. Assoc. 65:284, 1974.

GENERAL CONCEPT

Program planning is the development of a course of action to achieve predetermined objectives (Chapter 3) within a framework of implementation (Chapters 4 to 6) and evaluation (Chapter 9).

OUTCOMES

The student should do the following:

- State the purpose and value of careful planning.
- List, enumerate, and describe the legislation that created health planning activities in the United States.
- Describe the constraints to health planning.
- Discuss the actual way to overcome these constraints for effective planning.

The art of program planning

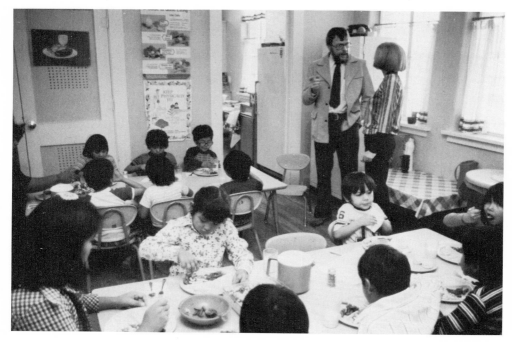

The midday meal at the Head Start program, Santa Ana Pueblo, New Mexico.

The nutritionist must be trained to function at the planning table. All too often the nutritionist has adequate technical ability but is not equipped to be effective as a planner. Nichaman and Collins[1] of the Preventable Diseases and Nutrition Activities at the Center for Disease Control, Atlanta, are firmly convinced that the nutritionist must also function as the planner if a nutrition program is to be effective:

Somehow there must be developed an understanding and acceptance by the policy making and program planning groups that nutrition services must be included in the initial plan for programs designed to maintain optimum health.

This cannot be achieved if nutrition services are tied to categorical funding. Neither can it be done if the nutritionist is not involved in the planning process. Identifying nutrition as a separate unit does not automatically assure involvement in major planning.

The health administrator and the legislative groups must be supplied with definitive descriptions of the problems, a clear-cut plan of action including cost in time, personnel, and dollars, and a method for evaluating the outcome as it relates to the total health systems. Furthermore, Nichaman and Collins[1] remind nutrition professionals that:

Traditional plans that address only limited or specific age groups must be replaced by a comprehensive approach. Nutrition problems are not unique to any one group. Prenatal nutrition, growth and development, obesity, the hyperlipidemias, the problems of the aging such as possible hypervitaminosis, and inborn errors of metabolism are all problems that deserve attention of state health nutritionists.

Berg,[2] of the Brookings Institution, Washington, D.C., calls attention to the lack of nutrition planning:

. . . as things now stand, some of the major factors and policies influencing nutritional status—agriculture, income redistribution, transport, and so on—are outside the interest and reach of those

Table 3-1. U.S. Department of Health, Education, and Welfare Regional offices

Region	Address	Telephone	States in region
I	Regional Health Administrator John F. Kennedy Federal Bldg. Government Center Boston, Massachusetts 02203	(617) 223-6827	Connecticut, Maine, Massachusetts, New Hampshire, Rhode Island, Vermont
II	Regional Health Administrator 26 Federal Plaza, Room 1005 New York, New York 10007	(212) 264-2560	New Jersey, New York Puerto Rico, Virgin Islands
III	Regional Health Administrator Post Office Box 13716 Philadelphia, Pennsylvania 19101	(215) 597-6637	Delaware, District of Columbia, Maryland, Pennsylvania, Virginia, West Virginia
IV	Regional Health Administrator 50 7th Street, N.E., Room 404 Atlanta, Georgia 30323	(404) 526-5007	Alabama, Florida, Georgia, Kentucky, Mississippi, North Carolina, South Carolina, Tennessee
V	Regional Health Administrator 300 South Wacker Drive 34th Floor Chicago, Illinois 60606	(312) 353-5256	Illinois, Indiana, Michigan, Minnesota, Ohio, Wisconsin
VI	Regional Health Administrator 1114 Commerce Street Dallas, Texas 75202	(214) 749-1271	Arkansas, Louisiana, New Mexico, Oklahoma, Texas
VII	Regional Health Administrator 601 East 12th Street Kansas City, Missouri 64106	(816) 374-3291	Iowa, Kansas, Missouri, Nebraska
VIII	Regional Health Administrator 9017 Federal Office Building 19th & Stout Streets Denver, Colorado 80202	(303) 837-4461	Colorado, Montana, North Dakota, South Dakota, Utah, Wyoming
IX	Regional Health Administrator Federal Office Building 50 Fulton Street San Francisco, California 94102	(415) 556-5810	Arizona, California, Hawaii, Nevada
X	Regional Health Administrator Arcade Plaza Building 1321 Second Avenue Seattle, Washington 98101	(206) 442-0403	Alaska, Idaho, Oregon, Washington

who are supposed to be looking after their country's nutrition, and those who do formulate such policies do not specifically include nutrition needs as part of their planning equation. This is the crux of the nutrition planning dilemma.

Still, the question may arise: Why involve nutritionists in the planning process? Nutritional competency has already been described in Chapter 2. The senior professional nutritionist brings to the planning procedure a body of scientific knowledge outside the scope of other experts, experience with techniques required for identifying populations and individuals who are risking nutritional deficiency, ability to analyze the relevance and likely effectiveness of some of the total range of policy measures for reducing malnutrition, and familiarity with the network through which services are delivered.

Although many health disciplines can contribute to planning for nutrition services, the public health nutritionist and the program administrator should have major responsibility for developing a *written* plan for inclusion in the overall plan for health services. If there is no public health nutritionist in the agency or project, consultation should be obtained from public health nutritionists in state or local health agencies or regional offices of the Department of Health, Education, and Welfare (Table 3-1).

To obtain a comprehensive picture of community problems, resources, and attitudes relative to nutrition, inputs from a variety of individuals and groups are important. An advisory committee, with broad representation from nutritionists, dietitians, other health professionals who are knowledgeable about nutrition problems and resources, consumers, and interested lay persons can be helpful in planning and implementing nutrition services. Such a committee can provide a mechanism for the involvement of all community agencies concerned with nutrition services.

THE NUTRITIONIST AT THE PLANNING TABLE

The role of the nutritionist in the planning process begins with identification: Who is at nutritional risk (their geographic and socioeconomic distribution, age-sex category, numbers), what nutrients are lacking, and why. Some assessment needs also to be made of the evolution and of the nature and magnitude of the problem. (The reader will find a detailed discussion of nutritional assessment and surveillance in Chapter 7.) All stages of the planning process, from the identification of relevant measures through design and analysis, will require the joint efforts of nutritionists, statisticians, economists, and other health planners. It seems pertinent to pause here and review the history of health planning.

WHERE DID PLANNING BEGIN?

USE OF POLITICAL PROCESS

Most public health officials fail to take a full part in the political process—in assuring the implementation of their proposals—because they simply do not understand the dynamics of community decision-making. They do not know why proposals for some absolutely essential public health activities are cancelled, postponed, underfinanced, watered down or even ignored. And not knowing, they pass the baton to others, satisfied with the technical adequacy of their contribution and hopeful that someone else will transform their dreams into reality.

Kent Mathewson: Program planning in relation to the total Community in the executive process in public health administration, Ann Arbor, Mich., 1968, University of Michigan School of Public Health.

Planning is a comparatively new concept in the field of public health. Its evolution is an interesting one, since during most of public health's history, programs and activities developed in a highly unplanned manner. In the past, most public health programs were the direct result of some kind of a crisis, such as an epidemic or an earthquake. Unfortunately, this kind of an approach is still very evident in public health practice at the present time. Also, many programs were often dependent on the personal interests and former experiences of the individuals in charge rather than on broadly based or long-range planning.

In the early 1920s a committee of the American Public Health Association on Administrative Practice and Evaluation was the beginning of some serious attention to quality planning. Because of this effort, many short training courses were developed in schools of public health, and specific agencies began to participate in planning and evaluating aspects of public health.

WHY PLAN?
APHA Statement on Planning

The American Public Health Association addressed itself during recent years to the development of a formal statement on the subject of Health Planning. The statement as adopted presents the following useful list of the purposes or objectives of careful health planning.
1. Improved organizational patterns for health services.
2. Speed development of needed new health services, strengthen existing services and improve utilization.
3. Discourage programs not needed in the community.
4. Improve the quality of health care through better coordination.
5. Eliminate duplication of health services among official and voluntary agencies at all levels.
6. Reduce fragmentation of health services at the state and community levels.
7. Help to achieve better geographical distribution of health services with option utilization.
8. Establish priorities among new health programs and services, develop better balance among health programs and provide services more responsive to the special health needs of the area.

Guidelines for organizing state and area wide community health planning, Dec., 1966, American Public Health Association.

Several factors led to a greater consciousness about the importance of careful planning and programing to obtain results:
1. Legislation was passed to enhance public health activities.
2. Funds became more available for public health work.
3. Public demands for services increased.
4. Government and management in general became more sophisticated.

WHY ANALYSIS?

The tools of analysis are still fairly primitive. We are learning as we go along and the best they can now do is to clarify some of the consequences of choices, but the very process of analysis is valuable in itself for it forces people to think about the very objectives of government programs and how they can be measured. It forces people to think in an explicit way. It is an important tool in a fight against creeping incrementalism. "Ten percent to those with the most bureaucratic or political muscle, five percent to all others."

William Gorham: Notes of a practitioner, Public Interest **8:**4, Summer, 1967. Copyright 1967 by National Affairs, Inc.

5. Health agencies became more visible and began to be held more accountable for their work.

Three events solidified the turn to increased interest and activity in health planning among various organizations. These events have occurred in the past decade, creating more impetus in the field of public health than at any other time in its history. The first put forth by the Department of Defense, was the Programming Budgeting Systems (PPBS), which devised certain planning techniques. The success of this approach caused the President in 1965 to instruct his cabinet members to use similar techniques within their departments and agencies.

Public Law 89-749—the Comprehensive Health Planning and Public Health Service Amendments (1966)

The second event was Congress's passing of Public Law 89-749, the Comprehensive Health Planning and Public Health Service Amendments in 1966. As Hanlon[3] states, the importance was threefold:

1. It tended to move federal health assistance away from categorical grants toward block grants, and so made possible greater state and local program determination.
2. It encouraged and required more deliberate and more efficient program planning.
3. It reorganized the level on which potential involvement in social concerns occurred by requiring the establishment of state and local or regional (so-called area wide) planning

commissions. These were made up of members from a number of different professions, agencies, citizens' groups, and institutions.

Comprehensive health planning is a complex process that requires the active involvement of many segments of the community, including representatives of business interests, educators, medical providers, local officials, representatives of civic and minority groups, and others. Local officials, because they are responsible for allocating community resources and because they possess the potential capacity to motivate community leaders and coordinate community health-related programs (both private and public), must assume an active role in comprehensive health planning processes if plans are to be implemented and if programs are to serve the health needs of the community.

In 1968, W. V. Curran, Professor of Health Law, Harvard School of Public Health and Medicine, criticized P.L. 89-749 because of its very broad implications but mainly because these far-reaching amendments do not carry with them constitutional authority or power. For instance, there is no provision for federal involvement in private or public planning and little legal power to enforce federal interest. On the other hand, any aid given to local or area-wide planning agencies is from state or local government, and thus these agencies do not have autonomous authority either. State and local planning agencies do not have to be represented under these acts, or is there necessarily a review of federal funding by the local planners, who after all, are in the position to know best the situation and requirements of a particular area. As Curran[4] points out, there are many conditions and requirements for the state and local agencies but very little for federal activity, which is just the level where legislation could be most effective in terms of comprehensiveness and coordination.

Public Law 93-641—the National Health Planning and Resources Development Act (1974)

The third event to activate public health planning was the passage of Public Law 93-641 by the 93rd Congress on January 4, 1975. It is known as the National Health Planning and Resources Development Act of 1974. The law addresses the subject of nutrition in the national health priorities in that it intends to promote "activities for the prevention of disease including studies of nutritional and environmental factors affecting health and the provision of preventive health care services."[5] A document entitled "Community Nutrition in Preventive Health Care Services" has been prepared by the National Health Planning Information Center to address this nutrition priority.[6] This legislation was most significant because it developed a single new federal program for state and area-wide health planning and resources development. It replaces the former Regional Medical Program, the Comprehensive Health Planning Act, and the Hill-Burton Act. The organizational function and composition are shown in Fig. 3-1.

Health Systems Agencies (HSAs)

The Health Planning and Resources Development Act calls for the establishment of a national council for health policy, state health planning and development agencies, and local Health Systems Agencies. In addition to providing federal grant funds for the support and operation of state and local planning agencies, it includes technical and financial assistance for the development of health resources. The purpose of the act is to improve the health of the area residents by increasing accessibility, continuity, and quality of health services in the area by restraining increases in the costs of providing those services. The intent of the legislation is that the nation will be completely blanketed by the health services areas. Each area will have a Health Systems Agency (HSA) composed of a staff, a governing body of consumers and providers, and the community at large. (See Appendix 1 for Directory of Centers for Health Planning.)

The goals of the HSAs will be "the provision of effective health planning for its health service area and the promotion of development within its area of health services, manpower,

NATIONAL

```
Secretary  ───►  National Council
DHEW             on Health Policy
                 and Development
```

Functions

1. Designate and approve health systems agencies
2. Issue national guidance for health planning
3. Establish health planning information center
4. Approve State Medical Facilities Plan
5. Make loan and loan guarantees to nonprofit, private entities
6. Make development grants to HSAs
7. Review HSA and state agency budgets
8. Periodically evaluate performance of HSAs, state agencies, and SHCCs

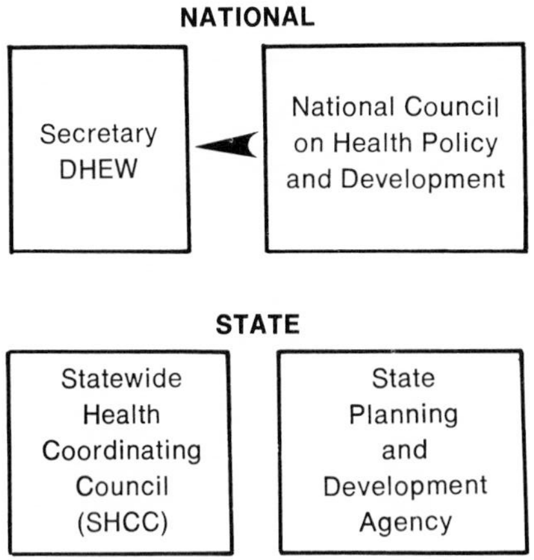

Functions

Advise the Secretary on policy guidelines

Composition

15-member body consisting of VA Chief Medical Director, Assistant Secretary for Health and Environment—D.O.D. and Assistant Secretary of Health—HEW, plus 12 members appointed by the Secretary

STATE

```
Statewide         State
Health            Planning
Coordinating      and
Council           Development
(SHCC)            Agency
```

Functions

1. Annually review and coordinate HSPs and AIPs of state health systems agencies
2. Approve State Health Plan based on health service plans of the HSAs
3. Review HSA budgets
4. Approve state plan and application by state for allotments to the states made under PHS, CMHC, and CAAPTR

Composition

16 to 40 persons appointed by Governor, 60% of which must be selected from HSA nominees; majority of appointees must be consumers

Functions

1. Prepare State Health Plan based on health services plans of the HSAs
2. Assist SHCC in reviewing state medical facilities plan
3. Administer certificates of need and Section 1122 review
4. Review every five years all institution services as to *appropriateness*

Composition

An agency of the State selected by the Governor and approved by the Secretary

Fig. 3-1. National Health Planning and Resources Development Act of 1974—P.L. 93-641, organizational functions and composition.

and facilities which meet identified needs, reduce documented inefficiencies, and implement the health plans of the agency."[7]

The roles, or duties, of such agencies are then as follows:

1. To gather, analyze and report its conclusions from the objective data that are available: statistics from a wide variety of sources, measures of all kinds, and so on.
2. To gather and similarly analyze and report its conclusions from the subjective data available: the things people see as problems and suggest as solutions based on their individual experiences.
3. To devise solutions to the problems, and ways of implementing them, taking into account the legal and financial limitations that may exist, and to test community sentiment about them.
4. To seek to implement the solutions which meet community acceptance, making use of all available resources including the interest of members of the community.
5. To increase community understanding of the long-range implications of individual actions in the health systems.[8]

The particular Health Services Areas will be proposed by each state's Governor, subject to the review of the nation's Secretary of Health, Education, and Welfare. Meetings were held in the spring, 1975, throughout the United States to inform provider groups, public agencies, and consumers on the specifics of the legislation, as well as to gather input for the area designation process. After this process the Governor of each state formulated recommendations to the Secretary regarding area boundaries. Each state has had a person selected by the Governor to coordinate the responsibility for area designation.

WHAT IS HEALTH PLANNING?

Health problems vary with time and place and so, too, does health planning. Planning may be international, national, regional, state, or local in character. Organizationally, it may encompass an entire community, a public or private agency, or it may pertain to a professional discipline such as nursing, so-

WHAT IS HEALTH PLANNING?

In practice, planning does not simply follow a series of textbook steps, but is rather an iterative process that resembles more the tango—four steps forward, three steps back, with an occasional turnaround. Objectives, for example, are not settled on early in the game. Sifting through the various proposals, the planner judges the worth of one objective against the worth of another. Having modified his objectives, he reexamines program proposals in a continual process of testing the desirable against the practical. In short, there is no simple formula, but a planning process does provide a framework that can help force clarification of nutritional objectives and identification of the better alternatives to achieve them.

Reprinted from *A. Berg, N. S. Scrimshaw*, and *D. L. Call*, editors: Nutrition, national development, and planning, Cambridge, Mass., 1973, M.I.T. Press, p. 248. By permission of The M.I.T. Press, Cambridge, Massachusetts. Copyright © 1973.

cial work, or hospital administration. In another dimension a plan may be concerned with a particular health problem (hypertension, lead poisoning, or birth defect) or with an environmental hazard to health (such as water or air pollution). Whatever the problems or the needs, the synchronizing of plans requires an overall design. Much confusion can be eliminated if every health plan is appropriately labeled as to scope, focus, geographic area, and the time to be encompassed.

Hilleboe and Schaefer[9] define health planning as an orderly process of the following:

1. Detecting and defining community health problems and identifying unmet health needs.
2. Assessing available and potential resources.
3. Establishing priority goals (by matching need and resources in considering alternatives and their consequences).
4. Formulating the necessary administrative action to achieve program goals.
5. Relating results to goals by periodic evaluative studies.

There are a variety of designs offered for health planning. Usually the nutrition planning sequence starts with a definition of the nature, scope, and trends of the nutrition problem, leading to a preliminary statement of broad objectives. Methodologies and programs relevant to the objectives emerge along with budgetary and resource allocations. The last step is evaluation. There is no one way. There are many variations—some have five steps, some have ten—but they all begin with problem identification and end with evaluation.

Public health administration

Public health administration has been defined as "the planned and organized social application of the knowledge and techniques of various and varying disciplines to the biological, physiological and sociological advantage of man." Even in this early definition there was emphasis on the planning within the total social context. Planning in public health should be seen as only one aspect of total social and economic planning.[10] Seipp,[11] too, relates health planning to the larger issue of economic development:

The essential planning problem is to maximize the contribution forthcoming from the provision of health services to the total national building efforts of society. Planning within the health sector thus is undertaken in the terms of the larger framework of national developmental planning . . . At the same time, the improvement of the health of the population represents an essential means or instrument for the developing society to attain its social and economic goals. It is when health measures are assessed from this instrumental point of view they can be recognized as productive in character. They represent a necessary element in the total process of development facilitating the obtainment of general goals of a society.

The daily problem facing health administrators is how to improve existing programs with limited funds and at the same time obtain additional resources to support new programs. Because competition for tax money is so stiff at every level of government, humanitarian considerations in themselves do not assure enough available money for health purposes.[12] Consequently, the majority of departments are on limited budgets and they have difficulty in maintaining even the bare

minimum services. Despite this, legislative bodies continually trust many new responsibilities without additional funding. Formal health planning may contribute to solving the twin problem, but the usual planning process followed in many health agencies often consists of only two phases. The first is to set some goals, and the second is immediately to implement the program for quick results—generally with little or no provision for evaluation of output.

However, limited budgets demand critical appraisal of nutrition programs as a continuous ongoing process. How much and what has been done toward the stated objective and what has been the cost in time, money, and materials to produce these results? The importance of asking these questions will be discussed further in Chapter 6. It should be noted here, though, that there are a large number of reference materials which have been developed on the subject of planning and the importance of its various aspects.[9,13]

CONSTRAINTS TO PLANNING

As the art of planning evolved, there were problems with public health administrators who were eager to maintain the status quo. Mathewson[14] testified to this when he said:

. . . to be completely frank I must say that many of the public health officials with whom I have come into contact have played a very limited role or have stayed completely outside of the dynamics of the community decision-making process. Of course, there are several understandable explanations for this. Many public health technicians who live with human suffering and whose days are filled with unending efforts to alleviate the suffering cannot conceive that the rest of the world needs more than a call for help to galvanize this into appropriate action.

New and different methods of health care delivery systems were developed to overcome the complacency of some public health administrators who frequently let the unique opportunities slip away.

Gorham,[15] who had a great deal to do with the development of the Planning-Programming-Budgeting-Systems (PPBS) in the Department of Defense and later in the Department of Health, Education, and Welfare, noted the problems of planning techniques in the government level. Leaders in government are influenced by political pressure groups, outspoken constituents, or perhaps a personal experience such as an illness, which might cause an official to favor a program aimed at a specific problem. Such decisions could be made without proper, planned consideration of costs, benefits, or efficiency.

The determination of specific goals, one step in the planning process, provides a foundation for actions necessary to obtain desired results and established standards against which these results can be measured. Some cautions about goal setting are essential, however. First, unless goals are based on full realization of the scientific technical aspects of the problem for which a solution is being planned, they may be impractical.

Second, unless goals are distilled from an analysis of need and resources, including community understanding, acceptance, and the support of the program, at a particular time and place, they may be neither relevant nor worth achieving.

Somers,[16] Professor of Community Medicine at Rutgers University and long concerned about health delivery systems, has stated that she sees no possibility of comprehensive health care for the individual without his understanding of and participation in the process. Kane[17] goes a step further and adds that there is no possibility of comprehensive health planning without the understanding and participation of the community. A discussion of the role of consumer participation in planning is discussed later.

Third, most health administrators do not perceive goal setting in broad terms of comprehensiveness, of social and economic aims, and of long-term benefits even though such awareness is helpful in deciding intermediate priorities. As Hilleboe and Schaefer[9] explain:

The health administration of a state agency, for example, is largely concerned with the extent and characteristics of those health problems that are within his jurisdiction. He faces the task of weighing the relative priorities of departmental programs involving human ailments and environ-

mental hazards. He will also be sensitive to the localized problems for which local health plans will be necessary as part of statewide planning. While he may be conscious of national health planning, he will probably view this national enterprise largely in relation to his needs for federal funds.

In good comprehensive planning it is more than the plan that is needed. A planner must be cognizant of the inherent problems when there are inadequate data, insufficient attainable resources, rapid scientific and technologic changes, and the scattered responsibility and authority in health matters.[9] Certain problems became clear after the comprehensive health planning program was in existence for five years. Roseman[18] picked out the most evident to be an avoidance of conflict in formulating policy and goals; failure to deal with basic causes of health problems; naivete regarding the need for political influence expertise both within and outside the health field; extremely inadequate funding for comprehensive health care because of expectations about health insurance funding.

To counterbalance these problems, Roseman finds it necessary to develop procedures for planned implementation of health care programs that are not bogged down by excessive concern for cost reduction, coordination, and allocation of resources. Because of these traditional concerns, the innovative planning role of comprehensive health programs has been limited thus far. Reevaluations and analyses such as Roseman's are important if programs are to be improved.

The National Commission on Community Health Services,[19] too, believes that planning is a vital part of any community health service if it is to be truly a helpful and quality service. The commission has emphasized the following:

Action planning for health should be community-wide in area, continuative in nature, comprehensive in scope, all inclusive in design, coordinated in function and adequately staffed. The responsible participation and involvement of all sections of the community, coordination of efforts and development of cooperative working arrangements are fundamental to effective action planning.

CONSUMER PARTICIPATION

A discussion on health planning would not be complete without reference to consumer participation in health programs, referred to briefly earlier. One of the confusing contributions of the poverty programs that were begun in the 1960s has been their emphasis on consumer participation in the planning of public programs. The confusion has stemmed from the lack of a clear-cut definition of both consumer and participation. Kane[17] offers a definition of consumer participation as "the process by which recipients of care in a health program or community, through a representative mechanism, exercise some degree of authority in designating goals for health planning and share in the ongoing evaluation of the services designed to meet these goals." A recommendation for the various steps in collaborative health planning with the potential contributions of both providers and consumers as proposed by Kane is shown in Fig. 3-2. It is suggested that the implementation of each step implies more trust than is presently enjoyed between provider and consumer groups. The hope is that by identifying more distinct and appropriate roles for both consumer and provider, each group may drop some of its defensiveness and develop a trust in the other's good faith. "Without this there can be no joint problem solving."[17]

Kane cautions that meaningful consumer participation must encompass some decision-making power. A definitive role for the consumers indicates that they are the appropriate group to decide what the desired direction and outcome of services should be. However, Kane advises that technical plans and details should not be a consumer responsibility. He raises interesting questions, and the reader is referred to his discussion of the topic dealing with the examination of pertinent questions. What is consumer participation? Why is it useful in health planning? After definition and purpose are considered, the following questions should be asked:

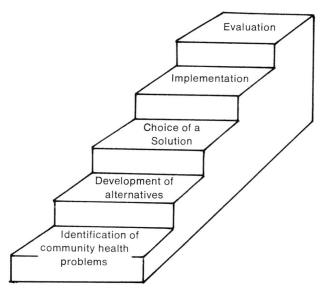

Fig. 3-2. Steps in collaborative health planning. (From Kane, R. L., editor: The challenges of community medicine, New York, 1974, Springer Publishing Co., Inc. Copyright © 1974 by Springer Publishing Co., Inc. Reprinted by permission.)

Whom does consumer participation benefit? What are the potential problems? Should the goal and method of implementing consumer participation be identical across different programs and population groups?

Consumer representation was an inherent part of federally funded activities such as the Hill-Burton program, which supported the building of hospitals, and of the community mental health center movement. The Office of Economic Opportunity's war on poverty went further by requiring a majority of consumers on boards. The advent of comprehensive health planning with its regional planning boards that were responsible for the coordination of all health activities in an area—preventive, environmental, and health services delivery—mandated consumer representation.

THE WAY TO PLAN

What types of factors must be considered when health administrators and nutritionists try to develop programs for achieving community goals? Hanlon[3] cites that they generally fall into three categories:

1. The plan, including programming, control and evaluation.
2. The money, including its acquisition, management and accountability.
3. The personnel, including their recruitment, training, organization, and management as well as relationship with other parts of government and with the public in general.

It should be pointed out that although planning appears to be only one of three considerations, everything in each of the other two factors is, in fact, involved in program planning. In other words a plan is incomplete if it does not include consideration of what resources exist and how best to use them, what method of evaluation will be used, and what results are hoped for.

In the United States' complex society, organizational and community planning approaches and the system analyses are not only most efficient but increasingly necessary to deal with the many different areas and kinds of problems throughout the country.

For instance, rarely, if ever, can a single individual or board make a decision having to do with either a conservation, research, or national immunization program. There are just too many interrelated considerations involved. What is most important is to find the common interests, concerns, responsibilities, and activities among various organizations and groups, and for this, planning is required.

In modern administration it is imperative to develop and use effective and objective approaches to program planning, establishment of program priorities, program control, and evaluations that efficiently coordinate all available resources.

ANALYSIS REQUIRED IN DEVELOPING A PROGRAM PLAN

The development of a program plan to achieve results can be one of the most gratifying tasks that a public health professional undertakes. The plan, graphically presented as a wheel, is shown in Fig. 3-3. In each of the seven major steps, evaluation must be considered. The question, What results will be obtained? must be considered throughout the planning process.

Each of the seven steps to be taken, depicted in the wheel, builds on the previous activity. These seven steps as shown are (1) determine the need; (2) develop a precise plan; (3) develop priorities for the plan; (4) develop an action plan or method to achieve the objectives; (5) design the method of participatory management so as to avoid personal insecurity; (6) consider the audience and critics; and (7) supply data to determine the specific evaluation. Each of these steps will be applied to the hypothetical community presented in the following chapters in which a plan is actually developed, implemented, and evaluated.

Step one, the determination of the need for a particular community, is often referred to as "community diagnosis," "needs assessment," and many other terms. This important first step actually identifies the problem. An examination of the community's charac-

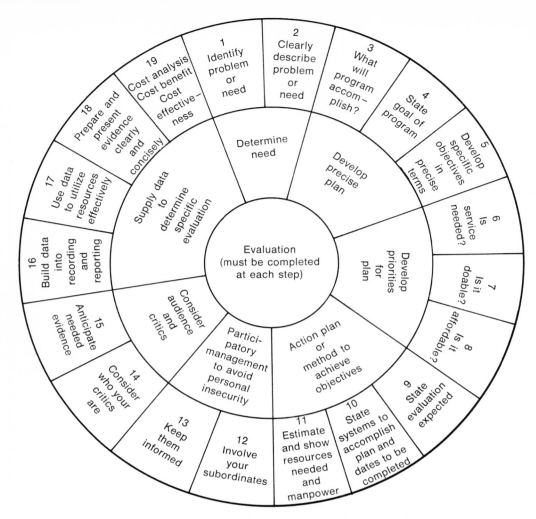

Fig. 3-3. Analysis required in developing a program plan.

teristics such as the vital statistics, population at the poverty level, and leading causes of death, to name a few, enables the planner to clearly describe the problem.

Step two, the development of a precise plan, can be translated into quantifiable goals and objectives. The planner must ask: "What will the program accomplish?" A statement of goals and specific objectives must follow. Objectives written in precise terms are the foundation of any program plan. Unless these are clearly stated, evaluation will be difficult to achieve.

Step three, the development of priorities for the plan, is one of the most difficult tasks in a program plan. Three questions must be examined at this step: Is the service needed? Is it doable? Is it affordable? The answers to these questions will allow the nutrition planner to determine what can be achieved with the existing or new resources in a specified time period.

Step four, the development of the action plan, is the "how to." A statement of evaluation expected can be made only if clear and concise objectives have been formulated. A statement of the systems to accomplish the plan and the dates for completion plus an estimate of the resources and manpower needed allow for realistic planning. The planner can then predict what is to be achieved, when, and by whom.

Step five, the consideration of participatory management so as to avoid personal insecurity among staff members, is a step that is often overlooked and yet it is a vital part of the plan. If subordinates are not informed of the plan, resistance may develop, affecting performance. The involvement of employees in the developmental and planning stage assures acceptance of the tasks. The expertise of employees is a valuable input.

Step six, the consideration of audience and critics, from the outset, will avoid problems with later integration. Questions about what type of evidence will make the point best are important to consider. To whom is the information being presented: to health officers, the legislation, the federal government, or a community group? The wise planner will not underestimate the ability of a lay or professional group to interpret the program plans and objectives.

The final and seventh step, the gathering of data for decision making, is the purpose of the evaluation process. The data collected must be relevant to the program's objectives. Too often there is a massive compilation of data that bears no meaning to the study. The collection of data should allow for the necessary recording and reporting so that the data can be utilized effectively and presented as evidence to fulfill the program goal and objectives.

As stated earlier, evaluation is an ever-continuing, ongoing process throughout all steps of the planning wheel, a vital part of each of the seven major steps with their nineteen specific components. Chapter 4 will build on the first three steps, components of one through eight of the wheel presented in Fig. 3-3. Chapter 6 will encompass the next three steps, components nine through fifteen on the wheel. The remaining components, sixteen through nineteen, will be referred to in Chapters 9 and 10.

SUMMARY

The need for planning ability on the part of the nutritionist should not be underestimated. He or she ought to be aware of the administrative activities necessary to a comprehensive health care program and how such activities are to be implemented. Both the nutritionist and the administrator should be supplied with a clear-cut plan of action, including a description of the problems, the cost in time, personnel, and dollars, objectives and goals, and a method for evaluating the outcome of the program. A certain amount of political awareness and expertise is invaluable as well.

A joint effort among nutritionists, statisticians, legislators, economists, administrators, and other health planners will provide the most effective and efficient health care program. When all participate, the health program becomes part of the total economic picture and functions smoothly within it.

In the past this has not always been the case, since most programs resulted from a specific catastrophe, such as an epidemic or natural disaster, or else were dependent on some legislator's or administrator's particular interest. However, recently legislation has become more sophisticated in dealing with the total picture, especially with the passage of the National Health Planning and Resources Development Act of 1974. This law, passed by Congress in 1975, includes provision for the study of nutrition and environmental factors that affect health. In other words, it provides for preventive health care services within a comprehensive health care program through the establishment of a Health Systems Agency.

Through this provision, federal grant funds are made available for the operation of local planning agencies and local quality health service. Particular service areas are designated through the offices of the Governor of each state. There is thus ensured some coordination between federal and local operations.

To have effective planning, it is important to have specific goal setting, an understanding of community needs, resources, and receptivity, an awareness of social and economic benefits in the long run, and a provision for a critical appraisal of the program. All these desired requirements are best fulfilled when the planning is done on an interorganizational level, where there is cooperation and coordination among various groups and programs.

The health planner is able to implement solutions once the health problems and health care resources are identified within a community. A typical United States urban community, Everywhereville, U.S.A., will be presented in Chapter 4, which will allow for the diagnosis of this hypothetical community.

REFERENCES

1. Nichaman, M. A., and Collins, G. E.: Nutrition programs in state health agencies, Nutr. Rev. **32:**66, 1974.
2. Berg, A., Schrimshaw, N. S., and Call, D. L., editors: Nutrition, national development, and planning, Cambridge, Mass., 1973, M.I.T. Press, p. 248.
3. Hanlon, J. J.: Public health administration and practice, ed. 6, St. Louis, 1974, The C. V. Mosby Co.
4. Curran, W. J.: Public health and the law. Comprehensive health planning: audacious law-making, Am. J. Public Health **58:**1100, 1968.
5. P.L. 93-641, National Health Planning and Resources Act of 1974.
6. Owen, Y. A.: Community nutrition in preventive health care services, Hyattsville, Md., 1978, U.S. National Health Planning Information Center.
7. P.L. 93-641, National Health Planning and Resources Act of 1974, Section 1503.
8. Health Systems Agency of New York City, 1976. Modified from a Department of Health, Education, and Welfare statement (mimeographed).
9. Hilleboe, H. E., and Schaefer, M.: Papers and bibliography on community health planning, Albany, 1967, Albany Graduate School of Public Affairs, State University of New York.
10. Hanlon, J. J.: Can accounting sell health? In Economic benefits from public health services, Public Health Service Publication No. 1178, Washington, D.C., 1964, Government Printing Office.
11. Seipp, C.: Health planning and economic development. John Grant Memorial Section, 91st Annual Meeting, Kansas City, Nov. 13, 1963, American Public Health Association.
12. Linnenberg, C.: Economics in program planning for health, Public Health Rep. **81:**1085, 1966.
13. Strauss, M. D., and DeGrout, I.: A bookshelf on planning for health, Am. J. Public Health **61:**656, 1971.
14. Mathewson, K.: Program planning in relation to the total community in the executive process in public health administration, Ann Arbor, Mich., 1968, University of Michigan School of Public Health.
15. Gorham, W.: PPBS, its scope and limits, Public Interest **8:**4, 1967.
16. Somers, A. R.: Comprehensive care and the consumer, J. Med. Educ. **45:**465, 1970.
17. Kane, R. L., editor: The challenges of community medicine, New York, 1974, Springer Publishing Co., Inc.
18. Roseman, C.: Problems and prospects for comprehensive health planning, Am. J. Public Health **62:**16, 1972.
19. National Commission on Community Health Services: Health is a community affair, Cambridge, Mass., 1966, Harvard University Press.

Appendix 3-1

DIRECTORY OF CENTERS FOR HEALTH PLANNING
June, 1977*

The National Health Planning and Resources Development Act of 1974, P.L. 93-641, authorizes the establishment of Centers for Health Planning to assist in the implementation of the Act. The organizations listed below have been selected to provide consulting and training assistance to Health Systems Agencies, Statewide Health Coordinating Councils, and State Health Planning and Development Agencies in specific DHEW Regions. The Centers also work together to help

*DHEW, Bureau of Health Planning and Resources Development, Hyattsville, Md., 1975.

meet National needs. Each of the Centers for Health Planning has both a Regional and a National Office DHEW Project Officer. All requests for assistance from the Centers should be coordinated with the Project Officers.

The Bureau of Health Planning and Resources Development, Health Resources Administration, Department of Health, Education, and Welfare, has the responsibility for national coordination of the Centers program. The National Coordinator of the Centers for Health Planning is Mr. Jeffrey Tirengel, Bureau of Health Planning and Resources Development, Center Building, 3700 East-West Highway, Hyattsville, Maryland 20782 —(301) 436-6730.

Regions and states	Centers for health planning	Regional project officer
Region I (Boston) Connecticut, Maine, Massachusetts, New Hampshire, Rhode Island, Vermont	Center for Health Planning Boston University 53 Bay State Road 4th Floor Boston, Massachusetts 02215 Director: Mathew Skinner (617) 353-3764	William McKenna DHEW Region I JFK Federal Building Boston, Massachusetts 02203 (617) 223-6441
Region II (New York) New York, New Jersey, Puerto Rico, Virgin Islands	Alpha Center for Health Planning, Inc. 1010 James Street Syracuse, New York 13203 Director: W. David Helms (315) 422-5365	Phyllis Lusskin DHEW Region II 26 Federal Plaza New York, New York 10007 (212) 264-4490

Regions and states	Centers for health planning	Regional project officer
Region III (Philadelphia) Delaware, Maryland, Pennsylvania, Virginia, West Virginia, District of Columbia	Center for Health Planning Health Planning Research Services, Inc. 550 Pinetown Road Fort Washington, Pennsylvania 19034 Director: Robert Pickard (215) 628-4428	Jay Halpern DHEW Region III P.O. Box 13176 Philadelphia, Pennsylvania 19108 (215) 596-6645
Region IV (Atlanta) Alabama, Florida, Georgia, Kentucky, Mississippi, North Carolina, South Carolina, Tennessee	Health Planning/Development Center, Inc. Center for Health Planning Suite 1010—Healey Bldg. 57 Forsyth Street, N.W. Atlanta, Georgia 30303 Director: Raphael Levine, Ph.D. (404) 524-4743	Earl Wright DHEW Region IV 50 Seventh Street, N.E. Atlanta, Georgia 30323 (404) 242-2316
Region V (Chicago) Illinois, Indiana, Michigan, Minnesota, Ohio, Wisconsin	Midwest Center for Health Planning 1 South Park Street Madison, Wisconsin 53715 Director: James Kimmey, M.D. (608) 255-5666	Gloria Kronewitter DHEW Region V 300 South Wacker Drive Chicago, Illinois 60606 (312) 353-1650
Region VI (Dallas) Arkansas, Louisiana, New Mexico, Oklahoma, Texas	Center for Health Planning Southwest Center for Urban Research 1200 Southmoore Houston, Texas 77004 Director: Hardy Loe, M.D. (713) 526-8801	Forrest Stokes DHEW Region VI 1200 Main Tower Room 1835 Dallas, Texas 75202 (214) 655-3932
Region VII (Kansas City) Iowa, Kansas, Missouri, Nebraska	Region VII Center for Health Planning 104 Lewis Hall Columbia, Missouri 65201 Director: Kenneth Bopp (314) 882-2211	Charles Jackson DHEW Region VII 601 East 12th Street Kansas City, Missouri 64106 (816) 374-2924
Region VIII (Denver) Colorado, Montana, North Dakota, South Dakota, Utah	PACT Center for Health Planning 90 Madison Street Suite 604 Denver, Colorado 80206 Director: Cyril Roseman, Ph.D. (303) 320-0917	Carolyn Rimes DHEW Region VIII 11037 Federal Office Bldg. 1961 Stout Street Denver, Colorado 80294 (303) 837-4051

Regions and states	Centers for health planning	Regional project officer
Region IX (San Francisco) Arizona, California, Hawaii, Nevada, Guam, Trust Territory of Pacific Islands, American Samoa	Western Center for Health Planning 693 Sutter Street—Suite 408 San Francisco, California 94102 Director: Joseph Hafey (415) 673-7266	Philip W. McClain DHEW Region IX 50 Fulton Street San Francisco, California 94102 (415) 556-3550
Region X (Seattle) Alaska, Idaho, Oregon, Washington	TAC/X Center for Health Planning 100 West State Street Boise, Idaho 83702 Director: John Cambareri, Ph.D. (208) 345-2777	James Van Hoomissen DHEW Region X 1321 Second Avenue Arcade Plaza Seattle, Washington 98101 (206) 442-0516

GENERAL CONCEPT

A profile of the community allows for health planning. Each element in the planning process is an important step in completing and implementing a plan that is workable, a plan where results can be demonstrated and measured.

OUTCOMES

The student should be able to do the following:

- Define community, community nutrition, and community assessment.
- List the six basic elements of effective program planning.
- Utilize the hypothetical community to develop a needs statement and a goal statement.
- Discuss in detail the factors to be considered in determining need, developing a precise plan, and developing priorities.

The community: assessment, elements in planning process, and setting priorities

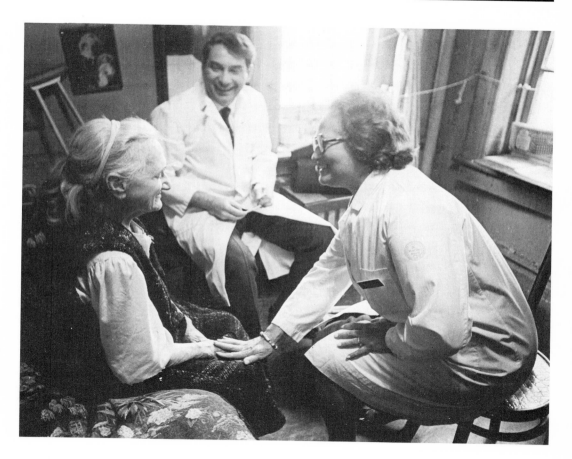

CHAPTER 4

WHAT IS A COMMUNITY? WHAT IS COMMUNITY NUTRITION?

Although efforts to improve the health and well-being of people have taken place under a variety of circumstances, the most important settings for nutrition improvement programs are communities. Community, as the term is used here, is defined by Deuschle[1] as a group of individuals or families living together in a defined geographic area, usually comprising a village, town, or city; it may represent only a few families in a rural area or may include heavily populated cities; it may range in size from less than a hundred to a few thousand people. Members of a community live and work together, feel a sense of loyalty to the community, and share a limited number of common interests.

Accepting Deuschle's definition of a community, what, then, is community nutrition? A definition which allows for flexibility and scope in both teaching and practice is that community nutrition is the academic discipline which deals with the identification and solution of health problems of nutritional implications within communities or human population groups.

WHAT IS COMMUNITY NUTRITION?

The meaning of the word "community" must be clarified. "Community medicine" is sometimes defined as health care of people in groups. Others take it to mean care of people in their environment, home or work, but outside of hospitals and institutional medicine. Concepts such as "family medicine" and "comprehensive care" are sometimes included in community health. "Comprehensive medicine" or "continuity of care" must supervise and support people throughout episodes of health and sickness, whether inside or outside institutions. Community nutrition must emphasize applied nutrition and in fact it is consumer-oriented. It cannot exclude individual nutrition or nutrition in institutions such as hospitals. Food sciences are essential but most of our knowledge of applied nutrition in communities derives from close observation of patients by clinicians and scientists as far as the consumer is concerned. . . .

"Community nutrition" is therefore the whole of the nutritional sciences applied to the consumer as groups or as individuals. It is the interface between food and people and probably some 90 per cent of all nutrition takes place in the home. Each culture has always had its special preferred food, food taboos, and food habits.

About 400 B.C., Hippocrates stated "The physician must know, and must be at great pains to know, what man is in relation to food and drink and habits generally, and the relation of each to each individual."

Cicely D. Williams: The foreword. In McLaren, D. J., editor: Nutrition in the community, London, 1976, John Wiley & Sons, Inc., p. xii. Reproduced with permission. Copyright © 1976, John Wiley & Sons Limited.

Since nutrition is both a science and an art, too often one is considered with disregard for the other. Nutrition practitioners have become aware of the past gap that exists between knowledge acquired and the implementation of that knowledge. Community nutrition bridges this gap. In the mid-1960s, war was declared on poverty, hunger, mal-nutrition, ignorance, and disease. In a cautious descent from the ivory tower, nutritionists recognized the flaws in the lack of practice of their expertise. The era of revelation gave way to the era of relevance. Nutrition students and medical students were demanding relevance. Community nutrition emerged as the conscience of nutrition as it related to real world problems. Its area of concern became problems of health among groups of people—health being defined in the sense of the World Health Organization definition of maximal physical, mental, and social well-being.[2] Such a concern with the health problems of populations leads inevitably to a broad range of interests—from the cause and prevention and control of disease to the organization, financing, and effectiveness of health care delivery.

WHAT IS COMMUNITY ASSESSMENT? HOW CAN ONE DIAGNOSE A COMMUNITY?

Community diagnosis is the attempt to identify as fully as possible what the health problems with nutritional implication are and what resources are currently available; it enables the practitioner of community nutrition to implement solutions. As early as 1927, Emerson[3] described the importance of community diagnosis. Labeling it public health diagnosis in an address that still has a contemporary ring, he called for periodic diagnosis of the community just as one would recommend the regular health assessment of an individual patient.

McGavran[4] has been one of the more articulate formulators of the analogy that the community is a patient and should be studied in a similar fashion.

As Tapp[5] suggests, community diagnosis need not be comprehensive. It may be the study of a part of a community, a partial community diagnosis looking at a piece of the community picture with several linking parts, without attempting to make all possible connections. This would contrast with the comprehensive community diagnosis, which represents an attempt to study all aspects of the community and to relate them to each other and then tries to arrive at some basis for establishing priorities. The actual process of establishing priorities goes beyond diagnosis and enters into the area of treatment. Data are necessary for cost-benefit and cost-effectiveness analyses on which priorities depend. To do such an analysis, a body of information must be established—the data base, the real description of the community.

This description of the community presents its background, its history, its geographic determinants. The people must be characterized—not just their demography but their culture and their ethnic differences. In addition, other major factors that contribute to the color and texture of the community map are the people's religion, taboos, education, interests and concerns, socioeconomic status, housing, schools, and other institutions. Too often in the past the knowledge, attitudes, and practices as related to values have been overlooked. Questions must be asked: What is the nature of health and disease patterns, food supply, and market places? How do the people generally approach living together?

Gathering existing data on these and other factors will help to determine whether the community's nutritional resources are adequate, what groups are potentially at high nutritional risk, and how well the community's nutritional and related health needs are being met by existing curative and preventative health programs. A unique method for monitoring trends in food utilization at the community level has been provided by Harrison and co-workers in their study of household refuse in Tucson, Arizona.

As Christakis[6] outlines, in effect, the community assessment paints a picture of the health of the community, its ecology, and the factors influencing the way its people live. To do this, demographic, epidemiologic, cultural, and geographic data must all be utilized. The community's entire health care capabilities and potential including medical, educational, and social welfare as well as nutritional must be surveyed.

There are existing sources of information on which community assessment relies.

COMMUNITY DIAGNOSIS: THE GARBAGE PROJECT

For two years, The Garbage Project of the University of Arizona has been collecting data on household refuse in Tucson, Ariz. The study of household refuse offers several advantages as a supplement to traditional methods of collecting data on patterns of food utilization at the community level: (a) it is a nonreactive measure of behavior; (b) it is relatively inexpensive and demands no time or cooperation on the part of the subjects; and (c) it offers the possibility of quantitatively estimating food waste at the household level. In a sample of about 300 households studied over periods of several months in 1973 and 1974, the average household wasted between $80 and $100 worth of food per year (exclusive of food waste which was poured down the drain, ground up in garbage disposals, fed to household pets, composted, or disposed of other than in the garbage can). Changes in food utilization and waste patterns from 1973 to 1974 are noted.

Gail G. Harrison, William L. Rathje, and *Wilson W. Hughes:* Food waste behavior in an urban population, J. Nutr. Ed. 7:13, 1975. Reprinted with permission from the Journal of Nutrition Education. © Society for Nutrition Education.

What is known about the community from its health records, vital statistics, morbidity, and mortality records? What is known about health services, number of professionals, number of health-related facilities? In addition to United States census studies data, which give the characteristics of the population group—sex, age, race, marital status, education, income, and housing—what is known from hospital records, public assistance records, and private, public, and social welfare agency statistics?

Jelliffe[7] suggests, as an oversimplification and as a rough guide to thinking, that the level of nutrition in a community, especially of its vulnerable young child population, may be considered as being due to the numerous complex, interacting ecologic molding forces, expressed in the following nonmathematical "equation" at the top of p. 76.

Each of the components of the equation affects the community nutrition level directly and by way of the other factors indicated. Each is, of course, shorthand for a complex situation.

$$\text{Community level of nutrition} \propto \frac{\text{Education level} \times \text{Economic level} \times \text{Food availability} \times \text{Aspects of health} \times \frac{\text{(Conditioning infections}}{\text{Preventive services)}}}{\text{Population size}}$$

The education level includes not only the formal level of schooling and the limited technical personnel available in a country, including those in extension services, but also literacy in general.

The economic level operates on a country basis, such as when governmental funds become available for social services, such as schools and health services, food stamp and supplemental food programs, as well as for specific nutrition programs directed at major problems. At the family level improved earning capacity means that there will be more money that can be used for the purchase of a greater range of foods.

Food availability in the community nutrition–level equation is shorthand, both for the food present in the country as a whole (and its distribution and cost) and also for the food within the reach of a family, especially to the young child, to pregnant and lactating women, and to the elderly.

Certain "aspects of health" particularly influence the community nutrition level, especially health services concerned with prevention.

It is becoming increasingly apparent that the level of nutrition in a community is related to the number of mouths to be fed—that, in fact, population size (including family size and the closeness of child spacing) is the "universal denominator" for all other components of the equation.

Although the collection of all these data describing the community may not be simple, in the long run it offers direct planning for nutrition programs that meet the needs of the community—programs that are realistic and meaningful.

With this data base in hand, it is now possible to formulate a problem list and consider a plan for problem management. Good questions to ask are: What results can be expected from alternative programing? What would happen if no treatment took place?

THE HYPOTHETICAL COMMUNITY

Community diagnosis is the attempt to identify as fully as possible what the health problems and health care resources are. It enables the health planner to implement solutions. Each element of the planning process, as shown in Fig. 4-1, steps 1 through 8, is an important step in completing and implementing a plan that is workable, a plan where results can be demonstrated and measured. The steps required in developing a program plan are shown: determine the need, develop the precise plan, and develop priorities for the plan. With each of these steps, evaluation (data gathering for decision making) is considered.

A hypothetical community, that is, a typical United States urban population with its variety of health care delivery systems and health and nutrition problems, has been designed to use as the model for the program planning that is being discussed here. The tools and methodologies needed to look at a community's specific health and nutrition problems will be presented with examples taken from the hypothetical community. This will show the student and practitioner how to proceed to solve the problems presented.

This community, the county of "Everywheresville, U.S.A." is different throughout the country, of course. The population structure, the family characteristics, the employment and economic situation, the educational profile, the transportation system, the programs available for specific population groups, the available health services, and the community health and nutrition problems are all factors that will vary east to west, north to south.

However, the six basic elements of effective program planning can be applied to any Everywheresville in the United States. This community will be studied so that the following information can be determined:

1. Definition of need

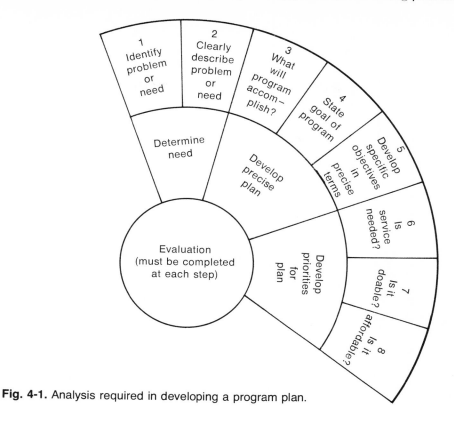

Fig. 4-1. Analysis required in developing a program plan.

2. Development of quantifiable goals and objectives, with a precise plan
3. Setting priorities
4. Development of an action plan, which is the method of *how to* implement a plan including participative management
5. Supplying data to determine effectiveness
6. Evaluation of achievements or accomplishments

All the available data concerning the community should be gathered and collated, as in this profile of Everywheresville.

HYPOTHETICAL COMMUNITY OF EVERYWHERESVILLE, U.S.A.—1977
A community diagnosis

Population characteristics
  Population—500,000
  Urban setting
  Population mix
    White—60%
    Black—20%
    Spanish American—15%
    Other—5%
  Age distribution of population
    Large percentage of population are 30 years of age and under
    15% of population are elderly

Employment and economic situation
  Industry—marketing and manufacturing
  Income levels
    Average—$10,000 to $12,000 per year for a family of 4 persons
    Poverty level—20% of population below poverty level
  Unemployment rate—10%
Family characteristics
  Family size
    Average—4 persons
    Low-income average—5 persons
  Working mothers—60% employed
Educational characteristics
  Educational level

High school graduates—75%

College and above—10%

Noneducated—15%

Educational resources

Elementary schools

High schools

Community colleges

Vocational schools

No mandatory health education in schools

School Lunch Program available in most schools

School Breakfast Program available in selected areas only

Transportation characteristics

No mass transportation; private automobiles provide transportation

Programs available for specific population groups

Day care facilities available for 50% of working mothers; other 50% of children cared for in private homes

Food and nutrition programs (other than schools)

Food stamps—serving only 25% of those eligible

Women, infants, and children—supplemental feeding program for pregnant and lactating women, infants, children

Case load—1,000 clients representing approximately 10% utilization*

Title VII—several congregate feeding sites for the elderly throughout major population centers

Health services available (other than private providers)—County Health Department

Personnel

Health director, M.D.—1

Pediatric nurse assistants—2

Sanitarians—3

---

*500,000

20% poor = 100,000

10% women, infants, and children = 8,000 to 10,000 (potential case load of 8,000 to 10,000 eligible for this program)

Nurses—15

Health educator—1

Nutritionist—1

Services for behavioral health

Services for planning environmental health

Social workers—2

Health workers—2 per clinic setting

Health worker trainees—2

Services available

General community hospital

Family planning clinics

Limited prenatal clinics for population requiring services (clinics staffed primarily by pediatric nurse assistants)

Equipment available for nutritional assessment

Outdated or inappropriate equipment available for measuring heights and weights

Limited facilities for biochemical determinations

Computer services at health department very limited

Health and nutrition problems in community

Health problems

Cardiovascular disease in adult population

Cancer

Accidents

Diabetes

Anemia in 17% of 1- to 2-year-old indigent population

Overweight in 19% of child population

Obesity in 40% total population

High incidence of women with complications in pregnancy

Short stature in 18% of indigent population (preschool-children and school-children)

Elevated serum cholesterol levels in large percentage of population 18 years of age and under; of these a large number had two or more additional cardiovascular risk factors

Poorly nourished elderly population

Widespread dental disease

DEVELOPING A PROGRAM PLAN

Program planning is defined as a process that includes the identification of a problem and its related aspects; the setting forth of a goal and objective toward which the program should be directed; and the development of alternative action plans, one of which is to be selected, implemented, evaluated, and updated.

Step 1. Determining need

The first step in the planning process is a description of the problem. What are the specific health problems with a nutrition component? What are the nutrition problems? How severe are they? Who is affected? What is the age distribution of the population? What age group is affected? What are the patterns of health and illness? This step usually consists of a straightforward collection of already available and easily obtainable hard data. (See Chapter 6, including Appendix 6-1.)

Identifying and describing the need for a particular effort is a difficult but necessary task. Before any program is conceived, this kind of clear description of what the need is and what problem it is going to solve is extremely important.

The term "need" may be described as a lack of something required or desired. The final achievement of all program planning is to meet a need, satisfy a want, or alleviate an existing condition. To determine a need, several criteria can be employed. Determination of a need may arise from the following:

1. General observation, that is, an expression of a "desire" for some particular program
2. Failure to achieve a predetermined standard
3. Result of surveys, studies, or surveillance information for baseline data

Collection of baseline data

The purposes of collecting data are to obtain factual knowledge about the problem, to permit an accurate diagnosis of its causes and systematic approaches to its solutions, and to help assess or evaluate changes that follow. Types of data that may be collected include the following:

1. Findings of anthropometric studies
2. Data from clinical nutrition surveys
3. Biochemical studies
4. Vital and health statistics
5. Result of special studies on local foods; review of marketplaces
6. Cultural—anthropologic and sociologic data, including material on food habits and food preference, "power structure" in local communities, the decision-making process, and leadership patterns
7. Role of women

Principles in data collection

According to Latham,[8] a recognized investigator in public health planning, certain principles should be observed if relevant information is to be found and used effectively:

- Studies and surveys should only be undertaken if their importance is relative to the sources available.
- Only data likely to be useful for planning and evaluation of the program should be collected. Appropriate time tables must be worked out.
- The data should be as objective as possible. In some cases subjective data also have to be used. However, the reliability of data must be carefully weighed and due importance given to quantitative studies that are factual.
- Statistical advice should be obtained on sampling procedure and to determine the statistical significance of changes recorded.
- A system of recording results in all aspects of the planning should be devised. This should aim to simplify both the collections and analysis of data.
- Small pilot studies may be necessary to train staff in data collection, to improve techniques, and to establish the optimum means of establishing good relations with the population.
- The community must always be prepared in advance to receive the study personnel.
- The tabulation and analysis of data collected must be carried out with care and a careful summary prepared.

If the need or want is not clearly identified and described, what to do about it cannot be considered. Problems arise in describing the need when the statement is one of the solutions rather than a clear expression of a need. For example, "We need to supply iron supplements to children" is really a solution whereas the *need* may be to reduce the rate of iron-deficiency anemia among 1- to 5-year-olds.

Examples: need determined by data collection

Everywheresville, the hypothetical community, indicates a particular area of need. For example, there is the problem of anemia in children; 17% of the children 1 to 2 years of age from the indigent population have iron-deficiency anemia and are at nutritional risk. There is the need to design a program to reduce iron-deficiency anemia in children.

Another example would be the prevalence of cardiovascular disease. The rate of cardiovascular disease in Everywheresville is 40% and has increased by 25% with decreasing age in the last ten years. Any rate above 50% is considered an epidemic. There is need to design a program to reduce cardiovascular disease risk.

Thus, in the process of need determination, or problem identification, the planner pinpoints the need. He now recognizes, for example, two specific nutrition problems in Everywheresville—iron-deficiency anemia in children and a prevalence of cardiovascular disease in an increasingly youthful population.

With an adequate description of the scope, nature, and victims of the nutritional problems of a community in hand, the next step is to begin to develop a precise plan. Here the planner determines what the program will accomplish, states the goal of the program, and develops specific objectives in precise terms.

Step 2. Developing precise plan
Stating goals and objectives

In the past, one of the most serious drawbacks in public health agencies and nutrition programs has been the vague determination of what goals and objectives are expected. Because of this, agencies were at a disadvantage when approaching providers of funds for adequate public health nutrition programs. Certainly one of the most serious lacks in effective planning has been due consideration of the communities' interests or needs, a necessary complement to professional input in developing goals.

The determination of goals and standards depends on a number of factors whose importance varies according to time and place. The first inquiry should be to find out what the government and the community have in mind as their purpose in creating programs. This is important whether or not the planner agrees with that purpose. Without this knowledge all intentions and efforts may fail.

One of the most common approaches in

determining goals and objectives is to collect and analyze statistical data, for example, births, illnesses, and deaths, or to conduct special surveys and studies. Information from these sources, if properly obtained and analyzed, indicate the problems that will suggest desirable goals and standards to be established, achieved, and maintained. (See Appendix 6-1, p. 160.)

An example of this approach was completed in the state health department in Arizona in 1969. For a new, developing public health nutrition program, very limited data were available on the nutrition problems in the community. However, *A Nutritional Status Survey: Selected Arizona Characteristics*[9] was available, giving data such as infant mortality, maternal mortality, causes of death, the vital statistics for the community that had nutrition implications, the amount and type of food programs throughout the state, and medical and nutrition services available to pregnant women, infants, children, and adults. These data were available without utilization of additional funds, since most of the information came from already existing sources. In fact, this publication was the springboard for obtaining funding from the legislature to combat the problem of a high incidence of anemia in the state. Without this information only a vague statement about the nutrition problems could have been developed!

All of these data collected should be studied in relative terms, that is, in relation to other times, in relation to other places, and in relation to each other. There may be a political climate that is right for certain programs, or there may be a funding source available for a problem that is not the nutritionist's number one priority. One of the difficulties in applied nutrition programs has been lack of funds to support adequate planning. Planning is often rushed after programs are launched without adequate baseline data, usually because of little resources and time. These aspects of planning must be taken into consideration before an effective program can be launched.

The program need not be elaborate; for

instance, it might be planned only to coordinate and strengthen existing activities related to improved food choices and modified intake. A pilot program should have clearly stated plans for later expansion. Such a program should establish coordinating committees at national, regional, and local levels; provide for additional nutrition training of staff if needed; and involve the community in its planning, execution, and evaluation, as suggested in Chapter 3.

A TOOL: STATISTICS TO MEASURE RESULTS

There is a fine distinction between the traditional activity counts—enumerations of nursing and clinic visits for various purposes or sanitary inspections of different types of establishments—and the kinds of statistics which focus attention on number of persons served and types and amounts of service received. With the traditional counts, quantitative evidence is being accumulated to describe how each public health worker spends his time—how much effort is being expended for each separate program. With the latter type of statistics, information is being collected on the results of that effort.

Measurements of results, then, is the key to what we want to achieve with service statistics. The term "service yield indices" is an apt phrase. Just as a farmer finds it necessary if he is to know whether he is operating at a gain or loss, to reckon the number of bushels of wheat or bales of cotton he gets per acre in return for the labor and expense of production, so the public health worker must calculate the service being rendered to the community in relation to the need for service.

E. Flook: The value of good service statistics in a modern health department, Public Health Rep. **68:**811, 1953.

Difference between goals and objectives

An arbitrary differentiation has been made by many people between goals and objectives, even though both imply a "results orientation" or what will be accomplished. However, to differentiate between the two terms, a goal, mission, or purpose is usually a statement of broad direction, general purpose, or interest. It may be somewhat unreachable, and it is seldom quantifiable. The following is one example of a goals statement: "To increase the health status and the quality of life for the citizens of the state."

Goals, or standards by which results may be judged, tend to be broad, all-encompassing ideals because they are derived from values. Values, in turn, originate and undergo revision according to an individual's experiences with his social and physical environment. Values may be defined as impressions of what is desirable or worthy; they are then utilized as criteria for choice of action.

Ranked values lead to a hierarchy of goals, many of which are widely accepted. A characteristic of a hierarchy of goals is that the concrete goals are at the lowest level (these are usually called objectives) and the more generalized, all-encompassing or abstract goals are at higher levels. The formulation of abstract goals is essential because many of the most important human goals can be adequately or meaningfully stated only in general terms.

The concept of a goal hierarchy, presented by Powell,[10] is illustrated by Fig. 4-2. At the top of the pyramid, the ultimate goal of comprehensive health planning has been declared by Congress to be "promoting and assuring the highest level of health attainable for every person, in an environment which contributes positively to healthful individual and family living . . ." Such an ultimate goal is of an abstract and long-term or permanent nature, but it is refined and given greater specificity by subdividing it into subgoals which appear at the next level in the hierarchy. These, in turn, are further divided and specified at subsequent lower levels. Level two contains those goals which relate to the four major concerns of comprehensive health planning: physical and mental health needs, environmental needs, and their ancillary, administrative needs. Level three is where goals are identified for particular program areas and serve as means for achieving the higher level goals. Level four involves the most specific subgoals of the hierarchy. These are the most tangible for a community and take the least time to accomplish. These are referred to as "objectives," which provide specific target dates for completing specific projects that are necessary for achieving level three (program) goals.[10] Thus, in planning

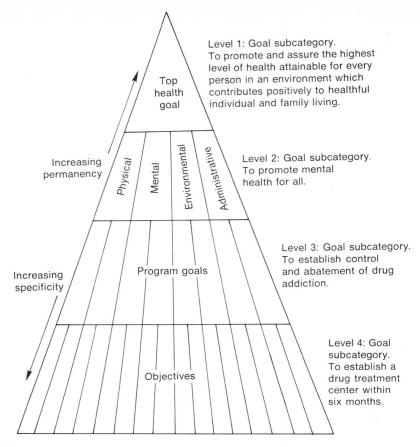

Fig. 4-2. Concept of goal hierarchy. (From Powell, M. D., Bodwitch, W. P., Fiedelman, B. P., and Winter, W. C.: Comprehensive health planning: a manual for local officials, Washington, D.C., National Association of Counties Research Foundation.)

terminology, one can see that objectives are highly specific. They must include expected results in qualitative and quantitative terms, within a given time frame.

Odiorne,[11] designer of the Management by Objectives System (MBO), has said:

Objectives often explain behavior better than any other contributing factor in a managerial situation and the understanding and control of objectives is more vital than other factors since they provide the main energizing and directive force for managerial action. Objectives are the focal point around which executives can concentrate their efforts and mobilize their resources.

This can apply to organization and management of a public health system, since the identical factors of money, manpower, resources and accomplishment, or results orientation are the ones that must be utilized, coordinated, and evaluated.

Benefits from writing sound objectives

Some of the benefits resulting from writing sound objectives are summarized by Drucker[12] as follows:

1. Objectives identify the basic ideas, principles and fundamental concepts of the organization and what it is trying to achieve. They give meaning and direction to the work of the people associated with the organization.
2. Objectives provide the basis for guiding,

leading and directing the organization. They stand as targets that people strive to reach together and provide a center along which managers can integrate and coordinate those efforts.

3. Objectives provide standards of performance that are essential to the control of human effort in an organization. Evaluation of individual performance is based upon the extent to which mutually agreed upon objectives are being achieved.

4. Objectives motivate people. They help provide a sense of unity, harmony, cooperation and concern for achievements which are essential for all organized endeavors.

5. Objectives help program planners in the following ways:
   a. Organize and explain the whole range of organizational phenomena in a few general statements.
   b. Test these statements in actual practice.
   c. Predict behavior.
   d. Appraise the soundness of decisions.
   e. Analyze their own experiences, and as a result improve their performance.*

Stating objectives effectively is the prime program responsibility. Developing meaningful written objectives of program statements is the basis of program management. A specific format for writing them follows:

To/action verb/desired result/time frame/
   resource required.
Example
To/reduce/anemia by 40% in those identified at risk/in one year/utilizing nutrition staff in fourteen countries.

Guidelines for writing objectives

The following five general guidelines for writing program objectives, stated by Loeb,[13] apply to formulating objectives for a person, unit, section, or department:

1. State objectives in terms of expected results, not in terms of activities or processes.
2. Specify results that will be tangible and recognizable so that all involved in planning, including advisory board and other agencies or groups of special interests, will

also recognize the objectives that have been accomplished.

3. State objectives so that expected results are very specific, not general.

4. State objectives in terms of results to be accomplished this month or this year (if the program is continued next year and the years thereafter, include specific time limitations).

5. Show how the objectives of a specific program help further the objectives of the organization, or department or unit and the mission and purposes of the statewide or national structure.

Common errors in setting objectives

Reif[14] alerts the planner to some of the most common errors in setting objectives:

- Common objectives are not clarified for the whole unit.
- Objectives are set too low to challenge the individual subordinate.
- Common objectives are not clearly shaped in small units to fit those of the larger unit.
- Individuals are overloaded with patently inappropriate or impossible objectives.
- Responsibilities are not indicated in the most appropriate positions.
- Methods of working are stressed rather than clarifying individual areas of responsibility.
- Areas that are familiar to planners are emphasized rather than achieving a more constructive job objective.
- Policies as guides to action are not available so that once results are presented ad hoc judgments are issued in correction.
- Objectives are accepted uncritically without a plan for their successful achievement.
- The very real obstacles that are likely to hinder the subordinate in achieving his objectives including numerous emergency or routine duties which consume time are ignored.
- Newer objectives or ideas proposed by subordinates are ignored by superiors and only those deemed suitable are imposed.
- Planning and action that would help subordinates succeed are lacking.
- Intermediate target goals and dates are not set to measure subordinate's progress.
- New ideas from outside the organization are not introduced nor are subordinates permitted or encouraged to do so, thereby freezing the status quo.

---

*Modified from Drucker, P.: Management: tasks-responsibilities-practices, New York, 1974, Harper & Row, Publishers, © 1973, 1974 by Peter F. Drucker.

- Subordinates are not permitted to seize targets or opportunities in lieu of stated objectives that are less important.
- Previously agreed upon objectives that have subsequently proved unfeasible, irrelevant or impossible are not scrapped.
- Successful behavior is not reinforced when objectives are achieved nor is incorrect unsuccessful behavior corrected when they are missed.

Method of writing objectives

Utilizing the basic formula to develop objectives—to/action verb/desired results/time frame/resources required—as applied to the hypothetical community Everywheresville, it is possible to develop sound objectives.

Earlier, two specific needs in the community were identified.

1. Seventeen percent of children ages 1 to 2 years from the indigent population have iron-deficiency anemia and are at nutritional risk.
   Example: To deal with the incidence of anemia, the following objective could be completed:

   To/action verb/desired results/time frame/resource required.
   To reduce the prevalence of anemia in 1- and 2-year-olds by 40% in those identified at risk in one year by utilizing the nutrition team in each of the fourteen counties.

2. The prevalence of cardiovascular disease in Everywheresville is 40% and has increased by 25% with decreasing age in the last ten years. Any rate above 50% is considered an epidemic.
   Example: To design an objective for the need in the cardiovascular disease area, the following objective could be completed:

   To/action verb/desired results/time frame/resource required.
   To reduce the prevalence of cardiovascular disease risk factors (hypercholesterolemia, obesity, hypertension, smoking, and inactivity) by 40% and obesity by 30% in the 10,000 people screened, utilizing

personnel and funds from the state appropriations and county health department nutrition staffs.

Step 3. Setting priorities

The relationship of possible goals and objectives to each other is of particular interest and concern to public health administrators. It necessitates the development of some means of determining the relative importance of various health problems and hence various public health activities. In this day and age of limited funds and resources, it is important to put in priority the objectives stated for any organizational unit. In establishing priorities three questions must be considered (Fig. 4-1):

- Are the services needed?
- Are the services doable?
- Are the services affordable?

In other words, priorities are established in relation to goals. At any given moment or place there are many public health problems, many more than can be treated adequately with what resources are available. Some problems obviously must take precedence over others. As previously indicated, the decisions too frequently are made on the basis of personal whims or interests or because of some political or public pressure groups rather than as a result of careful study and analysis.

In determining program priority, there are certain fundamental factors that should be considered. For example, generally a problem that affects a large number of people should take precedence over one that affects relatively few people, but not if the former is the common cold and the latter a smallpox epidemic. A disease that kills or disables should take precedence over one that does not, but only if an effective method of scientific attack is at hand. Similar factors should also be considered, particularly the existence of scientific knowledge and techniques, the availability of suitable personnel and funding, the propriety and legality of the contemplated action, and its acceptance by the community.

In addition, Nathan[15] has pointed out that

one should consider pressures and interests of special and local groups, expressed views of a chief executive, editorials in the local newspapers, official policies expressed by the legislature, and the opportunism that may appear when funds are available with regard to a particular problem. Also to be considered are sudden advances in knowledge or technique and/or the need for further research and demonstration.

Another approach to setting priorities is given by Hanlon,[16] who considers the following factors: the *size* of the problem, the *seriousness* of the problem, the *effectiveness* of the results and PEARL (P for propriety, E for economics, A for acceptability, R for resources, and L for legality).

According to Hanlon, the *size* of the problem is defined as the number of persons having the problem or being directly affected by it in rates per 100,000 population. Only those who may reasonably be expected to receive public health services, if they are made available, are to be counted among this population.

The *seriousness* of the problem may be determined by four factors: the urgency, severity, economic loss, and number of people who may be affected directly and indirectly.

The *effectiveness* of the results can only be positively determined when more accurate measuring devices and methods are discovered and used. Meanwhile, judgments about the values of the program should be made as it is actually being implemented and as it would be were it carried out under optimum conditions.

The components that make up PEARL are not directly related to a program's effectiveness or even the need for it but are important to decide if a program can be accomplished in a specific time, that is, its feasibility.

Two specific methods of establishing priorities might also be considered. One possible approach is to follow a version of the International Technical Assistance Programs of the United States Government that was developed several years ago and is now used

in some training programs in a modified form.[17] The first step in this method is for the key professional and management personnel of a particular project to meet together and to list every conceivable type of activity and program regarding a particular problem that is being engaged in, might be instituted, or has ever been requested. The number of items may easily number in the hundreds. Following this listing down one axis, across the other axis is listed every conceivable factor that might be considered in judging whether or not a particular activity or program should or could be engaged in at the moment or in the near future. Then there is discussion of each possible activity or program in terms of these many factors, resulting in a rating of each from 0 to 4 plus. By this means it becomes possible to consider existing or potential activities or programs from a broad overall objective yet relative point of view. From the consensus that develops, the results usually fall into three broad priority categories:

1. For activities or programs that are consistently rated 3 plus or 4 plus for every qualifying factor. The conclusion is that under all circumstances these particular activities should be carried out.

2. Of secondary importance are certain activities or programs that ordinarily might not merit attention without special precise explanation and justification because of reservations with regard to one or several qualifying criteria.

3. In the third category are certain activities or programs that are not justified and should not or cannot be engaged in. It is recognized, however, that in unusual circumstances certain nonhealth considerations might result in a decision to engage in one of these activities.

A second method that has been used in determining priorities is the use of a priority matrix. The purpose of the matrix is to measure each objective against all other objectives. The matrix is compiled in the following manner.

The twenty-two objectives developed for a particular program listed (A to V) are inserted

	A	B	C	D	E	F	G	H	I	J	K	L	M	N	O	P	Q	R	S	T	U	V	Horizontal
A		X									X	X	X	X	X	X	X			X	X	X	11
B											X	X	X	X	X	X	X			X		X	9
C				X	X	X	X	X	X	X	X	X	X	X	X	X	X	X	X	X			17
D					X		X	X			X	X	X	X	X	X	X	X	X	X	X	X	15
E							X	X			X	X	X	X	X	X	X	X	X	X		X	13
F							X	X	X		X	X	X	X	X	X	X	X	X	X		X	14
G								X	X		X	X	X	X	X	X	X	X	X	X		X	13
H									X		X	X	X	X	X	X	X	X	X	X		X	12
I																							0
J											X	X	X	X	X	X	X	X	X	X	X	X	12
K												X	X	X	X	X	X			X			7
L													X	X	X	X	X			X			6
M																X				X			2
N															X	X	X			X			4
O																X	X			X			3
P																	X			X			2
Q																							0
R																			X	X		X	3
S																				X			1
T																							0
U																						X	1
V																							
Total vertical spaces	0	0	2	2	2	4	4	2	2	9	1	1	1	2	2	2	1	10	2	17	10	10	
Total horizontal X's	11	9	17	15	13	14	13	12	0	12	7	6	2	4	3	2	0	3	1	0	1	0	
Total	11	9	19	17	15	18	17	14	2	21	8	7	3	6	5	4	1	13	11	2	18	10	
Rank order	10	13	2	6	7	4	5	8	21	1	14	15	19	16	17	18	22	9	11	20	3	12	

Fig. 4-3. Responsibilities of a nutrition program.

on the vertical and horizontal axes of the priority matrix (Fig. 4-3).

A. Complete screening.
B. Make and record referrals.
C. Write patient care plan; include behavioral objectives.
D. Intervene on underweight.
E. Intervene on obesity.
F. Intervene on high-risk pregnancy.
G. Intervene on anemia.
H. Intervene on CVD risk.
I. Intervene on short stature.
J. CNW routine training.
K. CNW modular training.
L. In-service for other health personnel.
M. Training for nutritionists.
N. Training for personnel in aged, group care, and educational facilities.
O. Training for the public by use of media.
P. Training for the public by group presentations.
Q. Training for the public by individual session (telephone or office).
R. Submitting monthly, quarterly, and annual reports.
S. Identify nutrition needs and resources to community and governmental agencies.
T. Develop materials and evaluate existing materials.
U. Complete voucher issuance and records.
V. Monitor grocer relations.

A priority list of these twenty-two objectives can be established in the following manner:

1. If the objective in the left column is more important than the objective across the top, put an X in the box. If not, leave blank.
2. Work only to the right of the diagonal line.
3. Sum the Xs on each horizontal line and transfer these sums to the bottom of the page where it says "Total Horizontal Xs."
4. Sum the blank spaces above the diagonal line in each vertical column.
5. Total the vertical spaces and horizontal Xs for each objective.
6. Assign rank order to the objectives, with the first priority being the objective with highest total.

Utilizing this matrix, the following priority listing occurred:

1. Community nutrition worker routine training.
2. Write patient care plan, include behavioral objectives.
3. Complete voucher issuance and records.
4. Intervene on high-risk pregnancy.
5. Intervene on anemia.
6. Intervene on underweight.
7. Intervene on obesity.
8. Intervene on cardiovascular disease risk.
9. Submit monthly, quarterly, and annual reports.
10. Complete screening.
11. Identify nutrition needs and resources to community and governmental agencies.
12. Monitor grocer relations.
13. Make and record referrals.
14. Community nutrition worker modular training.
15. In-service training for other health personnel.
16. Training for personnel in aged, group care, and educational facilities.
17. Training for the public by use of media.
18. Training for the public by group presentation.
19. Training for nutritionists.
20. Develop materials and evaluate existing materials.
21. Intervene on short stature.
22. Training for the public by individual session (telephone or office).

Methods for setting priorities may vary from agency to agency and project to project. It is important that the nutritionist, as administrator, become knowledgeable and comfortable in the practice of setting objectives and adopt that method which works in the specific setting.

SUMMARY

To develop a program plan that answers the needs of a community's health problems, a community diagnosis or analysis is necessary. This diagnosis must try to discover data such as general population characteristics, family characteristics, employment and income situations, educational resources, transportation facilities, health programs and services already available, and of course, the health problems within the community. The first step then is to determine and clearly identify the need for a particular program, and this is done through the collating and interpretation of available and relevant data.

The next step in formulating a program plan is to develop a precise plan by stating the program's goals and objectives. Although both goals and objectives refer to the expected results of a program, goals are usually designated as the overall, long-term purpose, whereas objectives are the more immediate and specific hoped-for results. Goals may be ranked in a hierarchy according to their value, those with the most permanent and abstract purposes at the top, and those projects with the most immediate and short-term objectives at the bottom. Objectives should be stated in terms of expected results rather than activities or processes.

The third step is to evaluate and compare goals and so establish priorities for possible programs. When setting priorities, one should consider the size and seriousness of a problem, how many people are affected directly and indirectly, how effective the program will be, and other factors such as resources of personnel and funding, receptivity by the community, and the general feasibility of implementing the program. A method of evaluation should also be part of the plan.

A nutrition plan is only as good as its implementation. Success in implementation depends on strong leadership, sound organization and administration, extensive training and research, and continuous planning. The next step will be to formulate an action plan, or a method to achieve objectives, which will be discussed in Chapter 6. However, it is significant to first study some programs that are on-going at the local level. Thus Chapter 5, on community nutrition programs: strategies at the local level, follows.

REFERENCES

1. Deuschle, K. W.: Organizing preventive health programs to meet health needs, Ann. Am. Acad. Political Soc. Sci. **337:**36, 1961.
2. Constitution of the World Health Organization, Geneva, 1948.
3. Emerson, H.: Public health diagnosis, Chicago, 1927, Fifth Sedgewick Memorial Lecture.
4. McGavran, E. G.: Scientific diagnosis and treatment of the community as a patient, J.A.M.A. **162:** 723, 1956.
5. Tapp, J. W.: Community diagnosis. In Kane, R. A., editor: The challenges of community medicine, New York, 1974, Springer Publishing Co., Inc.
6. Christakis, G., editor: Nutritional assessment in health programs, Am. J. Public Health **63**(suppl.): 1, 1973.
7. Jelliffe, D. B.: Epidemiology of undernutrition. In McLaren, D. J.: Nutrition in the community, London, 1976, John Wiley & Sons, Inc.
8. Latham, M. C.: Planning and evaluation of applied nutrition programmes, Rome, 1972, FAO/UN.
9. Spendlove, G., Yanochik, A., and Maruna, D.: Nutritional status survey, selected Arizona characteristics, Phoenix, 1968, Arizona Department of Health.
10. Powell, M. D., Bodwitch, W. P., Fiedelman, B. P., and Winter, W. C.: Comprehensive health planning: a manual for local officials, Washington, D.C., National Association of Counties Research Foundation, pp. iv-49.
11. Odiorne, G. S.: Management by objectives: a system of managerial leadership, New York, 1965, Pitman Publishing Corp.
12. Drucker, P.: Management: tasks-responsibilities-practices, New York, 1974, Harper & Row, Publishers.
13. Loeb, A. M.: Evaluation of programs. Proceedings of a Workshop on Program Planning Implementation and Evaluation in Public Health Social Work, Berkeley, Calif., Jan., 1975, School of Public Health Social Work Program, University of California.
14. Reif, W.: Management by objectives notebook, Tempe, Ariz., 1975, Arizona State University.
15. Nathan, M. R.: Some steps in the process of program planning, Am. J. Public Health **46:**68, 1956.
16. Hanlon, J. J.: Public health administration and practice, ed. 6, St. Louis, 1974, The C. V. Mosby Co.
17. Hanlon, V. V.: The design of public health programs for underdeveloped countries, Public Health Reports **69:**1028, 1954.
18. Anonymous: Responsibilities of nutrition program.

GENERAL CONCEPT

Every health care program, from the federally funded to the state operated, to those on the local level, should allow for the vital nutrition component if it is to successfully be a part of the increasing trend to preventive health care. It is the function of the nutritionist to approach the program with creativity and courage to be innovative in serving the surrounding population.

OUTCOMES

The student should be able to do the following:
- Identify the role of the nutritionist in the variety of health care services at the local level.
- Name various services under the Department of Agriculture Child Nutrition Program and Family Food Assistance Program.
- Identify other programs aimed at specific population groups.
- Indicate particular risk factors and health problems for each age group in the life cycle and describe the skills necessary to deliver the nutrition services.

Community nutrition programs: strategies at the local level

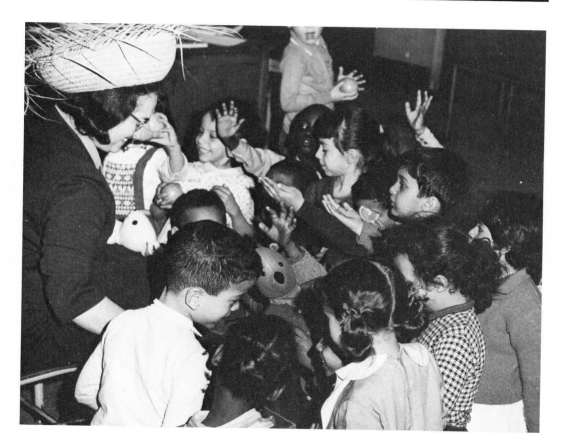

Most health agencies and many community health projects employ nutrition personnel to plan, direct, and carry out nutrition services. At the present time in the United States, an estimated 2,000 nutritionists, professionally trained in the art and science of nutrition, are involved in the delivery of nutrition services in health care programs at the local level. Each year, Congress appropriates funds for a variety of grant and contract programs designed to improve the distribution and effectiveness of health services, particularly for those populations who are underserved or disadvantaged. Although nutrition is not always visible in the titles of these health programs (e.g., Maternal and Child Health, Migrant Health Projects, Apalachian Health Program, National Health Service Corps projects, Indian Health Services), it is usually an important and integral part of them.[1] The nature and extent of the nutrition service provided in these health programs will, of course, vary with program needs, resources, and priorities.

An earlier discussion in Chapter 2 listed the specific competencies and responsibilities of the public health nutritionist whose task it is to assess needs, plan, implement, and evaluate the nutrition component of health services. It was also stated that at the local and community level the nutritionist, diet counselor, or community dietitian acts as a specialist in a specific program serving a particular population group. In a specific setting—a maternity and infant care program, an adolescent clinic, a drug rehabilitation house, a geriatric center—the nutritionist provides direct service to an individual client or population group. Here specific skills are combined and coordinated to meet individual and family needs, and they should include at least the following essential services: assessment of food practices and dietary status; nutrition education and counseling to meet normal and therapeutic needs; and provision of, or referral to, resources for appropriate food service, special feeding equipment, and/or supplemental food assistance.

The nutritionist employed in such a position, that is, as one who functions as the implementer of nutrition services at the local level, is often a person with a baccalaureate degree. Faculty from ten institutions indicated that the students enrolled in their programs (community nutrition, community dietetics, and/or public health nutrition) must, on graduation, demonstrate competence in the following aspects of nutrition-related service[2]:

- The individual assumes responsibility for the nutritional care of individuals and families, as a nutrition counselor.
- The individual contributes to and is utilized by the health care team in the provision of health care to individuals and families.
- The individual plans, implements, and evaluates nutrition education lessons for a group of well people.
- The individual plans, implements, and evaluates educational programs for groups of people who are under the care of a physician.

- The individual can describe the nutrition component of community health programs, including the intent of past legislation and current legislation.
- The individual communicates effectively, orally and in writing.
- The individual engages in selected continuing education.

NEW ROLE FOR DIETITIAN FOCUS ON COMMUNITY POPULATION

The impact of rapidly changing forces on the health care delivery system has mandated that the various health professions engage in self-study and prepare for differing roles and competencies that may be required. For dietetics, such deliberations have led to the suggestion that not only will dietetic practice in the future be altered in several ways, but the setting in which it will be practiced will expand . . . The American Dietetic Association's Position Paper on education for the profession of dietetics calls for dietitians to enlarge their sphere of practice to the "vertical" or community population.[*] Other Position Papers suggest that dietitians should be employed in health maintenance organizations, physician group practices, ambulatory care clinics, neighborhood health centers, and well-baby clinics.[†] To practice in these settings, however, dietitians will need to be competent in providing nutritional care services of a different dimension from those they have traditionally given. Dietetic services will be directed more to health needs in contradistinction to the needs of the acutely ill. The focus will be on consumer education, establishing or changing of food habits consonant with health and with disease prevention, and managing nutritional problems for the non-hospitalized person in the community. There will not be the constraints imposed by the procedures and organizational structure required of the acute care setting—nor will the role of the dietitian necessarily be as well defined . . . Sixty-eight role functions for nutritional care dietitians and dietetic technicians who practice in ambulatory care settings were developed, based on observations in ten health care delivery settings. These functions, categorized under major roles of manager, consultant, educator, diet therapist-counselor, and advocate, were identified and validated by a panel of experts.

Mary Ann Scialabba: Functions of dietetic personnel in ambulatory care, J. Am. Diet. Assoc. **67:**545, 1975. Reprinted by permission. Copyright The American Dietetic Association.
[*]ADA Position Paper on Education for the profession of dietetics, J. Am. Diet. Assoc. **59:**372, 1971.
[†]ADA Position Paper on the Nutrition component of health services delivery systems, J. Am. Diet. Assoc. **58:**538, 1971; ADA Position Paper on Nutrition services in health maintenance organization, J. Am. Diet. Assoc. **60:**317, 1972.

The community nutritionist is a person with the scientific knowledge of the principles of nutrition, who disseminates nutrition information and is concerned with the nutritional implications of policies relating to food production, marketing, utilization, and consumption. But it is most important that this health professional, when functioning at the community level, be a behavioral scientist and a change agent. In the past, too often and most unfortunately, the enthusiasm "to do" and to provide services has led to neglect in planning a course of action necessary to achieve predetermined objectives, as was discussed in Chapter 4. There is a need to plan within a framework of implementation as has been described in Chapter 4, where a list of specific nutrition programs available for specific population groups was presented, including day care facilities, supplemental feeding programs, and congregate feeding sites for the elderly. Specific health problems also have been discussed, including cardiovascular disease, cancer, accidents, diabetes, anemia, overweight, as well as specific recommendations for designing a program plan to deal with these problems (Chapters 3 and 4, Fig. 3-3).

COMMUNITY DIETITIAN, R.D.

The community dietitian, R.D., with specialized community dietetic preparation, functions as a member of the community health team in assessing nutritional needs of individuals and groups. The community dietitian plans, organizes, coordinates, and evaluates the nutritional component of health care services for an organization.

Responsibilities

1. Develops and implements a plan of care based on nutritional needs and available sources and correlates with other health care.
2. Evaluates nutritional care and provides follow-up for continuity of care.
3. Utilizes human effort and facilitating resources effectively.
4. Compiles and uses pertinent operational data to assure provision of quality nutritional care.
5. Interprets, evaluates, and utilizes pertinent current research relating to nutritional care.
6. Utilizes appropriate tools in providing nutritional care.
7. Communicates appropriate dietary history and nutritional care data through written record systems.
8. Counsels individuals and families in nutritional principles, diet, food selection, and economics and adapts teaching plans to the individual's life style.
9. Provides consultation and works with community health team members to coordinate nutritional care with the total health care for individuals and groups.
10. Provides consultation to and works with community groups.
11. Evaluates foodservice systems, making recommendations for a performance level that will provide optimal nutrition and quality food.
12. Develops nutritional care and foodservice standards for provision of food to groups.
13. Conducts or participates in in-service education and consultation with professional staff and supporting personnel of own and related organizations.
14. Plans or participates in development of program proposals for funding.
15. Identifies and evaluates needs to establish priorities for community nutrition programs.
16. Plans, conducts, and evaluates nutrition education programs for the public.
17. Publishes and evaluates technical and lay food and nutrition publications for all age, socioeconomic, and ethnic groups.
18. Plans, conducts, and evaluates dietary studies and participates in nutritional and epidemiologic studies with a nutritional component.
19. Maintains effective verbal and written communications and public relations.

Recommended minimum annual salary: $14,600.*

Position paper on recommended salaries and employment practices for members of The American Dietetic Association, J. Am. Diet. Assoc. **71**:641, 1977. Reprinted by permission. Copyright The American Dietetic Association.

*It is important to emphasize that the recommendations are *national* minimums. Salary levels for dietitians vary greatly in different areas of the nation and even between suburbs and inner city for a variety of reasons. There are differences in the number of qualified persons available, the general earnings level, and the cost of living. In New York and California, where dietitians' salaries are highest, the recommended minimum will be substandard. It should be attainable in other cities.

The nutrition program at the local level should relate to the seven stages, steps 1 to 19, shown in the analysis required in developing a program plan. (See Fig. 3-3.)

GUIDELINES FOR POPULATION GROUPS IN COMMUNITY NUTRITION: THE LIFE CYCLE

Although the design or plan for various community nutrition programs may be similar, there are slight variations based on the risk factors and problems for each age group of the life cycle. Specific guidelines have been developed for determining risk, standard criteria, a statement of the problems, and intervention techniques with behavioral objectives and referral sources for pregnant women, infants and children, adolescents, adults, and the elderly, as shown in Tables 5-1 to 5-5.

Pregnant women	Table 5-1
Infants and children	Table 5-2
Adolescents	Table 5-3
Adults	Table 5-4
Elderly	Table 5-5

The findings of this type of assessment will delineate the specific problem on which to focus as the following discussion indicates. Once behavioral objectives are stated and records adequately kept with follow-up, change and outcome can be measured. Such data will determine future funding!

GUIDELINES FOR POPULATION GROUPS IN COMMUNITY NUTRITION: MATERNAL AND CHILD HEALTH (Tables 5-1 and 5-2)

Legislative provisions for health services for mothers and children were first initiated in Title V of the Social Security Act of 1935. Formula grants were provided to states for maternal and child health services. Although studies in the 1930s and 1940s established the contributions of nutrition in pregnancy to the health of the mother and condition of the infants at birth, it was the 1970 report of the National Research Council Committee on *Maternal Nutrition and Course of Pregnancy*[3] that more clearly defined the nutritional needs and negated earlier widespread practices of dietary restriction of calories and so-

dium during the prenatal period. This report specified the importance of the mother's nutritional status prior to conception, outlined the need for and role of various nutrients during pregnancy, and also identified the pregnant teenager as being at particularly high nutritional risk, since she adds the nutrient needs of the fetus to those of her own growing body.[4]

In 1974 the Social Security Act required that each state develop a state plan providing five projects: Maternity and Infant Care, Intensive Infant Care, Health Services for Children and Youth, Dental Health for Children, and Family Planning Services. The goal is to provide comprehensive health care, continuity in health management, and supervision of care to low-income and high-risk population groups. A multidisciplinary approach is emphasized with services in the fields of medicine, dental care, nutrition, nursing, and social work.

THE INFANT'S NUTRITIONAL INTAKE

The science, art, and craft of nutrition is important to everyone, but especially to the young who must achieve good growth and development.

The ultimate value of nutrition programs lies in their application. What matters is the food that the mother puts into the spoon that goes into the child's mouth, and the child's ability to utilize it. No amount of scientific investigation, knowledge of biochemistry or analysis of food will achieve adequate nutrition for an individual or a community until the application of the art of nutrition receives more serious consideration.

Cicely D. Williams: Grassroots nutrition—or consumer participation, Martha Trulson Memorial Lecture, 1972, J. Am. Diet. Assoc. **63:**128, 1973. Reprinted by permission. Copyright The American Dietetic Association.

The role of nutrition in each of the preceding projects can be better understood by reviewing the objectives of the legislation.[5] In the case of the Maternity and Infant Care Project, the objective is to find the vulnerable patients early in pregnancy and to provide them with comprehensive multidisciplinary health care to prevent adverse outcomes. Too often women in low-income families receive poor, late, or no prenatal care,

Text continued on p. 101.

Table 5-1. Guidelines for population groups in community nutrition—pregnant women

Determining risk	Standard criteria (technique/equipment/standards)	Problem	Intervention		Referral sources
			General guidelines	Sample client behavioral objectives	
Anthropometric Height Prepregnant weight	Steel tape measure Balance scales	Short stature Underweight	Promote adequate weight gain and nutrient intake	Client will identify difference between nutrient needs during pregnant and nonpregnant states	Maternal and Infant Care Project
Weight gain	Follow pattern of National Academy of Sciences weight gain grid	Weight loss or inadequate weight gain		Participant will plot and determine the components of her weight gain during pregnancy	Prenatal care WIC Program Food stamps
Biochemical Hemoglobin Hematocrit Urine	Center for Disease Control Standards adjusted for altitude Stick test for sugar, ketones, protein	Anemia Diabetes Toxemia	Promote regular and early use of prenatal services	Participant will identify reasons for early use of prenatal services and relationship to outcome of pregnancy	Regional perinatal programs
Clinical Obstetric history Blood pressure Smoking, alcohol, and drug intake questionnaire	Questionnaire Sphygmomanometer	Repeated pregnancy and lactation at intervals of less than 1 year Previous problem pregnancies High parity Mothers 19 or 35 years old Smoking, alcohol, and drug use increase risk of low birth weight or birth defects Pica and allergies	Encourage decision on breast or bottle feeding during last trimester	Participant will identify reasons to *breast feed* or *bottle feed* an infant	Title XIX Maternal and Child Health Services
Dietary 24-hour recall or food frequency	24-hour recall or food frequency form				

Table 5-2. Guidelines for population groups in community nutrition—infants and children

Determining risk	Standard criteria (technique/equipment/standards)	Problem	Intervention		Referral sources
			General guidelines	Sample client behavioral objectives	
Anthropometric Height Weight Head circumference (to 2 years of age) Skinfold thickness (over 5 years of age)	Balance scales, steel measuring tape, infant measuring board, calipers; National Center for Health Statistics (NCHS) growth grids Triceps skinfold according to Seltzer and Mayer, Postgrad. Med. **38:** A-101, 1965	Poor growth (ht/age <5th percentile, wt/ht <5th percentile, head circumference <5th percentile)	Rule out child abuse or neglect Check diet for energy and nutrient adequacy	Parent will plot and interpret screening values for height, weight, and head circumference on growth grids	Private physician WIC Program Children and Youth Crippled Children's Services Regional center for high-risk newborns Title XIX (Early Periodic Screening, Diagnosis and Treatment Program) Head Start
		Failure to thrive (drop in position on growth grid)	Check feeding environment	Parent will explain relationship between weight/height and health problems	
		Obesity (wt/ht >95th percentile)	Aim for child to "grow into" ideal weight range rather than lose weight	Parent will identify ideal weight for his/her infant	
Biochemical Hemoglobin Hematocrit Serum cholesterol	Center for Disease Control Standards; adjusted for altitude Cyanmethemoglobin method for hemoglobin Wybenga method on microsample	Anemia	Identify cause of anemia (malabsorption, dietary, bleeding)	Parent/participant will identify causes, symptoms, and consequences of anemia	Child Abuse and Neglect Center Food Stamps Commodity foods
		Elevated serum cholesterol (>160 mg/dl)	Investigate other cardiovascular disease risk factors	Client/parent will identify cardiovascular disease risk factors and state those which can be modified	

Clinical				
Birth weight	Sphygmomanometer with child-size cuff; quiet environment	Birth weight <5½ lb.	Monitor low birth weight infant to determine catch-up growth rate	Parent explains meaning of systolic and diastolic readings
Blood pressure		Diastolic blood pressure for 3- to 12-year-olds greater than 90 mm/Hg	Caution should be exercised in labeling children as hypertensive because of psychosocial and economic implications; use of term "high normal blood pressure" is appropriate during evaluation and follow-up*	Parent explains factors that contribute to hypertension
Dental caries				
Dietary				
24-hour recall or food frequency	24-hour recall or food frequency form	At risk of nutrient and energy intake inappropriate to age according to RDA	Identify key nutrients, function, and food sources	Parent will explain factors affecting weight gain during infancy
Feeding development			Describe introduction of foods and food preparation	Parent will identify eating problems occurring during infancy leading to obesity
			Discuss weaning	Parent will identify appropriate feeding skills for their infant or child

*Report of the Task Force on Blood Pressure Control in Children, Pediatrics Supplement, vol. 59, May, 1977.

Table 5-3. Guidelines for population groups in community nutrition—adolescents

Determining risk	Standard criteria (technique/equipment/standards)	Problem	Intervention		
			General guidelines	Sample client behavioral objectives	Referral source
Anthropometric Height Weight Skinfold thickness	Balance scales, steel measuring tape, calipers NCHS growth grids for ht/age and wt/age and wt/ht before puberty	Teenage pregnancy	Concentrate on fact that mother is still physiologically developing, as well as supporting growth of fetus	Client will identify reason for increase of nutrient and energy needs due to (1) her own physiologic development, and (2) her pregnant state	Prenatal care WIC Program Maternal and Infant Care Project
		Obesity (wt/ht >95th percentile in prepuberty)	Explain relation between between weight, self-image, and peer acceptance	Client will explain how obesity relates to social problems in adolescence, hypertension, diabetes, cardiovascular disease risk, and obesity as an adult	Weight Watchers International, Inc. Physical fitness programs and recreational facilities
Biochemical Hemoglobin Hematocrit Serum cholesterol	Center for Disease Control Standards; adjusted for altitude Cyanmethemoglobin method for hemoglobin Wybenga method on microsample	Anorexia nervosa	Concentrate on psychological factors and influence of entire family	Client will identify ideal weight for age and sex and identify health risks associated with rapid weight loss	Physician, psychologist, or guidance center
Clinical Blood pressure Dental caries Drug and alcohol abuse and venereal disease questionnaire	Sphygmomanometer; quiet environment	Alcohol and drug abuse	Investigate social environment in terms of peer pressure and peer acceptance	Client will state energy/nutrient requirements and explain how substance abuse affects satisfying these requirements	Drug treatment centers Alcoholics Anonymous Free clinics Neighborhood health centers Nontraditional, alternative health centers
Dietary 24-hour recall or food frequency	24-hour recall or food frequency form				

Table 5-4. Guidelines for population groups in community nutrition—adults

Determining risks	Standard criteria (technique/equipment/standards)	Problem	Intervention		
			General guidelines	Sample client behavioral objectives	Referral sources
Anthropometric Height Weight Skinfold thickness	Balance scales Steel tape measure, calipers Metropolitan Life Insurance Height and Weight tables Triceps skinfold according to Seltzer and Mayer, Postgrad. Med. **38:** A-101, 1965	Obesity (>20% over ideal weight for height)	Relate obesity to chronic health problems Develop personalized intervention plan on desirable life-style modifications that include diet and exercise	Client will explain association between obesity and chronic health problems Client will identify which disease risk factors he has and how he can modify them	Weight Watchers International, Inc. Physical fitness program and recreational facilities
Biochemical Hemoglobin Hematocrit Serum cholesterol and other lipids Blood glucose	Center for Disease Control Standards, adjusted for altitude	Anemia Diabetes Elevated cholesterol (>200 mg/dl) Hyperlipidemias, Types I to V Hypertension (blood pressure >140/90 mm Hg)	Concentrate on personal diet modifications using diabetes exchange list	Client will describe relation between insulin, physical activity, and diet intake and importance of reaching and maintaining ideal weight to control diabetes	Food stamps
Clinical Blood pressure Cardiovascular disease risk factor questionnaire; family history, diabetes, smoking, physical activity, stress	Sphygmomanometer Treadmill, lung function test	Risk of heart attack, stroke, and certain cancers (lung, esophagus, bladder); increases with number and severity of risk factors such as overweight, fat intake, hypertension, elevated cholesterol, smoking, inactivity, and stress			Stop smoking clinics Alcoholics Anonymous
Dietary 24-hour recall or food frequency	24-hour recall or food frequency form	Alcoholism and drug abuse	Investigate causal factors in substance abuse and suggest coping mechanisms	Client will state energy/nutrient requirements and explain how substance abuse affects satisfying these requirements	

Table 5-5. Guidelines for population groups in community nutrition—elderly

Determining risk	Standard criteria (technique/equipment/standards)	Problem	Intervention General guidelines	Intervention Sample client behavioral objectives	Referral source
Anthropometric Height Weight Skinfold thickness	Balance scales Steel tape measure, calipers Metropolitan Life Insurance height and weight tables Triceps skinfold according to Seltzer and Mayer, Postgrad. Med. **38**: A-101, 1965	Obesity (20% over ideal weight for height)	Increase nutrient density of diet to adjust for decreased energy need Stress importance of food in social environment	Client will identify own decreased energy needs and name specific foods high in nutrients, low in calories Client will identify food/social programs for which he is eligible and which are available in his community	Weight Watchers International, Inc. Title VII Congregate meal site Meals on Wheels Food stamps
Biochemical Hemoglobin Hematocrit Serum cholesterol and other lipids	Center for Disease Control Standards, adjusted for altitude	Anemia Diabetes Elevated cholesterol (25 mg/dl, with elevated proportion of low density to high density lipoproteins)			
Blood glucose Clinical Blood pressure	Sphygmomanometer	Hypertension (blood pressure 140/90 mm Hg)			
Cardiovascular disease risk factor questionnaire; family history, diabetes, smoking, physical activity, stress	Treadmill; lung function test	Risk of heart attack, stroke and certain cancers (lung, esophagus, bladder); increases with number and severity of risk factors such as overweight, fat intake, hypertension, elevated cholesterol, smoking, inactivity, and stress Osteoporosis			
Dental Socioeconomic status Dietary 24-hour recall or food frequency	24-hour recall or food frequency form	Inadequate food intake due to poor dentures, low income, and deprived social environment			

NUTRITION PROGRAMS: MATERNAL AND INFANT CARE

The Maternity & Infant Care and Children & Youth Project brought to Boston a level of comprehensive health care for pregnant women and children heretofore unavailable to the poor. Among the innovative aspects of the program is the opportunity it has provided to develop a community nutrition program focused on health promotion and the prevention of disease. . . .

In this project, nutritionists work largely within one geographic area serving a population with a number of definable characteristics, needs, and goals. The nutritionist must know the community she serves in order to meet its needs and improve the life style of the residents to the fullest extent possible. . . .

The Nutrition Service has developed a good working relationship with the local welfare offices, with the result that allotments for pregnancy and other conditions requiring special diets are generally approved without difficulty. One can only speculate about the underutilization of this benefit in other parts of the state where the individual may have no advocate. Nutritionists have recently been invited by the Welfare Department to help in planning a revision of policy concerning special diet allotments. . . .

Working in the community, one becomes aware of clusters of need and of problems of special interest groups. One such need is for programs to control overweight and obesity. The group method of weight reduction and control has had wide appeal. Although the expressed purpose of one group, generally called a "Slim Club," is weight loss, meetings serve as a forum for the discussion of many matters related to food, consumer education, household management, and a variety of other topics. . . .

Largely in response to requests from the nursing service, materials are developed in English and Spanish for use with and by mothers. These materials have the acceptance of both pediatricians and nurses in the units where they are used. They are comprised of single sheets, each of which discusses pertinent facts about one food group or a common problem in pediatric nutrition. One or more of the small sheets, printed on one side, may be given to the mother at one visit for posting in her kitchen for easy referral. . . .

A final area which deserves comment is the role of auxiliary personnel in community nutrition programs. It has long been felt that nutrition aides could, under supervision, assume some of the tasks now performed by the nutritionist, as well as some of those left undone. These might include food demonstrations, work with small groups, and intensive work in the homes of selected families. . . .

Jeanne P. Goldberg: Some community services in a Boston Program, J. Am. Diet. Assoc. **62**:537, 1973. Reprinted by permission. Copyright The American Dietetic Association.

which leads to a high incidence of complications during pregnancy, high mortality, and premature delivery two or three times more frequently than that in women receiving good maternal care. The infants are subject to high risks for developing brain damage, neurologic disability, and mental retardation.

Maternity and Infant Care Project

The Maternity and Infant Care Project should include the following features of nutritional services:

1. The nutritionist participates as a member of the team to develop a program and procedures for maternity services such as clinic services, home visits, hospitalization, group classes, special school for pregnant teenagers, supplemental feeding and provision of nutrient supplements (iron and/or vitamins).

2. There is consultation with physicians to establish routine procedures for nutritional care for both normal and high-risk patients.

3. There is in-service education to health professionals and paraprofessionals and staff of cooperating agencies.

4. There is nutritional counseling for prenatal patients about therapeutic diet modifications, breast feeding, and infant feeding.

5. There is group education for expectant parents.

6. There is nutrition education as a part of a school health program for pregnant teenagers.

7. Evaluation and preparation of references, resources, and teaching aids to be used in the maternity service by both health workers and clients are available.

8. The coordination and direction of the Special Supplemental Food Program for Women, Infants, and Children is an integral part of the maternal and child health service.

9. An inventory or information and referral mechanism of related food, nutrition, and health services that may benefit health agency clients such as Food Stamp Program, Expanded Nutrition Education Program, and homemaker services should be readily available and employed.

10. Evaluative studies, surveys, and re-

search in areas of applied public health nutrition and dietetic practice related to maternity care are an essential part of the program.

Infant and Child Health Program

The importance of proper nutrition for growth in infants, young children, and adolescents is second only to prenatal needs. Whether infants are breast or bottle fed, mothers need to know when to add solid foods to the infant's diet, keeping in mind that too early introduction of solid foods is niether necessary nor advisable. Overfeeding infants and too rapid weight gain are now considered to be predisposing factors to lifelong obesity. Meeting basic nutritional needs, controlling weight gain, and developing sound eating practices are the primary elements of nutrition education for parents of infants and young children.

FAMILY INTERVIEWS

Family interviews are conducted with the mother or the family member responsible for the child's care. During this person-to-person communication, nutritionists learn about the family's food habits, particularly the diets administered to the child during the weaning period and after, as well as during illness. These interviews afford an excellent opportunity to obtain information about local availability of foods, popular ways of preparing them, and beliefs about which foods are best for children, both in health and disease. Such information is essential when attempting to improve the general diet of the family.

Susana J. Icaza: The nutritionist caring for malnourished children, J. Am. Diet Assoc. **63**:131, 1973. Reprinted by permission. Copyright The American Dietetic Association.

Crippled Children's Services Program

State crippled children's services locate children who have crippling conditions and provide them with medical, surgical, corrective, and other services, including inpatient services. Children with handicapping or crippling conditions need special nutritional care for their regular growth and development and also help in treatment and intervention procedures. If a child must undergo surgery,

THE NUTRITIONIST IN DAY CARE

You may ask, "How can I, a dietitian, effect a positive influence in day care by changing a feeding service to a nutrition education program?" The answer is not simple. First, we must know what is happening in our own communities. We must educate day care directors to the need for and benefits of nutrition education. Inviting them to joint meetings with regional dietetic associations and offering nutrition education workshops are two approaches.

Let's assume that you have already taken the introductory step. You are functioning at the policy-making level in a day care program, and your responsibilities include food service. Interpreting nutrition for a full-day program, especially for prekindergarten children, requires more than an extension of the regular school lunch. Foods suitable for older children are, more often than not, inappropriate for the very young.

Food must be of the best quality to be effective as an educational vehicle . . .

Food service and nutrition education cannot be administered separately if either program is to be effective. Their relationship is symbiotic. Food service, therefore, must be embraced by the educational arm of the day care organization. Too often, the philosophy of feeding is inappropriately delegated to the fiscal division, where the chief responsibility is to balance the books, not to educate children . . .

Young children learn through first-hand experiences—their world is a laboratory. The day care curriculum should be planned for active participation, and equipment should be especially chosen to meet this purpose. Food-oriented activities, other than at mealtime, can be used to supplement nutrition learning, as well as to involve many aspects of the curriculum.

Nutrition and nutrition education are factors of utmost significance in the child's total growth and development and in the provision of a totally adequate environment. Professionals in nutrition education and dietetics must find ways to expand their roles in well rounded day care programs which include these important factors. More and more, the interdisciplinary approach must be used if the total needs of the child are to be met.

Loretta Juhas: Nutrition education in day care programs, J. Am. Diet. Assoc. **63**:135, 1973. Reprinted by permission. Copyright The American Dietetic Association.

---

his nutritional status prior to surgery is of vital importance in enabling him to withstand the trauma of such treatment. In situations of orthopedic handicap, nutrition education is helpful in the ideal weight for best mobility. Even in cases of a speech defect, proper nutrition can aid the work of the speech therapist in improving his ability to communicate. Furthermore, often handicapped children have difficulty with the mechanics of eating, and guidance from the nutritionist and other team members will help to achieve independence in eating.

As a member of the health team serving the infant and child health program and all ill or handicapped children, the nutritionist's role includes the following:

1. Consultation with physicians, nurses, and other health professionals and paraprofessionals.
2. Counseling to mothers on infant or child feeding regarding both nutritional needs and emotional impacts of food.
3. Monitoring of nutrition and health data.
4. Provision of nutrition education classes, exhibits, and teaching aids.
5. Dissemination of information through articles for newspapers, programs for radio and television, and answering of inquiries.
6. Participation in planning, reviewing data and following up on referrals from the Early Periodic Screening, Diagnosis and Treatment Program for children eligible for Medicaid. Low-income children are a particularly high risk for malnutrition, and these screening procedures offer a built-in nutrition surveillance system.
7. Coordination of the Special Supplemental Food Program for Women, Infants and Children to be an integral part of the infant and preschool child health programs. This can provide foods most needed to correct nutritional health problems.
8. Consultation with professional staff and parents on the special needs of handicapped infants and children.

The increase in child day care facilities makes specific requirements and standards regarding nutritional needs, special diets, and food service management and sanitation essential in these facilities. Nutritionists should participate in writing standards, training and assisting personnel, and especially in planning and preparing the meals. Group programs are helpful in reaching staff from a large number of centers as well as providing for useful exchange of practical ideas. Day care programs concerned with child development such as Head Start programs frequently conduct ongoing education programs in which the nutritionist should participate and contribute educational articles as well as for newsletters and newspapers.

Intensive Infant Care Program

The objective of the Social Security Act of 1974 regarding infant care is to reduce infant mortality and morbidity by providing intensive care for one year to infants who have any health condition or are in circumstances that increase the hazards to their health. The use of high-quality medical services delivered by the intensive care centers has already reduced the mortality of high-risk infants, especially in cases of prematurity and conditions detrimental to normal growth and de

---

NEWBORN INTENSIVE CARE FOR STATE OF INDIANA

Management of the premature and critically ill newborn infant presents complicated problems requiring special expertise, frequently involving nutritional factors . . . Since most babies who die succumb in the first day of life, the need for rapid diagnosis and therapy is obvious. To speed this process, a hotline—24-hr. telephone consultation service—is available to any physician who has a problem involving the mother-to-be, her unborn, or newborn infant. This very successful aid has been instrumental in reducing perinatal mortality in our area. Frequently, as a result of these telephone conversations, a decision is made to transfer the child to the Riley perinatal unit. When the newborn is in extreme jeopardy, a specially trained medical team is dispatched from Riley Hospital by helicopter or by a mobile newborn intensive care ambulance. Approximately 350 babies a year are evacuated in this fashion from their place of birth; no deaths in transit have occurred since the program was begun over three years ago.

Karyl Rickard and *Edwin Gresham:* Nutritional considerations for the newborn requiring intensive care, J. Am. Diet. Assoc. **66**:592, 1975. Reprinted by permission. Copyright The American Dietetic Association.

---

velopment such as cardiopulmonary failure. The feeding of these small, often premature babies requires expert nutritional care both during the hospitalization and follow-up periods when the infant returns home. Many opportunities exist for the nutritionist to improve the care of these infants.

The role of the nutritionist within newborn intensive care is yet in the formative stages. As a member of the medical team, the nutritionist is able to determine nutrient needs of high-risk infants and recommend formulas and vitamin/mineral supplements as well as offer nutrition counseling that can be used by the parents when the baby returns home. Growth charts plotting both heights and weights, diet histories, and applicable laboratory tests are necessary assessment tools.

GUIDELINES FOR POPULATION GROUPS IN COMMUNITY NUTRITION: ADOLESCENTS (Table 5-3)
Health Services for Children and Youth

Similar to the infant and maternal health care programs, the primary objective of the children and youth program, as legislated by the Social Security Act of 1974, is to establish programs to provide comprehensive health services for children of low-income families by offering a full spectrum of care, including case finding, preventive health services, diagnosis, treatment, correction of defects, and

---

NUTRITION SERVICES—DEFINED

Before discussing some of the existing child health programs in greater detail, I would like to define nutrition services. As defined in the comprehensive health services projects for children and youth, nutrition services in comprehensive health care for children include:

(a) An assessment of the child's nutritional need and status.
(b) Initial and follow-up nutritional counseling in normal and/or modified diets.
(c) Assistance in obtaining foods, necessary dietary supplements, or equipment for self-help feeding when necessary to maintain or improve dietary intake.
(d) Nutrition education.
(e) Food service based on acceptable nutritional standards when health care is purchased in a hospital or other group care facility.
(f) Guidance in home management practices . . .

Child health programs and delivery of nutritional care

Using this definition of nutrition services, let us examine some of the existing child health programs and how they are being used to deliver nutritional care to children and their families . . . There are the fifty-five Maternity and Infant Care programs and the fifty-nine Comprehensive Health Services projects for children and youth designed primarily for low-income families and located in specific target areas with major health needs and problems and limited resources . . . The Maternity and Infant Care and Children and Youth programs are unique in that they focus on comprehensiveness and continuity of care, including screening, diagnosis and preventive services, treatment and correc-

tion of defects, as well as after-care services. In 1970, an estimated 128,000 mothers and over 400,000 infants and children were registered for care in these 114 comprehensive health programs.

Basic premises in these comprehensive health services projects for mothers and children include:

(a) Child health programs should start with the health of the mothers and be family-centered.
(b) Services should be comprehensive—focuses on health supervision and maintenance, as well as treatment and rehabilitative services, and provide for continuity of care.
(c) All relevant disciplines should be involved, as well as a variety of facilities and health care delivery systems.
(d) Services should be readily available and accessible to all families.
(e) Supervision from a qualified physician should be provided.

Health care is provided by a multidisciplinary team, including nutrition personnel with varying levels of training. In addition to nutritionists, dietitians, and home economists, projects use auxiliary level personnel, such as nutrition technicians, home management and community health aides, as well as volunteers. Positions for nearly four hundred nutrition personnel are budgeted in the Comprehensive Health Care projects for mothers and children . . . As you can see, nutrition personnel in these projects not only have considerable responsibility for initiating and developing all elements of the nutritional care plan, but actually carry out and provide the nutrition services needed.

CHILDREN AND YOUTH PROJECTS
A profile of C & Y

There are fifty-nine projects—actually sixty-seven separate reporting units located in central city areas (67 per cent), in peripheral urban or rural areas (23 per cent), and some in two locations (9 per cent).

Over three million children of eligible age live in the geographic areas served by the projects. An estimated half million of these will be served by projects. Features common to most of the projects include the following:

a. Use of a multidisciplinary team to deliver care, with each contributing as appropriate to the care process. Nutrition is considered a fundamental discipline on the core team. Auxiliary workers, such as community health aides and family health workers, are also involved in the team.

b. Participation of community and families in organizing the projects, developing needed resources, and marshaling approaches to specific community problems, e.g., a significant number of the projects have a board which formulates policy and involves community participation.

c. Concern with total environment of the child in the delivery of care, which means that the health team becomes involved in such problems as adequacy and safety of housing, provision of day-care services, availability of food assistance programs, and so forth.

d. Outreach efforts to enroll eligible families in the system and improve follow-up and continuity of care through use of mass media, community aides, satellite clinics, and various other means.

Linkage and cooperation with other existing community agencies insures a coordinated service system which can make the most effective use of existing resources.

Mary C. Egan and *Betty J. Hallstrom:* Building nutrition services in comprehensive health care, J. Am. Diet. Assoc. **61:** 491, 1972. Reprinted by permission. Copyright The American Dietetic Association.

NUTRITION AND LIFE-STYLE:
THE ADOLESCENT

The Door, A Center of Alternatives, is a multiservice youth center in New York City's Greenwich Village . . . to help young people constructively meet the challenges and difficulties of being young and of growing up in an urban environment. It is oriented in particular toward disadvantaged and troubled youth and those not easily reached by traditional institutions.

The Door combines the features of a free medical clinic, a community mental health center, a community youth center, a cultural center, and a therapeutic drug and delinquency rehabilitation center. It conducts ongoing psychiatric, drug, court diversion, and youth advocacy programs . . .

In addition to providing professional counseling and care to young people in immediate need, the programs, services, workshops and seminars of The Door are intended to help young people find real, positive alternatives to life styles presently characterized by aimlessness, apathy, alienation, destructiveness, drug abuse, and crime . . .

The Nutrition Counseling Service serves young people who, out of ignorance, apathy, youthful rebellion, or the deprivations inherent in a ghetto or street existence, have acquired unhealthy eating habits or developed nutrition-related medical problems. It also serves young people who are aware of the detrimental effects of many eating patterns in our society and who are attempting (often in a misguided way) to find a healthier, more natural diet . . .

The Nutrition Counseling Service has two main functions. First, it provides nutrition education aimed at increasing the awareness among young people of nutritional requirements and of the role of eating habits in promoting health. Second, as part of The Door's Medical Clinic, it provides therapeutic nutritional counseling, helping to deal with health problems related to nutrition and adding the dimension of nutrition to the health team approach . . .

Another function of the Nutrition Counseling Service is the presentation of Youth Awareness Seminars in Nutrition. These have dealt with a variety of topics of relevance to young people, including attitudes about food; interior ecology—what makes a balanced diet and the need for and function of macro- and micro-nutrients; issues surrounding chemical additives, environmental contaminants, and processed vs. "natural" foods; diets associated with a life philosophy—vegetarianism, yoga diet, and macrobiotics. Guest speakers are occasionally invited to present a seminar. The visit of Frances Lappe, author of "Diet for a Small Planet," drew a record attendance by the youth and staff.

"Rap groups" are conducted about the young peoples' nutrition-related interests. The nutritionist leading such a group must be knowledgeable about a variety of subjects, including herbalism, fasting, organic gardening, the Green Revolution, Bulgarian yoghurt cultures, food cooperatives, Choate's report, yin-yang, chemical preservatives, mega-vitamin therapy, Adelle Davis, Dr. Atkins' revolutionary diet, and, above all, the biochemistry of nutrition and the behavioral aspects of eating . . .

The nutritionists of the Nutrition Counseling Service and the entire staff of The Door feel that at least as important as the information transmitted is the warmth and concern expressed, for these give the young people a reason to listen.

Reva T. Frankle, Betsy McGregor, Judy Wylie, and *Mary B. McCann:* The door, a center of alternatives—The nutririonist in a free clinic for adolescents, J. Am. Diet Assoc. **63:**273, 1973. Reprinted by permission. Copyright The American Dietetic Association.

aftercare both medical and dental. Here the multidisciplinary approach involving preventive and medical care includes not only physical examination and medical and laboratory services but nursing, social work, nutrition, dental, and other health services as appropriate. Success of projects is measured in part by reduction of hospital admission as children receive regular health supervision. Average annual cost per child has been about $125, as of 1976. The projects are to maintain close working relationships with other health programs in their communities.

Dental Health Program for Children

Nutritionists working with dentists and dental hygienists should develop education programs around concepts of caries control and become proponents of water fluoridation as a public health measure to prevent caries in a community-wide approach.

The primary objective of the Dental Health Program for Children, as legislated by the Social Security Act of 1974, is to increase availability and to improve quality of services necessary to prevent dental disease and restore and maintain oral health in children from low-income families where dental care is often not within reach. Factors contributing to inadequate dental care are family income, educational level of parents, effectiveness of dental health education, and community organization of a dental program for children. Ninety to ninety-five percent of children entering school require dental attention. The average child has eleven teeth decayed, missing, or filled by the time he reaches 11 years of age.

NUTRITION EDUCATION IN DENTAL PROGRAMS

The dietary counseling program at the Public Health Service Hospital, San Francisco, was conceived out of a desperate need to affect change in the eating habits of the children who were brought here for dental care. The dental decay rate was very high in the children, and even more distressing was the fact that on subsequent recall visits the children were experiencing a large number of recurrent dental caries. There was no time to design a formal clinical study as the need was now . . .

Objectives. The nutrition counseling program developed is patterned after that described by Nizel.* The program objectives are: (1) to provide a personalized nutrition counseling program for children and their parents with emphasis on the influence of nutrition on dental health; (2) to instill positive attitudes in both parents and children toward good nutrition and dental health; (3) to emphasize the need for continuous evaluation of eating habits and the need for adjusting these habits as necessary; (4) to develop audiovisual aids to carry the important message of good nutrition and dental health to a large number of patients as a supplement to counseling.

The program consists of three or more visits to the Nutrition Clinic. Prior to the first visit, the pedodontist introduces the program to the parent and child, stressing the need for the program and encouraging them to accept it. These introductory remarks help to moti-

vate the parent and child to view the counseling as an integral part of the child's dental treatment. The pedodontist emphasizes the important relationship of the child's eating habits and food selections to dental health and the role good nutrition plays in the prevention of dental caries. The dental auxiliaries counsel the patients and their parents in oral hygiene at the time of the dental appointment. The parent and child are then given directions (a small printed map of the hospital) to the Nutrition Clinic for dietary counseling.

Evaluation. Although we have not yet collected sufficient data to document the effectivenss of the program, we feel that we have fulfilled our original objective. We have provided a personalized nutrition counseling program for parents and children to assist them in achieving an optimal state of good nutrition and dental health. Direct education through counseling and indirect education by means of audiovisual instruction reinforce each other.

Our final objective is to encourage others to develop similar programs in their health care facilities. A similar counseling program could be used in the private dental office, in school health classes (both elementary and secondary) and in health programs held by school and community groups. It might become an integral part of the education and total health care of any child admitted to a hospital pediatric department.

Lois G. Robinson, Audrey Paulbitski, Alice Jones, and *Michael Roberts:* Nutrition counseling and children's dental health, J. Nutr. Ed. **8:**33, 1976. Reprinted with permission from the Journal of Nutrition Education. © Society for Nutrition Education.

*Nizel, A. E.: The science of nutrition and its application in clinical dentistry, ed. 2, Philadelphia, 1968, W. B. Saunders Co.

Family Planning Services Program

The primary objective of the Family Planning Services Program as legislated by the Social Security Act of 1974, is to increase the accessibility of family planning services to areas with low-income families and high mortality for infants and mothers. The goal is to provide families the freedom of choice in the number and spacing of children so that the health status of the mothers and children improves and maternal and infant mortality decreases.

Nutrition services in family planning are directed toward improving the nutritional status of women at childbearing age, either preconceptionally or intraconceptionally. Emphasis should be on underweight or overweight, since these are risk factors in health for daily living as well as during pregnancy. However, special attention should be given to the increased chances of iron-deficiency anemia in cases where an intrauterine device is used. It is also believed that the use of oral contraceptives may alter metabolic needs for several nutrients, even though as yet there are no definitive recommendations for nutrition supplements.[6]

Nutritionists in family planning programs should participate in the following services:

1. Program planning for the family planning center to include nutrition education and diet counseling services
2. Consulting with physicians and the health team regarding nutritional needs of women using contraceptives and of young women in general
3. Education on food, nutrition, and diet to professional and paraprofessionals including community health workers working in family planning programs
4. Counseling in clinics, schools, and community groups
5. Dissemination of nutrition and weight control information through exhibits, posters, newspaper articles, and radio and television programs

School health: nutrition education

In addition to being the means by which various federal feeding programs operate, schools also can provide health screening, possible correction programs, and health education. (A discussion of federal food programs follows.) The nutritionist can plan with the school health coordinator, school physicians, teachers, nurses, and food service personnel about how and where to insert the nutrition component in children's education from preschool and kindergarten to Grade 1 through high school. The nutritionist as the

---

NUTRITION EDUCATION IN THE SCHOOLS

Tax dollars spent to give consumers a sensible, scientific guide as to how to spend their food dollars is an investment as well as an expenditure. It is an investment in our schools, our children, our system of health care, in ourselves, and in life itself . . .

Any national health insurance system should reimburse schools for nutrition services to children, including nutrition education. Nutrition must be conceptually integrated with health care, for neither can be as effective separately as both could be together . . .

We have the energy, the expertise, and the resources to start in the classroom. We can make the school lunchroom a laboratory for nutrition education. Nutrition education is among the most practical subjects the schools can teach. It is a skill that all Americans could apply every day . . .

Senator George McGovern: Child Nutrition Act of 1977, Congr. Record **123:**114, June 30, 1977.

---

technical consultant may act as the resource person and the coordinator of nutrition-oriented activities including teaching aids, curriculum plans, and field trips.

On Peck's[7] suggestion that the nutrition community come to an agreement on the functions and educational background needed for nutrition education specialists working in school districts, the Society of Nutrition Education surveyed administrators of state departments of education, of whom forty-two responded. Results showed that only a few of the respondents had a well-defined image of the person who should serve as coordinator of nutrition education programs in schools at the state or district levels.[8]

The key competencies necessary for the nutrition education specialist, as outlined by

Poolton,[9] indicate five essential categories: nutrition and food, education, communications, behavioral science, and government. An important first is for the well-qualified nutrition specialist to sell the education community on the importance of nutrition as a vital subject in the school curriculum. Once this becomes a reality, the recommendation of the White House Conference on Food, Nutrition and Health that a comprehensive and sequential program of nutrition education become available in the schools will have been met.

Other school-provided services are screening programs, consistent individual records of health and growth, and possibly laboratory

tests and treatment. Dietary intake records, too, are particularly helpful for individual follow-up and surveillance. The school nutritionist may be especially adept at noting and treating dietary-related problems, such as obesity, diabetes, hypertension, allergies, dental caries, and anemia.

Schools may also be able to offer information to parents individually or through parent-teacher groups. This kind of education

NUTRITION EDUCATION IN THE FIFTH GRADE CLASSROOM

At the present time, the basic premise is that by learning to choose foods from each of Four Food Groups, the public will be able to plan balanced meals and adequate intake will be assured. However, a nutrient, rather than food group, approach could well be a more effective means of teaching nutrition, given contemporary eating patterns and increased ability of students to cope with scientific knowledge. The new nutrition labeling regulations established by the Food and Drug Administration, represent an important resource for nutrition education programs, especially if a nutrient approach were employed . . . The purpose of this study was to develop and test a pilot nutrition education unit at the fifth grade level which utilized a nutrient approach and a nutrient abacus (nutri-planner) developed at Colorado State University as a basic teaching tool. In addition the unit was designed to:

- Capture the interest of students
- Relate nutrition to the science curriculum
- Utilize the School Lunch Program
- Be easily understood and used by teachers not necessarily trained in nutrition . . .

An abacus-centered nutrient approach . . . is colorful, unique, and allows for student initiative and decision-making. It can be integrated into biology, mathematics or other curricula. Perhaps the greatest strength of the nutrient abacus approach for nutrition education lies in the fact that it allows students to understand why certain food choices or combinations of foods are better than others . . .

Linda Dee Meyers and *G. Richard Jansen:* A nutrient approach in the fifth grade, J. Nutr. Ed. **9:**127, 1977. Reprinted with permission from the Journal of Nutrition Education. © Society for Nutrition Education.

NUTRITION EDUCATION IN THE GRADES 5, 7, AND 10

When the Department of Food Science at North Carolina University received a grant in 1970 to carry out a comprehensive survey of the school lunch program in the state, interest had already been aroused in nutrition. Earlier that year from state funds the Board of Health had undertaken a survey to document the nutritional status of North Carolinians . . .

The major objective of this program was to determine whether nutrition education for elementary, junior, and/or senior high school students would contribute to any changes in food habits or acceptability of the foods served in the school lunch room . . .

Nutrition education was introduced in two elementary, two junior high, and one senior high school. Five matched schools in the same geographical area were used for obtaining control data . . .

Before introduction of nutrition education in the classroom, preliminary data obtained from all control and experimental students included: results on a nutrition test; acceptability ratings of school-served food for 10 days; and plate waste measurement for five days. Dietary recall records were obtained from experimental and within-school control students . . .

Elementary and secondary students were involved in a study which included determining the influence of nutrition education on acceptability and consumption of school-served food, dietary habits, and knowledge of nutrition . . .

Three-day dietary recall data showed that diets of seventh grade improved significantly after nutrition education . . . Plate waste from school lunch from fifth graders decreased significantly after the nutrition education program. Acceptability ratings of school-served food increased among fifth grade experimental groups more than among other groups.

The amount of change decreased progressively at higher grade levels . . .

Mary K. Head: A nutrition education program at three grade levels, J. Nutr. Ed. **6:**56, 1974. Reprinted with permission from the Journal of Nutrition Education. © Society for Nutrition Education.

ought to include information about special programs, as well as dietary facts. The Child Nutrition Act of 1977 (S. 1420) authorizes the Secretary of Agriculture to carry out a program of nutrition education as part of the food programs operating under the National School Lunch Act and the Child Nutrition Act.

Pregnant adolescents

During the 1960s and early 1970s, the number of infants born to adolescent girls (17 years of age or under) steadily increased from 189,188 in 1960 to over 200,000 reported births in 1973.[10] During adolescence a girl's nutrition requirements are at their highest, and pregnancy increases them further. Indeed, girls are at biologic risk if they become pregnant before they have reached full growth. In addition, surveys such as the Ten State Nutrition Survey, have shown that this age group had the least satisfactory nutrition status.

In response to the needs of this group, a shift in state and federal policy has permitted pregnant adolescents to continue to attend school, and a number of multidisciplinary programs have been established. A 1971 editorial in the *Journal of School Health* emphasized the need for such programs.[11] These generally include prenatal and infant care, psychological counseling, possibly home economics education, academic education, and nutrition information. Such programs are in effect in large cities such as San Francisco[12] and New York City[13] and also in areas such as rural Louisiana (the Cooperative Extension Service),[14] Minnesota (The Moorhead Area Learning Center),[15] Syracuse (The Young Mothers' Educational Development Program),[16] New Brunswick (Family Learning

---

NUTRITION AND THE PREGNANT ADOLESCENT

The subjects were twenty-nine pregnant girls, ages fifteen to nineteen years, who attended the Family Learning Center, a special school operated by the New Brunswick Board of Education for girls who become pregnant while attending regular school. Twenty-seven were black; two were white. In addition to course work, they received instruction in health (including pregnancy and events attending delivery), nutrition and child care. Antenatal care was given primarily at the clinics of the two local hospitals; in a few cases, girls were under the care of private physicians. Lunches were prepared at the school by the girls, and milk and fruit were available for snacks throughout the day. The atmosphere at the school is informal, pleasant, and accepting . . . This study indicates a benefit to both the students and their infants . . .

Christian M. Hansen, Myrtle L. Brown, and *Marie Trontell:* Effects on pregnant adolescents of attending a special school, J. Am. Diet. Assoc. **65:**538, 1976. Reprinted by permission. Copyright The American Dietetic Association.

NUTRITION AND THE PREGNANT ADOLESCENT

It is sometimes necessary to establish priorities for nutritional services in busy prenatal clinics with limited staff. When such priorities are set, teen-agers—particularly those under sixteen years of age—should always be included. A structured interview with the stated objective of completing a nutritional history and assessment is routine nutritional service for each teen-ager . . .

Many of the younger girls live with mothers who usually help provide food at this time. Older girls who may be living on their own often lack cooking skills and rely on the snacks which are available. These girls are interested in simple meal plans and snacks. We may suggest such foods as sandwiches made with cold cuts, peanut butter on crackers, juices instead of carbonated beverages, hard-cooked eggs, and other snack foods, such as raw fruit and vegetables with cheese dips. Suggestions for more elaborate meals with the use of simple recipes, such as baking one or two pieces of chicken, are well received. Foods which store well and are easy to prepare, i.e., instant mashed potatoes, fast-cooking rice, ready-to-eat breakfasts for evening snacks, macaroni and cheese, and other box dinners, have usually not been explored by these girls . . .

All of the Hartford clinical nutritionists believe the interview should be with the patient alone. Often when the mother accompanies the girl and is a part of the nutritional interview, the girl is quiet, distant, and difficult to reach . . .

The nutritional care plan is the core of the matter . . .

The development of a nutritional care plan should include opportunities for the patient to make choices, to have alternatives, and to be provided with a measure of self-determination . . .

Norma I. Huyck: Nutrition services for pregnant teen-agers, J. Am. Diet. Assoc. **69:**60, 1976. Reprinted by permission. Copyright The American Dietetic Association.

Center),[17] and Hartford (The Maternity and Infant Care Project),[18] among many others. All these programs stress the importance of proper nutrition to achieve optimal growth, development, and health maintenance.

NUTRITION (FOOD ASSISTANCE) PROGRAMS SUPPORTED BY THE U.S. DEPARTMENT OF AGRICULTURE

The National Nutrition Policy Study undertaken by the U.S. Senate Select Committee on Nutrition and Human Needs indicated that publicly supported food assistance was necessary either to maintain nutritional adequacy or to achieve socially desirable goals. This is especially true for the poor—people for whom the federal food programs are a matter of daily survival—or for those whose nutritional status is vulnerable in a rapidly changing and highly complex society, that is, schoolchildren and the isolated elderly.[19]

WIC: Supplemental Food Program for Women, Infants and Children (U.S. Department of Agriculture)

WIC is a special food program for pregnant and lactating women and for infants and children up to the age of 5 years who are at a high nutritional risk and are eligible for free or reduced price medical care because of low income. For nearly 8 years the U.S. Department of Agriculture has operated a Supplemental Food Program aimed at providing special supplemental foods for this group of people to obtain or maintain optimum health. In 1972 a $40 million pilot program was authorized, which was designed to determine if there was a better way of assisting this special group. This program has evolved into the WIC Program. The pilot program aimed (1) to determine the nutritional impact of supplemental food intervention and (2) to test the means of delivery using direct food assistance of vouchers redeemable for specific supplemental foods at retail markets.

The WIC Program was extended in 1973 with an appropriation of $100 million, and in October, 1975, the "pilot" preface was dropped and the program became the nation's primary supplemental food assistance program with a funding level of $250 million a year. It costs the federal government about $20 a month per recipient (in 1976) to provide iron-fortified infant formula, iron-fortified cereal, fruit or vegetable juices high in vitamin C, fortified milk, cheese, and eggs. As of April, 1976, there were about 600,000 recipients in the WIC Program.[20] Unlike the original Supplemental Food Program, since October, 1975, the WIC Program has become more than a food delivery program and has nutrition education as a major feature (Public Law 94-105).

Regulations that appeared in the August 26, 1977, *Federal Register* and took effect September 26, 1977 contain some notable changes from earlier regulations. These revised regulations establish a system of five priorities to determine which persons should be enrolled when a WIC sponsor reaches its

---

A WIC PROGRAM: NUTRITION EDUCATION

The first two-month educational program was devoted to an explanation of the program and the vouchers, on a one-to-one basis for the first month and to single clients or groups of two or three for the second month . . . During the next four months programs focused on a specific WIC food each month and included: a topic that was relevant to infant and child care; a quiz or handout that further emphasized the monthly topic; and recipes . . .

At the end of six months it was possible to make the following comments on the potential of the program at a local level:

Distribution of printed material was largely valueless unless the material was partially read and discussed with clients. Those distributed without comment were often discarded before the client had left the facility . . .

It was essential to have samples of the dishes recommended, utilizing WIC foods, for clients to taste, otherwise they were unwilling to spend money on unfamiliar foods . . .

An unexpected positive result of the WIC Program was the introduction to participants and their families into a health care delivery system . . .

Elizabeth Gaman: A WIC pilot program with nutrition education, J. Nutr. Ed. **8**:157, 1976. Reprinted with permission from the Journal of Nutrition Education. © Society for Nutrition Education.

"maximum participation level." Pregnant and breast-feeding women and infants with medically documented needs receive first priority; infants (up to 6 months of age) of WIC recipients receive second priority. Third in line are children with medically documented nutritional needs. Fourth priority is given to other pregnant and nursing women and infants in nutritional need "because of an inadequate dietary pattern, as documented by a person qualified in such assessments." A fifth priority is for children in nutritional need because of an inadequate dietary pattern; postpartum women in nutritional need have lowest priority. The regulations also allow infants born to WIC recipients to qualify automatically for benefits but do not place them in any priority category.

The need for a national priority system has grown as increasing numbers of WIC sponsors hit their budget ceilings. In the interim many states have implemented their own priorities. Such a system would be unnecessary if Congress provided the WIC Program with "performance funding," as in school feeding programs, making enough funds available for all eligible participants.

The final rules eliminate the term "recertification" and state that participants must be certified every 6 months. However, they allow recipients to remain in the program as long as there is a possibility of "regression in nutritional status" without the supplemental foods.

The regulations require local agencies to assure that participants are enrolled in a health care system. The Department of Agriculture relaxed that proposal, stipulating that recipients only be encouraged to participate. Changes occur often in the WIC Program, and therefore it is important to know current legislation.

Under a contract with the School of Public Health at the University of North Carolina, the Department of Agriculture has a detailed medical evaluation of nineteen projects.[21] Whereas the overall goals of the WIC program's nutrition education efforts are set at the national and state level, actual implementation and practice is carried out by the local agency delivering the program. It is the state agency, however, that is required to develop a plan for providing nutrition education to participants in accord with the following national guidelines.

- Proper nutrition is essential to the total concept of good health, with special emphasis on the nutritional needs of the WIC target audience.
- Assist the individual at nutritional risk to obtain positive changes in dietary habits.
- Maximize the effective use of the WIC food package considering ethnic, cultural, and geographic preferences.

Measuring the effectiveness of nutrition education is difficult but essential for future program planning and accountability. State agencies have been asked to monitor and evaluate their nutrition education efforts. Primarily the success of the WIC education program will depend on the ability of the nutrition educators to bring about voluntary changes in behavioral patterns of the target population.

According to a recent study, there are certain principles that can serve as supplementary guidelines for program development, implementation, and evaluation. Namely, they are the integration of nutrition education into the overall WIC Program; understanding of the recipient's household lifestyle; introduction of changes that are marginal, not radical; and lessons that are simple, concrete, and applicable to the clients' situations.[22]

Child nutrition programs (U.S. Department of Agriculture)

Among the public programs funded by the government at the local, state, and federal level are school feeding programs, including (1) school lunches, (2) school breakfasts, (3) their summer counterparts, (4) the nonfood assistance program, and (5) the special milk program, which are all child nutrition programs funded by the Department of Agriculture. The federal cost of these programs from 1970 to 1976 is summarized in Table 5-6.

A WIC PROGRAM: THE NUTRITION AIDE

As part of her orientation to the WIC system, the WIC *nutrition aide* is learning to distribute vouchers, screen and register clients, and make referrals. She is visiting other WIC sites to observe their methods. A night course in basic nutrition provides formal background to the informal, on-the-job discussions that occur during clinic hours. During distribution hours she is now conducting short, frequent talks on various topics such as WIC cereals and "stretching" WIC juices and is making herself available to interact with clients.

Lynn Ann Classen: An ongoing WIC Program, Feb. 1975–Aug. 1976, J. Nutr. Ed. **8**:159, 1976. Reprinted with permission from the Journal of Nutrition Education. © Society for Nutrition Education.

A WIC PROGRAM: DENTAL NUTRITION EDUCATION

How heartening it is to see nutrition education integrated into dental health services! . . . One goal of our Department's WIC Supplemental Food Program is to link up participants with as many other health services as possible and appropriate. One of the more successful of these efforts has been to provide fluoride supplements or prescriptions for fluoride to participants who live in unfluoridated water districts and are interested in obtaining fluoride . . .

Now that this part of the dental health program for WIC families has been implemented, we plan to go on to integrate dental health education (including nutrition!) more fully into the WIC program. The dental education component will include information on the importance of fluoride, effective oral hygiene technique for the removal of plaque, and dietary practices leading to good dental health.

Anne Hanford: Dental nutrition Education in WIC Program, J. Nutr. Ed. **8**:159, 1976. Reprinted with permission from the Journal of Nutrition Education. © Society for Nutrition Education.

POSITION PAPER ON CHILD NUTRITION PROGRAMS*

An adequately nourished body is essential to physical and emotional health and contributes to readiness for learning. All children need adequate food and educational opportunities to learn good food habits.

Model for child nutrition program

Any child nutrition program should consist of the following interrelated components:

(a) Assessing the nutritional needs of the child.

(b) Meeting the needs of the child through foods served and the environment in which it is served.

(c) Providing educational opportunities for the child to learn about food and its relationship to life, both physically and socially.

(d) Planning educational activities about food and nutrition for parents of the children.

Assessment of the nutritional needs of the child

The food needs of a child in a child nutrition program will depend on:

(a) His nutritional needs considering his age, stage of physical development, physical activity, and specific problems related to diet, e.g., overweight, underweight, diabetes.

(b) Amount and kind of food eaten away from the setting of the child nutrition program.

(c) The time he spends in the setting in which the child nutrition program operates.

(d) Cultural, ethnic, and environmental influences on his eating behavior.

Food services

The nutrition program should be planned to meet the child's nutritional needs and should be executed in such a way that positive contributions are made to the emotional and social development of the child.

(a) The foods served and times of service should be based on the needs of the child.

(b) At least one nutritionally adequate meal per day should be available to each child. This meal should provide a laboratory for the practice of learning about food and nutrition acquired by formal or informal instruction in the child care program.

(c) The environment in which food is served to the children should be conducive to optimal consumption of the food and to the formation of healthy attitudes toward food and eating, including the importance of food as a focal point for social and emotional interaction.

(d) The quality of the food served to the child should be of the highest order.

(e) Only those foods which make a significant nutritive contribution to the diet should have a place in the child nutrition program.

(f) All foods provided in child nutrition programs should be approved by a person or persons qualified by formal training and experience to judge the nutritional merits of the food.

Nutrition education

An understanding of the role of nutrition and its application in daily living can be regarded as preventive medicine and is in the interest of the child's future health.

A nutrition education program should be sequential from the preschool years and integrated into appropriate school courses, such as family living, sociology, health, and science, or provided informally as the setting dictates.

As a consequence of nutrition education, a child should:

(a) Increase his ability to make wise food choices throughout life.

(b) Understand the relationship between food and health.

(c) Gain knowledge of nutrients and their roles in the body.

(d) Develop the ability to evaluate advertising and other claims made about food and nutrition.

(e) Understand the influence of emotional and cultural factors on food choices.

(f) Become aware of the role food can play in aiding him to reach goals he sets for himself.

(g) Gain knowledge of career opportunities in the field of food and nutrition. Children, parents, and staff should all be involved in nutrition education programs.

Administration

Child nutrition programs should be coordinated at all levels by qualified staff with training in food, nutrition, and institutional food service management. Each agency charged with responsibility for child nutrition programs should adopt and promote standards for employment of state, district, and local food service personnel to develop and coordinate child nutrition programs.

The mandated curriculum for elementary and health teachers, directors of day care programs, specialists in special education, and other child centered institutional personnel should include courses incorporating basic nutrition concepts and their application to child nutrition.

Undergraduate and graduate training in food service management and nutrition education for dietitians and institution management majors should be made relevant to the needs of child nutrition programs.

Specific plans are needed at state, district, and local levels to provide for continuing renewal of the nutrition education curriculum and the child nutrition program. To assure continuance, it is essential that professional assistance on a regular basis be available to the district and the state.

Coordination with home and community

Effective child nutrition programs require a cooperative effort of the home, the institution, and the community. Specific plans should be developed by the institution (school, child care center) for involving parents in decisions regarding both delivery of food to the child and nutrition education activities. It is necessary to interpret child nutrition programs and needs to the community to obtain understanding, support, and improved child nutrition programs.

Coordination of all involved groups

The efforts of all groups involved in child nutrition programs, including nutrition education, should be coordinated at the federal, state, and local levels to achieve maximum effectiveness and avoid duplication. Such groups include, but are not limited to, child nutrition program directors, home economics educators, health educators, health department nutritionists, community nutritionists with other agencies, health education administrators, Extension Service nutritionists, and industry service organizations.

Coordination with industry

Government, the profession, higher education, and industry need to work together to provide nutritious foods that are accepted by children, efficiently served, and contribute to the nutrition education of the child.

Implementation

Legislation to establish an operating framework, program standards, and authorization for appropriations needs to be continually updated to implement comprehensive child nutrition programs.

Legislation is needed at the national, state, and local levels to promote implementation of nutrition education programs in child care centers, schools, and other child serving institutions, as well as to set standards for foods to be served. In all child nutrition programs, legislation is needed to provide funding authorization for research and development, teacher training, resource materials, and personnel to develop and coordinate child nutrition programs.

Summary

Achievement of comprehensive child nutrition programs will require reordering of certain priorities. The child nutrition program must focus on meeting the child's nutritional, physical, psychologic, and social needs through food, while serving as a vehicle for the child's learning about such interrelationships. Emphasis should be placed on the preventive aspects of nutrition and on active involvement of the child in his education about food and nutrition.

Position paper on child nutrition programs, J. Am. Diet. Assoc. **63**:520, 1973.

Table 5-6. U.S. Department of Agriculture food programs, family feeding, and child nutrition programs, federal cost (50 states and District of Columbia only), 1970-1976*

								1977	
Item	1970	1971	1972	1973	1974	1975	1976	I	II[1]
					Million dollars				
Food stamps									
Total issued	1,925	3,103	3,615	4,049	5,868	7,680	7,825	1,951	1,851
Bonus stamps[2]	1,104	1,699	1,980	2,209	3,498	4,602	4,658	1,168	1,086
Food distribution[3]									
Needy families	275	261	225	152	87	11	8	3	3
Schools[4]	234	311	275	253	355	364	444	201	97
Other[5]	34	37	39	48	36	33	32	14	12
Child nutrition[6]									
School lunch	337	628	785	939	1,137	1,340	1,503	526	392
School breakfast	14	22	28	43	67	94	119	44	36
Special food[7]	15	34	43	52	87	116	240	29	41
Special milk	96	92	91	63	90	134	150	46	38
WIC[8]	—	—	—	—	33	106	181	57	55
Total[9]	2,109	3,084	3,466	3,784	5,390	6,800	7,335	2,046	1,719

*Modified from U.S. Department of Agriculture: National food situation, Washington, D.C., Sept., 1977, Government Printing Office. [1]Preliminary. [2]Includes Food Certificate Program. [3]Cost of food delivered to state distribution centers. [4]Includes Special Food Services. [5]Includes supplemental food, institutions, elderly persons. [6]Money donated for local purchase of food. Excludes nonfood assistance. [7]Includes child care and summer food programs. [8]Special Supplemental Food Program for Women, Infants and Children begun January, 1974. [9]Excludes those food stamps paid for by the recipient. Do not add due to rounding.

Costs of these two programs increased in the fall of 1977 because of increases in the reimbursement rates for meals served and more meals served at the reduced price. The national average payment per lunch will be increased from 13.25 to 14 cents for a free meal. Reimbursement rates for breakfasts will increase from 10.75 to 11.25 cents with a 21-cent reimbursement for reduced price meals and 28 cents for each free meal. Part of these increases may be offset with the initiation of the new choice system. If a participant does not like all of the items offered with the meal, he need not be served them. The price of the lunch will remain the same while hopefully waste will be reduced.

National School Lunch Program

The largest of the child nutrition programs, the National School Lunch Program, begun under the administration of the Department of Agriculture in 1946, enables public and nonprofit private grade and high schools to provide nutritious lunches at a reasonable cost to children, or at reduced or no cost for the neediest. Every school lunch is a form of subsidized lunch, since the federal government pays 12.25 cents in cash plus an average of 11 cents in donated commodities for every school lunch served regardless of a student's ability to pay. States receive 54.5 cents more for each free lunch and 44.5 cents for each reduced price lunch, as of January, 1976.

All schools serving lunch are bound by law to offer a balanced, nutritious "Type A" lunch, which must contain a specified amount of milk, protein foods, vegetables, and/or fruits, bread, and butter or margarine. In 1977 specific guidelines were established to outline the amounts of foods to serve children of various ages (Table 5-7).

In the mid-1960s a study was initiated to determine the quality of the National School Lunch Program. It was conducted in forty-five communities across the nation under the sponsorship of the National Board of the Young Women's Christian Association, the National Council of Catholic Women, National Council of Jewish Women, National Council of Negro Women, and the interdenominational Protestant Church Women United. However, instead of focusing on the food provided, the study noted how poor children watched rich children eat and the numbers of slum schools without kitchens. The Committee on School Lunch Participation charged the Department of Agriculture with the major responsibility for the failure of the program and Congress for the insufficient appropriation of funds.[23]

In fiscal year 1975, nearly 80% of the nation's schools (88,500) took part in the pro-

Table 5-7. School lunch pattern requirements as of September, 1977—amounts of foods listed by food components to serve children of various ages*

Food components	Preschool children		Elementary school children		Secondary school boys and girls Group V (12 years and over)
	Group I (1 and 2 years)	Group II (3, 4, and 5 years)	Group III (6, 7, and 8 years)	Group IV (9, 10, and 11 years)	
Meat and meat alternates					
Meat—a serving (edible portion as served) of cooked lean meat, poultry, or fish, or meat alternates:	1 ounce equivalent	1½ ounces equivalent	1½ ounces equivalent	2 ounces equivalent	3 ounces equivalent
Cheese	1 ounce equivalent	1½ ounces equivalent	1½ ounces equivalent	2 ounces equivalent	3 ounces equivalent
The following meat alternates may be used to meet only ½ of the meat/meat alternate requirement:					
Eggs (1 large egg may replace 1 ounce cooked lean meat)	1 egg	¾ egg	¾ egg	1 egg	1½ eggs
Cooked dry beans or peas (½ cup may replace 1 ounce cooked lean meat)	¼ cup	⅜ cup	⅜ cup	½ cup	¾ cup
Peanut butter (2 tablespoons may replace 1 ounce cooked lean meat)	1 tablespoon	1½ tablespoons	1½ tablespoons	2 tablespoons	3 tablespoons
Vegetables and fruits					
Two or more servings consisting of vegetables or fruits or both; a serving of full strength vegetable or fruit juice can be counted to meet not more than ½ of the total requirement	½ cup	½ cup	½ cup	¾ cup	¾ cup
Bread and bread alternates					
A serving (1 slice) of enriched or whole-grain bread; or a serving of biscuits, rolls, muffins, etc., made with whole-grain or enriched meal or flour; or a serving (½ cup) of cooked enriched or whole-grain rice, macaroni, or noodle products	5 slices or alternates/week	8 slices or alternates/week	8 slices or alternates/week	8 slices or alternates/week	10 slices or alternates/week
Milk, fluid					
An option to fluid whole milk or flavored milk must be offered	½ cup	¾ cup	¾ cup	½ pint	½ pint

*From School lunch requirements, Federal Register, vol. 42, no. 175, Sept. 9, 1977.

gram, which was available to nearly 88% of the children enrolled in the nation's schools. About 25 million children (nearly 57% of the enrollment) participated. The program has been continually updated and improved.[24]

In late 1977 the House and Senate passed bills (H.R. 1139, S. 1420) further amending and improving the quality of the School Lunch and Child Nutrition Acts.

School Breakfast Program

The Child Nutrition Act of 1966 created the National School Breakfast Program. A pilot program was launched in poor areas and in areas where children travel long distances. Later the program was expanded and made available to all schools with free and reduced price breakfasts to children from families with low income as well as standard price breakfasts. No reduced price breakfast may cost more than 10 cents.

Like the school lunch program the breakfast program must conform to nutritional standards set by law. The guidelines intend that children who participate in both programs will receive two thirds of their daily nutritional needs. Unlike the lunch program, which must be operated by educational institutions, the breakfast program may be run by a church or some community action agency, for example, orphanages, homes for the mentally and physically handicapped, temporary shelters for abused children, hospitals for children who are chronically ill, and other places where special groups of children are offered shelter and treatment. The Department of Agriculture's Food and Nutrition Service (FNS) is seeking to do a 2-year nutritional evaluation of the school breakfast program and has $1 million for pilot nutrition education programs. The breakfast study undertaken in 1978 will examine the factors affecting student participation, nutritional content, and the effects of breakfasts on school lunches.

The school breakfast program has been

SCHOOL LUNCH

The project involved sampling of school lunches and laboratory analyses of nutrients in lunches as served and as eaten . . .

Meals were immediately transported by car from the schools to the laboratory. The temperature during the brief transit time, less than 30 minutes, was below freezing. These procedures were utilized to minimize nutrient losses during the transfer. Laboratory analyses conducted by a reputable Chicago firm Rosner-Hixon Laboratories, included determination of proximate composition and content of the specific vitamins and minerals required on nutrition labels—vitamins A and C, thiamin, riboflavin, niacin, calcium and iron. In six of the seven schools, representative samples of the children's leftovers were taken, so that average plate waste was calculated and subtracted from the meal as served. In this way, an average intake could be calculated . . .

The range of lunch acceptance as measured by percent waste (kcal served—kcal consumed/kcal served) varied fivefold in the six schools studied. A school which provided a monotonous cold sandwich menu had 50% of the calories left on the plate. A parochial school serving a hot lunch in a setting where teachers ate with the children, and in which some nutrition education had been conducted, showed only 10% calories on the trays. Waste was also relatively low (20%) in the only school which used on-site preparation . . .

I assisted the reporters in interpreting the results of the school lunch investigation. The results—together with data obtained from interviews with school personnel and from the literature were reported in a four-day series of articles in the *Chicago Tribune* . . . The articles received prominent front-page space for three out of the four days, and the series attracted considerable attention . . .

Information from the series has received more than statewide attention. Staff members from the Senate Select Committee on Nutrition and Human Needs and persons from the Food Research and Action Center (FRAC) have included these findings in their analyses. Representatives from agencies in other states have contacted me for additional information regarding the study. Concurrent investigation and press coverage of school lunch quality in other areas of the country was fortuitous, adding to the national interest. *Newsweek* included information about the project in a short article about school lunches.

Jane Voichick: School lunch in Chicago, J. Nutr. Ed. **9:**102, 1977. Reprinted with permission from the Journal of Nutrition Education. © Society for Nutrition Education.

criticized for its slow growth over the past ten years and its inadequate nutrition. Currently, the Department of Agriculture requires only ½ cup of juice, ½ pint of milk, and 1 slice of whole grain or enriched bread or ¾ cup of whole grain cereal. Some nutritionists believe that this breakfast needs additional protein, such as an egg or peanut butter.[25]

As in the lunch program, the federal government reimburses schools for each meal served according to whether the student receives a free, reduced price, or full price meal. In fiscal year 1975 about 2 million children in 14,000 participating schools were served breakfasts, of which nearly 80% of them (1.6 million) were free or reduced price meals.

Summer Food Program

In 1968 the National School Lunch Act was expanded to include a Summer Food Program that would provide a full, balanced diet especially for those children from low-income families. Any nonprofit tax-exempt institution or recreational program was made eligible to be a sponsor of this program if it served an area or group in which at least one third of the children were eligible for free or reduced price school meals.

In fiscal year 1975 the summer program served 1.8 million children, and total federal expenditure was over $105 million. In October, 1975, the National School Lunch Act and Child Nutrition Act (1966) was separated into the Summer Food Service Program and the Child Care Food Program. The first provided free meals as just described, whereas the Child Care Food Program extended services to include day care centers, Head Start centers, and generally all family and group day care centers rather than merely camps and recreational organizations.

Special Milk Program

Under the provision of the Special Milk Program, organizations are reimbursed at

---

NUTRITION: FAMILY ORIENTED

Current interest in comprehensive child care should alert nutrition educators to the importance of well-integrated nutrition components in child care programs. Syracuse University's Family Development Research Program has demonstrated a multifaceted approach to child development by offering a wide variety of services and activities to its families in a family-oriented comprehensive child care program. The major goal of this program is "to provide experiences for young children and their families which will foster in the child maximal cognitive and psychosocial functioning during the time he is associated with the program and throughout late life." Nutrition education and service are included in all phases of this preschool educational demonstration.

The Family Development Research Program includes approximately 100 families with first- or second-born children and mothers expecting their first or second child. It was assumed that these families would be more receptive to parent education than those where childrearing practices had been more firmly established . . .

Female Child Development Trainers (CDT's) recruited from the same neighborhoods as the families they serve were trained to provide information regarding cognitive development, health, and nutrition to expectant mothers and to mothers of young children.

From the sixth month of pregnancy, the CDT's make regular weekly visits to each family assigned to them and continue their visits as long as the child is in the program . . .

When the infant is six months old, the home visiting program is supplemented by a half-day program at the Children's Center . . . The program reinforces the trainer's teaching by providing emotional relationships between caregivers and infants through the use of tactile stimulation and food, which help establish basic trust in the infant. Periods of structured play and nutritionally adequate lunches and snacks are provided as well as an opportunity for the child to see and have contact with and eat with other young children close in age and ability . . .

We have indicated some of the ways that nutrition education can be integrated into a comprehensive child development program. It is important that the nutritionist be responsible for both direct service as well as consultive-type service. The center's meals must reflect good nutrition practices, while the home visit program emphasizes the importance of effecting change in the home when change is necessary.

Marjorie V. Dibble and *J. Ronald Lally:* Nutrition in a family-oriented child development program, J. Nutr. Ed. **5**:200, 1973. Reprinted with permission from the Journal of Nutrition Education. © Society for Nutrition Education.

least 5 cents for every ½ pint of milk served free to children in schools, child care centers, summer camps, or settlement houses. In 1975 nearly $123 million was spent for 2.1 billion ½ pints of milk.

In fiscal year 1975 federal expenditure for all the child nutrition programs totaled $2 billion.

Family Food Assistance Programs

The Department of Agriculture Family Food Assistance Programs, including the Food Stamp Program and the Food Distribution Program, differ from the child nutrition programs in that they are family oriented and include all age groups. These programs, too, emphasize participation rather than the availability or quality of food products themselves.

Food Stamp Program

The Food Stamp Program is under the auspices of the Food and Nutrition Service (FNS) of the Department of Agriculture and has regional offices throughout the United States. It is an outgrowth of a "food coupon program" begun in 1939 as an agricultural subsidy program that lapsed in the 1950s. In 1961 President Kennedy initiated a pilot program, which resulted in the Food Stamp Act of 1964. The goal was to guard and raise health standards in the nation through nutrition, and by 1971 the need to alleviate hunger and malnutrition in low-income households was recognized.

The procedure for the sale of food stamps varies among states and even among counties; however, all are subject to Department of Agriculture regulations. Each state submits a plan that must meet federal requirements, which is then administered locally. One requirement that must be upheld is allowing for the purchase of food stamps at least twice a month to provide for households without a great deal of ready cash at any one time. In all areas the purchaser pays a certain amount of money for food stamps, which have a higher value than the amount paid. These ratios, as well as other aspects of the program, such as eligibility abuse control and nutrition education, are reviewed and revised periodically.

Between 1972 and 1975 the program served over 15 million people annually. In 1975 it served over 20 million people, with federal funding at $4.4 billion.

Food Distribution Program

By 1977 the direct distribution of food to needy families had been phased out entirely, with Indian reservations being the last groups to receive such assistance. The packages of food staples have given way to the nationwide Food Stamp Program.

Expanded Food and Nutrition Education Program (EFNEP)

The Department of Agriculture since 1968 has also been funding the EFNEP, which was specifically designed to hire and train "nutrition aides" who live in low-income areas. Such paraprofessionals have been found to be most effective for disseminating nutrition information because they actually practice what they have learned amid the society that is in need of such dietary information. Being of the same ethnic background and neighborhood, the aide understands local eating patterns and can help to determine the best ways of introducing new patterns and effecting behavioral changes—including the purchase, preparation, and storing of specific foods.

OFFICE OF CHILD DEVELOPMENT

Through the Office of Child Development or other means, such as the Department of Agriculture, states may initiate or expand nonprofit food services for children in day care or other programs. Under the Office of Child Development the following programs have been initiated.

Head Start

The Head Start project offers basic education for disadvantaged children to prepare them for school. One third of Head Start children suffer from illness or physical handicaps, thus health and nutrition are vital parts of all these programs. In 1974, 379,000 children were enrolled in Head Start programs and 660 physicians actively served as medical consultants to these projects.

CHANGING NUTRITIONAL BEHAVIOR BY AIDES IN TWO PROGRAMS

The EFNEP was organized nationally through the Extension Service of the land grant universities and funded by the U.S. Department of Agriculture beginning in 1968 . . .

The launching of the Family Aide Program in two western Maryland counties in 1972 was the result of an assessment of the evidence of the aide's effectiveness as a teaching agent and local educational agencies' desire for cooperation in educational outreach. The program provides educational services to disadvantaged families in nutrition education, consumer education and child development. Its aim is to bridge the educational needs between the school, home and community . . .

The main interest here was the effectiveness of aides as change agents in nutritional practices. A 24-hour recall of the foods eaten "yesterday" was recorded by the interviewer . . . A nutritionist rated the food recall on a four point scale of 0 to 3, with zero being the lowest rating. The meals were rated as "clearly inadequate or not provided," "not well balanced," "fairly well balanced," and "well balanced . . ."

It may well serve both the program and the clients to initiate pilot programs on aide training modeled after the practical nurse program which would, in effect, enable aides to become educational technicians. While the initial investment is large, the benefit is larger. A better trained aide should be able to contact more than two families in an eight-hour day. She is likely to be more self-reliant and more successful as a change agent in health education, child development, consumer education or even nutrition. Once trained, the cost for maintenance could be considerably less than the present scheme of support.

Virginia Li Wang: Changing nutritional behavior by aides in two programs, J. Nutr. Ed. **9:**109, 1977. Reprinted with permission from the Journal of Nutrition Education. © Society for Nutrition Education.

Parent and Child Centers

Thirty-three Parent and Child Centers help low-income parents and children who enter Head Start programs with physical, mental, and/or language problems dating from infancy and early childhood.

National Center for Child Abuse and Neglect

The National Center for Child Abuse and Neglect provides three-year demonstration projects that offer preventive social and medical services to families and children at risk.

Developmental Disabilities Act

The Developmental Disabilities Act authorized grants to states for planning, administration, services, and construction of facilities for the developmentally disabled, such as those with mental retardation, cerebral palsy, epilepsy, or autism. The state Developmental Disabilities Planning Council should be contacted for further information.

Projects authorized under Title XX of the Social Security Act

The Social Security Act allocates money to social services according to local needs. For example, emergency shelter for an abused child may be provided. The local state Human Services Agency office will have the full plan for the area.

Projects authorized under Title XIX—Medicaid

The Medicaid program brings together existing programs of medical assistance for the blind, the disabled, and members of families with dependent children who receive public assistance payments or are eligible to receive them under Title XIX. States may receive federal matching funds to pay for comprehensive health care for children up to 21 years of age if they are from families unable to pay for this care.

Early Periodic Screening, Diagnosis, and Treatment (EPSDT)

EPSDT is required under the Social Security Act, since it can greatly improve child health services for the poor. Early recognition and treatment of illness and handicapping conditions contribute to efficient social welfare programs. To date there has been wide variance in the extent and effectiveness of such state screening agencies.

COMMUNITY FOOD AND NUTRITION PROGRAM (CFNP)

The Community Services Administration is able to fund local CFNP programs under provisions of the Economic Opportunity Act. In 1977 the emphases for local agencies in applying for such aid constituted several types of activities.

PROJECT HEAD START

There has been an almost phenomenal development of nutrition education activities through which public health nutritionists are adding their efforts to break the poverty cycle early in a child's life. As members of the multidisciplinary public health team, nutritionists are able to move in and help to bridge the gap between the child and his family and the home and the center.

Working with the children

Although working with children of this age group in a direct educational program may be a new experience for some nutritionists, difficulties usually may be overcome rather early if a few guidelines are followed. These are: (1) The content of the presentation must be simple and clear; (2) the approach of teaching must be relaxed and informal; (3) the nutritionist must be visibly enthusiastic in order to generate an enthusiastic response from the children; and (4) creativity and flexibility are essential. The visuals used must be easily understood by the children and relate to their everyday experiences. In addition to these guidelines, all the principles of developing effective visual aids should be followed.

To give leadership to Head Start Centers, public health nutritionists of the New York City Department of Health have introduced many innovations into Project Head Start, such as the use of imaginative techniques and activities including puppets, games, "fishing for breakfast," "touch and tell," and tasting parties of raw fruits and vegetables. The most successful are the puppet shows, songs, and games in which the children can actually participate.

Working with the parents

Most requests received by nutritionists from both staff and parents are for informal discussion groups. Several approaches are open to the nutritionists to acquire the background information needed to make presentations meaningful and encourage parents' participation. For example, the meal served at the Center can be used as a basis for planning family meals. A simple flannel board, a slit card (a folded piece of cardboard with slits cut in one side for displaying food models), or paper food models can be used to show how to plan the breakfast and evening meals for the family. If a series of discussions is planned, the program can be greatly expanded to include the planning of nourishing home meals, cultural patterns, food likes and dislikes, and limited food budgets . . .

Reva T. Frankle, Miriam F. Senhouse, and *Catherine Cowell:* Project Head Start: a challenge in creativity in community nutrition, Am. J. Home Economics **59**: Jan., 1967.

Advocacy projects

Advocacy projects are designed to expand access to the participation in various federal food projects, such as the WIC Program or school lunch and breakfast programs. They include plans for program evaluation and recommendations, implementation, legal help for participants, and also plans for changes in existing programs.

Self-help projects

Self-help projects are designed to help an indigent community directly by providing access to food distribution and production in terms of community-control, community-developed resources and by providing lower cost food to such communities. The aim is to make communities self-sufficient through a specific plan that includes eventual phasing out of federal funding such as, for example, cooperative programs for production and distribution of food.

Supplemental projects

Supplemental projects are designed to fill gaps in federal programs, such as for services that are tangential but necessary to the operation of food programs. There is also funding for pilot programs, but under this rubric, funding is not available on a continuing basis.

Crisis relief projects

Crisis relief projects are designed to meet emergency needs of households through direct provision of food when other programs do not or cannot fulfill these needs. Such relief is temporary.[26]

GUIDELINES FOR POPULATION GROUPS IN COMMUNITY NUTRITION: ADULTS— FAMILY HEALTH (Table 5-4)

It has been found, especially among poor rural and urban populations, that health services and particularly improvements in nutritional status, are most effective when aimed

FAMILY HEALTH

In December 1973, a one-year nutrition program was initiated in the Daniel Hale Williams Neighborhood Health Center in the Model Cities area of the Near South Side of Chicago which has a population of approximately 101,000. Twelve individuals, ranging from twenty to thirty-six years of age, were recruited from the neighborhood and trained to serve as family health workers. This project was made possible through the cooperation of the American Medical Association (A.M.A.) and a $42,000 grant from the Education and Research Foundation of the A.M.A.

The purposes of the nutrition program were: (a) to help meet the nutritional needs of a community; (b) to demonstrate the value of a health center nutrition outreach service to health and welfare funding agencies in the hope that program continuation would result; and (c) to demonstrate to appropriate medical organizations that programs of this nature can be organized and funded with reasonable facility . . .

An analysis of 350 nutrition interview forms shows that 98 per cent of the patients and families had a desire to learn more about planning better diets. Modified diets had previously been prescribed for 50 per cent of the patients without adequate dietary instruction, and they had found it impossible to follow the diets. The most common modified diets were diabetic, low-salt, low-fat, and weight control.

Patients had no concept of the relationship between nutrition and medicine and the importance of nutrition in preventing certain diseases.

Herman Louise Dillon: Improvement of the quality of life through a food and nutrition project; J. Am. Diet. Assoc. **67:** 129, 1975. Reprinted by permission. Copyright the American Dietetic Association.

FAMILY HEALTH

In 1973 Dairy Council of California (DCC) began development of a new instructional program for use in teaching a basic set of nutrition-related skills to homemakers. It was planned that both professional nutrition educators and paraprofessionals would serve as instructors in the program.

The goal of this project was to develop an instructional program that could be used effectively by both professional nutrition educators and paraprofessionals to teach a basic set of nutrition-related skills to homemakers. Following pilot testing and revision of the newly developed program it was field tested in eight small-group workshops. Three nutritionists taught one workshop each for paraprofessional staff from programs (Headstart, Title 1) in low-income communities. Five of these paraprofessionals subsequently conducted one workshop each for homemakers from their own communities. Program effectiveness was assessed with a 35-item criterion test. Post test mean scores were 86% for the workshops taught by nutritionists and 81% for those taught by paraprofessionals. Corresponding pretest scores were 35% and 29%, respectively. Both participants and instructors had very favorable attitudes toward the program. The completed program is now being used with consumers and young adults in a variety of educational and health-related programs.

Howard J. Sullivan, Margaret Gere, Bettye Jo Nowlin, and *Beverly Kloehn:* Development of a nutrition education program for homemakers, J. Nutr. Ed. **8:**118, 1976. Reprinted with permission from the Journal of Nutrition Education. © Society for Nutrition Education.

FAMILY HEALTH

In 1968, the State Department of Health and the nutrition community conducted a nutritional status survey based on selected characteristics of Arizona's population generally considered to have a relationship to nutritional status . . .

Four sub-systems—the development of community nutrition workers, screening, referral, and monitoring— were developed in an attempt to establish a mechanism for an on-going surveillance of the nutritional status of Arizona residents and to deliver efficient comprehensive nutrition services to those in need . . .

A need for accountability and the limited availability of funds have perpetuated the trend toward the use of screening programs with a focus on preventive medicine . . .

Counseling and education usually took place in the home on a one-to-one basis. Instruction seemed to be better accepted in the family's own environment . . .

The community nutrition worker, who could relate to patients and their problems because of their own personal experience, is the most significant educational tool in this program . . .

The improvement in nutritional status in the population through this mechanism provided the grounds for establishing a state-wide nutrition care delivery system. The delivery system has now been expanded state-wide.

Anita V. Yanochik, Carol Irene Eichelberger, and *Suzanne E. Dandoy:* The Comprehensive Nutrition Action Program in Arizona, J. Am. Diet. Assoc. **69:**37, July 1976. Reprinted by permission. Copyright The American Dietetic Association.

THE COMMUNITY NUTRITION TEAM

The current desire among health professionals and the persons they serve to make the hospital more open toward its community is increasing the emphasis on the hospital as the focus of contemporary health care. Mount Sinai School of Medicine, New York City, which was established more than four years ago, acknowledges the need to devote attention to the study and treatment of the health problems of the community in addition to those of individual patients . . .

Three groups were identified and studied because of their high incidence of nutritional deficiencies: 100 multiproblem families, as identified by the Little Sisters of the Assumption (LSA), a family health care agency staffed by nuns who are either social workers or nurses; narcotic addicts, as identified by the Exodus House Drug Rehabilitation Center; and geriatric citizens living alone, as identified by the Stanley Isaacs Neighborhood Center.

Community Nutrition Team

A Community Nutrition Team (CNT), consisting of a medical nutritionist, a pediatrician, a dietitian, a medical student, and a staff member (usually either a public health nurse or a social worker) from one of the participating agencies, was developed . . .

The CNT makes home visits, develops storefront and church-affiliated nutrition and health clinics, and provides other consultative services as needed. The division's nutritionist and a "Little Sister" serve as the avant garde of the CNT, making an initial home visit and arranging for a follow-up visit by the CNT.

At the follow-up visit, all family members are nutritionally evaluated . . .

Drug Rehabilitation Center

Narcotic addiction is the most prevalent and significant public health problem in East Harlem. The division of nutrition worked with the Exodus House Drug Rehabilitation Center to establish a storefront nutrition and health clinic. More than 400 addicts in the rehabilitation center have been examined . . .

A preliminary review of our evaluation indicates that many addicts undergoing rehabilitation have unusual diet patterns following withdrawal. Many such patients exhibit an unusual craving for carbohydrates; some patients demonstrate low folate and vitamin B12 levels or bizarre adipose tissue fatty acid patterns, and nearly 50 per cent of the patients have abnormal liver enzyme levels . . .

Stanley Isaacs Neighborhood Center

Meeting the health-related needs of the aged and chronically ill living in their own homes in the community is a priority of comprehensive health planning. These needs, which are well documented, include ambulatory health care services, nutrition services, a broad spectrum of home care, environmental and social services, a wide variety of different modalities of day and night care centers, and provision of foster homes.

The CNT and the staff of the Stanley Isaacs Neighborhood Center identified many aged persons who were unable or unwilling to leave their homes yet who could benefit from nutritional and medical evaluation. Visits were made to these persons' homes, and recommendations for follow-up care were made to the Stanley Isaacs Center Staff. In some cases, these aged citizens, living alone, had not seen a physician in three years . . .

More important, this project has demonstrated that a hospital-based medical school can work with established community agencies to explore new methods of meeting the health needs of a community . . .

Hospitals now should actively seek and officially be assigned the role of organizational catalysts, referral centers, and professional monitors of the quality and quantity of care rendered not only on their own premises but also throughout the communities they serve. Nutrition services must be included in such efforts; the experiences related here illustrate their importance.

Reva T. Frankle and *George Christakis:* Community nutrition teams, Hospitals **47:**56, Dec. 16, 1973.

at the family unit. The decisions about what foods to buy, how much money to spend, preparation, and storage are often made by more than one member of the family. The sensitive nutritionist is one who is aware of the interpersonal relationships among family members, as well as the differing health requirements of each.

Various programs have been directed specifically toward the family such as The Daniel Hale Williams Neighborhood Project in Chicago,[27] the Dairy Council of California Instructional Program for Homemakers,[28] and the Comprehensive Nutrition Action Program in Arizona, which began in 1968.[29]

In New York, through Mt. Sinai Hospital's nutrition clinic, a community nutrition team, consisting of a medical nutritionist, pediatrician, dietitian, medical student, and public health worker, made home visits and follow-

HOSPITAL'S COMMUNITY SERVICE—LIBRARY EXHIBIT ON FOOD PRICES

With food prices the topic of everyone's conversation, the time for presenting a food budgeting project was "now." But where should one begin with so broad a subject and a community as diversified as ours? . . .

As Nutrition Education Coordinator for Divine Providence Hospital's Community Health Service, I approached the local librarian to learn whether the library would cooperate in setting up a special reference table featuring information on food budgeting . . .

The new task was to obtain large quantities of printed matter on food budgeting and general nutrition, for it was felt that the topics should be considered together. Local agencies, such as the gas company, electric company, the health department, a dairy, the local food cooperative, and the office of the state representative, all supplied free materials for general distribution. I also wrote to many consumer-oriented food companies to request their publications . . .

Radio and television coverage heightened interest during the two weeks the Food Budgeting Service Center was in operation. Eleven volunteers from local agencies and organizations with personnel working in nutrition or related areas manned the tables during library hours. The volunteers added the visible concern of people with a mutual interest in food and feeding the family on a budget. They listened to the consumers, encouraged questions, and offered suggestions.

They also aided us by asking the library patrons to fill out an evaluation form, which was devised to find out how much interest there might be in a follow-up course on food budgeting and good nutrition. We learned that over half of the two hundred people who attended were also interested in principles of low-calorie menu planning. Accordingly, I have developed an instructional unit on low-cost and low-calorie foods which has been presented to our patients on reducing diets and their spouses. Presently, I am planning a "mini-course" that will present this subject in greater detail and will be open to the public . . .

Leni C. Reed: Hospital's community service—library exhibit on food prices, J. Am. Diet. Assoc. **64:**286, 1974. Reprinted by permission. Copyright The American Dietetic Association.

NUTRITION SERVICES IN THE DRUG REHABILITATION CENTER

I am a nutritionist in a drug rehabilitation center—a place where former drug addicts come full of hope for a new life free of drug dependency, a place where concerned staff learn together how best to deal with one of the most overwhelming problems of society today.

What is it like to be a nutritionist in a drug rehabilitation center? . . .

Our dietary history form was designed to collect data about food intake prior to, during, and after addiction. The interview lasted about half an hour, never less. The dietary history included a 24-hr. recall of the present diet and a listing of the present weekly food intake. The form also provided for information on the person's use of drugs, his diet before, during, and after drug addiction, and information about life style affecting nutrition, such as who cooks and shops at the client's home, modified diets used, and religious and cultural food habits.

As stated, the client is first seen by the nutritionist and then the laboratory technician. After the laboratory encounter, the client is introduced to the physician who elicits a medical history and performs a physical examination.

A second appointment is made for two weeks after the first one, at which time the dietary, laboratory, and medical findings are shared with the patient, and follow-up plans are made when indicated. Once our client, who has been a resident of the rehabilitation program, moves out into the community, he finds the nutritionist is still available to assist him with food buying, menu planning, budgeting, and even "how to set up a pad."

A nutritionist in a drug rehabilitation center can be the pivotal person for a health care plan. However, the real help for the addict comes from the ex-addict who is his chief support and role model. It is the addict who changes himself. To assist, the health profession must change almost as radically as the addict. There is an obligation for health professionals to work cooperatively with community agencies whose basic objective is to re-orient, re-educate, and rehabilitate the former drug addict.

Reva T. Frankle: The nutritionist in a drug rehabilitation center: a medical school reaches out, J. Am. Diet. Assoc. **65:**562, 1974. Reprinted by permission. Copyright The American Dietetic Association.

up visits to families and generally offered comprehensive health care based on a preventive orientation. These teams have also worked with drug rehabilitation centers (Exodus House) and with elderly groups (through the Stanley Isaacs Neighborhood Center).[30]

Adult health

Proper preventive care during the adult years can help stave off many crippling and degenerative diseases—such as cardiovascular disease, hypertension, cancer, diabetes, and obesity. Although all of these are affected by nutrition, the majority of the adult population is unaware of the relationship. It is up to the nutritionist to help educate the public through articles, radio and television, fitness programs, health screening programs, and

---

MENTAL ILLNESS

Day-treatment centers, partial hospitalization, and day hospitals are becoming increasingly popular alternatives to institutionalization of patients with mental illness. The purpose of these new treatments is to reduce the expense of long-term custodial care and to aid the individual in returning to a productive life . . .

One such day-treatment center is located at the Veterans Administration Hospital, Salem, Virginia. The Center, started in March 1975, now has sixty-one clients who had formerly faced the prospect of continuous custodial care. Most of these clients have been hospitalized frequently over the years and would generally be diagnosed as chronic schizophrenics. Their ages range from twenty-five to sixty years. The major purpose of the Center is to help them adapt to the outside world with its rewards and frustrations.

A nutrition education program is a significant component of this program for helping individuals to again become contributing members of society. We realized early in the program that the clients, mostly men, had little experience or skill in buying and cooking foods, particularly the less functional clients in the Tuesday-Thursday group. Previous skills, if any, had been lost during long years of institutionalization. During that period, too, many had lost the support they had previously had from family members such as mothers or wives.

The nutritional program was inaugurated by the Coordinator of the Day Treatment Center (first author) and the Chief of Dietetics for the Salem, VA Hospital, who involved all members of the staff. These included a dietitian, a volunteer with a bachelor's degree in home economics, a registered nurse, a social worker, a clinical counselor, a secretary-receptionist, and a psychologist . . . The program consisted of two phases. The purpose of the first phase was to provide clients with basic knowledge of nutrition and the handling of foods, while in the second, the objective was to develop clients' skills in the actual preparation of foods. A secondary but extremely important objective in both phases was to increase the clients' skills and confidence in social situations and to provide meaningful experiences to support an improved self-image.

Claudia A. Johnson, Cecelia E. Haney, Bryna Flowers, and *Loyd D. Andrew:* Dietitians help mental patients make it on the outside, J. Am. Diet. Assoc. **70:**515, 1977. Reprinted by permission. Copyright The American Dietetic Association.

also individual dietary counseling. Difficult though it may be, the emphasis should be on the wellness and health maintenance through modification of behavior and life-styles. The usefulness of proper dietary procedures in such modification has also been demonstrated in the work of nutritionists with mental health patients in a Veterans Administration Hospital in Salem, Virginia, as described in the accompanying article by Johnson and colleagues.

Migrant health

During the 1960s, federal migrant health legislation began to provide grants to states and local areas for comprehensive family health and medical services to seasonal farm workers and their families through special clinics geographically accessible and open during convenient hours. This group of itinerant farm workers has for some time suffered severely from lack of health care, housing, and education. In addition, people in this situation were ineligible for health and social service programs for which there were residency requirements.

In some states with warm winter growing

OBESITY

A nutritionist and a social worker co-led weight reduction groups for women for a 1-year period in order to assess the value of having nutrition education and counseling techniques taught in tandem. Good nutrition taught within a flexible diet plan was enhanced by the implementation of a behavior modification approach. Meal preparation and grocery store shopping were integral parts of the program since many group members had never been exposed to attractive and varied food preparation or wise food purchasing techniques. Daily exercise was constantly stressed as one of the important ways to lose excess weight and stay healthy. The groups were successful in that most women lost weight by changing meal patterns and were able to control their weight after the groups ended by continuing to reinforce themselves with nonfood rewards.

Bonnie M. Orkow and *Judy L. Ross:* Weight reduction through nutrition education and personal counseling, J. Nutr. Ed. **7:**65, 1975. Reprinted with permission from the Journal of Nutrition Education. © Society for Nutrition Education.

seasons, such as California, Arizona, Florida, and Texas, there are numbers of seasonal farm workers who do not travel out of the state. In these home base states migrant health services are usually conducted around the year, whereas migrant farm workers live in temporary housing and require health services on a short-term care basis.

All health planning undertaken for migrant workers should have a nutrition component. Many workers are Spanish or Mexican-American, and the nutritionist should provide teaching materials in Spanish that are meaningful to their cultural food habits. They should also be introduced to relevant programs, such as the Department of Agriculture's nutrition education program, school services, and financial aid program. High priority populations for nutrition services would be pregnant women, infants and children, and those persons with chronic diseases.

Indian health

The Nutrition and Dietetics Branch of the Indian Health Services (Department of Health, Education, and Welfare) attempts to provide comprehensive nutrition service for 517,000 American Indian and Alaskan natives. It offers in-hospital food services and nutrition counseling at health stations and home visits. It also conducts research into the special dietary needs of this population and aims to train individuals from these groups for nutrition-related careers.

Various studies, such as a survey of the nutrient intake and food patterns of Indians on the Standing Rock Reservation in North and South Dakota, indicate that typical intake is much below acceptable recommendations. There was a prevalence of fried and starchy foods and sugar; few vegetables, fruits, and protein foods were eaten, even though most families received government commodities.

MIGRANT HEALTH

For nearly two decades, the Division of Health, Florida Department of Health and Rehabilitative Services, through its associated county health departments, has provided health care, including some nutritional services, to migrant agricultural workers . . .

This eighteen-month program was designed to: (a) determine the nutritional status of a selected population of migrant agricultural workers and their families and (b) design, apply, and evaluate an intervention program to correct the major food and nutrition problems identified . . .

During the project period, families were observed through two winter seasons. Many appeared to live from day to day without future planning. Families depending on public assistance were observed to eat better at the beginning of the month. The children became independent early in life, and their eating habits reflected this. When parents went to work early, children either prepared their own breakfasts, skipped the meal, or bought a snack or soda on the way to school. Most school children received a free or reduced-price lunch, and for many, this was the most nutritious meal of the day. An entire family sitting together at the evening meal was uncommon . . .

During the six-month period between the end of the survey and the start of the nutrition education program, educational materials and approaches were developed and tested. Younger children enjoyed food coloring books, nutrition songs, and food games. Adolescents responded to participation skits, food grouping games, nutrition bingo, and other games. Adults enjoyed tasting parties, participation skits, slide presentations, films, food grouping games, and discussion sessions. Posters, charts, and other visual aids were used extensively.

After the three-month nutrition education program, a resurvey was made to evaluate its effect on the farm workers identified by the survey as having one or more biochemical abnormalities. The resurvey included selected parameters used in the initial survey—hemoglobin, hematocrit, serum iron and iron-binding capacity, plasma carotene and vitamin A, urinary riboflavin, height and weight, 24-hr. food recall, and family food frequency recall.

Expanded nutrition education and dietary counseling are clearly indicated as a part of family health programs and of maternity, family planning, child, and school health services. Short-term intensive instruction had limited effect in changing the food habits of adults established throughout a lifetime. Nutrition education for seasonal farm workers should be comprehensive and long-term with cooperation and consistency between programs in the schools and the community.

Mildred Kaufman, Eugene Lewis, Albert V. Hardy, and *Jo-anne Proulx:* Florida seasonal farm workers: follow-up and intervention following a nutrition survey, J. Am. Diet. Assoc. **66:** 605, 1975. Reprinted by permission. Copyright The American Dietetic Association.

INDIAN HEALTH

Ninety-four Indian women, living on Standing Rock Reservation in North and South Dakota, were interviewed to determine: their nutrient intake and meal patterns; the use of government commodities and traditional Indian foods; and attitudes toward food, weight, and health . . .

There was no typical day's menu, and food items in meals lacked variety. Breakfast consisted of hot or cold cereal, bread and/or fried potatoes, and sometimes fried eggs. Coffee was a favorite beverage. Most women had bologna sandwiches, potato chips, and carbonated beverages for lunch; a few reported boiled meat soup, fried potatoes, and bread. Chopped meat or other meat and fried potatoes were usually eaten at the evening meal.

Wojapi and fry bread are the traditional Indian foods eaten most frequently. Wild fruits and turnips, although available, are no longer used extensively. Frying and the traditional boiling are the most common food preparation methods.

Most of the women were overweight, but believed that they were healthy. Only nineteen could define a calorie, although forty-eight believed it was something that made one fat.

Seventy-four per cent of the families received government commodities; all except bulgur were used. The 44 per cent who had gardens met the recommended allowance for ascorbic acid and had higher intakes than the other women. Buffalo, fish, and wild game animals contributed to the food supply but were not a major source of food.

Mary A. Bass and *Lucille M. Wakefield:* Nutrient intake and food patterns of Indians on Standing Rock Reservation, J. Am. Diet. Assoc. **64**:36, 1974. Reprinted by permission. Copyright The American Dietetic Association.

INDIAN HEALTH

The Indian Community School is a private school organized by the Indians themselves to help the children who could not remain in public schools. One objective of the program is to get the children back into the public school system, if at all possible. The school opened with only two children in 1971; presently, seventy-two are enrolled . . .

We started working immediately, planning meals, adapting recipes to the tastes of these Indian children, surveying the need for equipment and utensils, and most of all searching for more food supplies. Milk was available under the Central City Citizens School Breakfast Program, and some surplus foods from USDA were available. All other foods were donations of church groups or individuals.

The nutrition project at the Indian Community School brought to light numerous health problems, such as obesity, diabetes, anemia, malnutrition, and suspected pregnancies.

Classes are held in an abandoned Coast Guard building, where breakfast and lunch programs were established. Food, dishes, and equipment came from numerous and unexpected sources. The menu was developed by a compromise between the eating habits of these Indian children and the USDA–donated foods available. Nursing students working with nutrition problems in the school opened the way for a health screening project carried out in 1973. Health problems of Indian children which required adjustment in food intake were brought to light.

Sister Brendan McCormick: Improving nutrition in the Indian Community School, Milwaukee, J. Am. Diet. Assoc. **64**: 405, 1974. Reprinted by permission. Copyright The American Dietetic Association.

The need for effective nutrition education is clearly apparent.[31]

GUIDELINES FOR POPULATION GROUPS IN COMMUNITY NUTRITION: THE ELDERLY (Table 5-5)

The Administration on Aging (AoA) was created in 1965 with the passage of the Older Americans Act that initiated Titles III, IV, and V programs. The AoA was originally within the Department of Health, Education, and Welfare and later was incorporated into the Office of Human Development. In the late 1960s the acts were amended, giving the states more power in the development of programs. Title III is a services delivery strategy that calls for state agencies to fund social service projects. In the early 1970s the concept of revenue sharing was introduced, making Titles III and IV funding in the form of block grants to states. In 1972, Title VII (Public Law 92-128), the National Nutrition Program for the Elderly was enacted, with special attention to congregate meal sites, home-delivered meals, and supportive services.

Title VII nutrition programs

Title VII authorized the Administration on Aging (AoA) to make formula grants to states

NUTRITION: THE ELDERLY

Because the population of older Americans is rapidly increasing throughout the United States, there is an urgent need for the dietetic profession to deliver adequate nutritional care to our elderly. Dietetic education should prepare all dietitians to function in many types of government and non-government programs and agencies developed to serve people throughout their entire life cycle . . . Reciprocal objectives for both the food systems management program and the Title VII Nutrition Programs were established . . .

Throughout Missouri, there are nine area Offices of Aging where Nutrition Project Directors assume responsibility for the Title VII Nutrition Programs. The number of nutrition programs or sites where the congregate meals are served and social services provided to the elderly in each Nutrition Project ranges from seven to sixteen. The personnel included in the training project were the Nutrition Project Directors and the site managers, head cooks, and volunteers at the nutrition programs or sites . . .

Agenda: Foodservice clinic for personnel in Title VII Nutrition Programs in Missouri

8:30 A.M.	Welcome by faculty and students
9:00 A.M.	Do you know what you know? (questions to give you an idea of today's topics)
9:30 A.M.	Standardized quantity recipes
10:15 A.M.	Food portion control
11:00 A.M.	Coffee break
11:15 A.M.	Food quality control
12:30 P.M.	Lunch
1:30 P.M.	Food product specifications
2:15 P.M.	Food safety

3:00 P.M. Putting your ideas in order (questions to show you how much you have learned today)

These survey findings revealed that more emphasis was given to technical skills for quality control than those for fiscal control throughout Missouri. Given the composite objectives of Title VII Nutrition Programs . . . equal emphasis should be given to both areas. These findings disclosed areas for emphasis in future training sessions.

Recommendation for research studies

Two inferences can tentatively be made from this feasibility study: (a) Senior dietetic students in food systems management enhanced the educational opportunities for personnel in Title VII Nutrition Programs in Missouri and (b) the students demonstrated that they can contribute to the nutritional care of the elderly in Title VII Nutrition Programs in Missouri. Controlled, evaluative research projects are needed to determine how to engage students in general, administrative, clinical, community nutrition, and graduate dietetic programs across the nation in meaningful participation in programs for aged persons. Dietitians have a future professional role in many community and government programs; active participation of dietetic educational programs in both community- and government-sponsored social programs, such as the Title VII Nutrition Program for the elderly, should facilitate meaningful contributions to society . . .

Nan Unklesbay: Students in food systems management contribute to nutrition programs for the elderly, J. Am. Diet. Assoc. 70:516, 1977. Reprinted by permission. Copyright by The American Dietetic Association.

for nutrition projects that provide low-cost, nutritious meals served primarily in congregate settings with supportive social services. Five major goals of the program include providing (1) low-cost, nutritious meals, (2) an opportunity for social interaction, (3) auxiliary nutrition and homemaker education and shopping assistance, (4) counseling and referral to other social and rehabilitative services, and (5) transportation services.

In addition to promoting better health among the elderly through improved nutrition, the Title VII nutrition program is of sociologic significance, since it is aimed at reducing the isolation of old age and offers older Americans an opportunity to live their remaining years in dignity.[32-34]

The need for this program is becoming increasingly more evident. In 1974 one in every ten persons in the United States was 65 years of age and older; one third of all older persons lived alone or with nonrelatives. At 65 years of age, the life expectancy is 13 years for men and 17 years for women. At 1974 death rates, the older population is expected to increase by 40% to 31 million persons by the year 2000.[35] Watkin[36] predicted that more people with physical impairments will survive so that the magnitude of the problems associated with old age and disability will increase rather than diminish with time.

Congregate meal sites

One of the primary responsibilities of Title VII elderly nutrition programs is to provide at least one hot meal a day, five days a week

REACHING THE ELDERLY

Concern for the nutritional problems of the elderly brought about the enactment of Title VII of the Older Americans Act. Under this legislation, congregate feeding centers have been established for the elderly. In addition to providing meals, supportive services include nutrition education programs. Circumstances that create the need for nutritional assistance, such as decreased mobility, poor health or diminished incentive, might also prevent older people from participating in nutrition education programs. This situation challenges nutrition educators to find ways of reaching these older people . . .

There are several advantages to using television public service announcements (PSAs) to reach the elderly rather than using half-hour or hour programs. PSAs are broadcast on commercial stations watched by a majority of the elderly, the audience is already established, and the PSAs are brief and to the point and can be repeated many times . . .

The effectiveness of a low-cost television advertising campaign as a means of nutrition education for the elderly was evaluated. Four PSAs about nutrition aimed specifically to people over 60 years old were produced at Iowa State University (ISU) by students in Telecommunicative Arts . . .

On the basis of comparison of PSA recall scores with nutrition knowledge scores, nutrient contributions of specific food sources and changes in mean nutrient intakes of the entire sample, the PSA campaign had no measurable impact on the eating behavior of the elderly subjects studied . . .

PSAs may be most useful to fill an immediate need, such as to provide publicity for a nutrition program, to offer further sources of nutrition information or to provide money-saving tips. The PSA messages that alluded to better health through an adequate diet might have been too general and distant to appeal to the elderly, even though this group expresses concern for their health. The PSAs may be most useful as part of a total nutrition education campaign.

Further research into the use of television PSAs combined with other nutrition education methods to reach the elderly would be useful. A better understanding of factors that will motivate modifications in eating patterns of this age group is necessary.

Judy J. Fitzgibbons and *Pilar A. Garcia:* TV, PSAs, nutrition and the elderly, J. Nutr. Ed. **9:**114, 1977. Reprinted with permission from the Journal of Nutrition Education. © Society for Nutrition Education.

to any senior citizen 60 years of age or older in a "congregate" setting—such as a church, school, or community center—where companionship, entertainment, and social services are also available.

The meals served must contain at least one third of the recommended daily dietary allowances, and menus must be certified by a registered nutritionist. Project sites are also required to tailor their menus, where feasible and appropriate, to meet the particular dietary needs arising from the health requirements, religious requirements, or ethnic backgrounds of eligible individuals. Each project must serve at least an average of a hundred meals daily. The expertise of the nutritionist is vital to assure nutritional quality and acceptability of meals, as well as to develop a series of appropriate group sessions for nutrition education.

Home-delivered meals (Meals on Wheels)

An integral part of the Title VII elderly nutrition project is the home-delivered meals requirement of the program. Title VII grantee organizations are required to furnish home-delivered meals to eligible persons who are unable to leave their homes. This nonprofit program of home-delivered meals is a community service administered by an official or voluntary or welfare agency. The service is provided to ill, disabled, and elderly persons whose physical, emotional, mental, or social conditions handicap their ability to obtain or prepare meals for themselves. Such services often make it possible for individuals to remain in their own homes, reducing institutional care, or to obtain special diets that they could not prepare. Support is usually from local sponsorship and income generated from the meals. Senate Hearings on the National Meals-On-Wheels Program describe the system used in Cook County, Chicago.[37] The program is an excellent way to reach the elderly home bound.

Supportive services

Local Title VII grantees are required by law to provide, in addition to their food service, recreational activities, information on and referral to other existing sources of social services (e.g., housing, legal services, etc.), and health and welfare counseling. Federal regulations provide for the following supportive social services as well:

1. Transportation of individuals and personal escort services to and from the congregate meal sites
2. Health and welfare counseling
3. Nutrition education
4. Shopping assistance
5. Recreation activities incidental to the project

These regulations also specify that not more than 20% of a state's allotment for any fiscal year, excluding funds necessary for administering the state plan, shall be used for supporting services. Unfortunately, lack of adequate funds has meant that these services are not being fully provided, and grantees have determined that the limited money available is better spent on more meals.

It has been estimated that about one fourth to one third of persons over 65 years of age have a health problem requiring prescribed dietary modifications as part of medical treatment. The interactions of drugs taken by the aged for multiple health problems may influence appetite and nutrient availability and produce side effects. It may make eating and food preparation difficult and influence choices of foods that are easy to prepare and eat but may not be the most nutrient dense. Compounding health-related nutrition problems such as chronic disease, dental status, and handicapping physical conditions are fixed and low incomes, which leave little money available for food; housing with inadequate facilities for storing and preparing food; and unavailable or inaccessible transportation to food markets. Too often, the elderly who are in search of renewed health fall prey to promoters of nutrient supplements, fad diets, and popularly called "health foods."

Medicare (Social Security Act, Title XVIII) has expanded the availability of health services to the elderly by covering hospital and nursing home care and home health services. The nutritionist should counsel elderly patients on normal and therapeutic nutritional needs with appropriate consideration to their health/disease status, long-established food patterns, budget, and availability and acces-

THE NUTRITIONIST AND THE VISITING NURSE

The Visiting Nurse Association (VNA) of Metropolitan Detroit, a member of the United Community Services and United Foundation, covers a tri-county area of some 1,300 sq. mi. with a population of 3.7 million. The agency provides multiple health services in the home through professionally qualified public health nurses, licensed practical nurses, and home health aides, with consultants in the fields of nutrition, maternal and child health, physical and occupational therapy, social work, speech pathology, mental health, and medical-surgical nursing. The Visiting Nurse Association is a certified Home Health Agency for Medicare and Medicaid.

Nutrition has been an integral part of the VNA program in Detroit since 1936. The service was established to provide both consultation to the staff and direct dietary counseling for patients and families in the home according to the prescribed nutritional care plan . . .

It is the responsibility of the public health nurse to plan with the physician and family, and, when special services are indicated, with the consultants. The public health nurse has the opportunity to evaluate and give nutritional guidance to patients and families and to help establish realistic goals for improving their dietary practices. It is one of the roles of the nutrition consultant to work with the nurse, provide her with sound nutrition information, and help her to develop skills and techniques in adapting her teaching to meet the individual social, cultural, and economic needs of patients and families.

In addition, the nutritionists provide direct service as specialists, ready to give instruction about normal or modified diets to patients when indicated. . . .

Shirley O'Connell: The nutrition consultant for visiting nurses, J. Am. Diet. Assoc. 68:247, 1976. Reprinted by permission. Copyright The American Dietetic Association.

sibility to food supplies and food preparation facilities. Time and effort spent in realistic counseling to elderly patients regarding food and nutrition needs can promote health and independence and prevent or delay costly institutional care.

NUTRITION EDUCATION

Nutrition education has a vital role in all approaches at all age levels of the life cycle in obtaining an optimal nutritional status within any community. By definition, nutrition education in the community is the application of the science of nutrition to the everyday lives

THE NUTRITIONIST AND HOME CARE

In my position as Nutrition Consultant with Home Health Services of Louisiana, Inc., a Medicare Providor Agency in New Orleans, I give direct patient and family dietary instructions.

I also participate in the training and orientation of home health aides. In-service training in nutrition is provided for the staff, including consultation with other staff members and participation in their orientation. I am a member of the committee which makes periodic multidisciplinary review of the progress of patients with Home Health Services. I am also a member of the Utilization Review Committee and of the Professional Services Staffing Conference . . .

Advantages of home counseling

The advantages of dietary counseling in the home, from my point of view, are:

(a) The diets can be personalized to meet, when possible, the patient's eating patterns, food likes and dislikes, and food allergies.

(b) Assessments can be made of the surroundings to determine if proper food handling techniques, such as adequate refrigeration and storage, are available and if cooking appliances can be safely used.

(c) Assessments can be made of the family or friends involved—will they be a hindrance or a help in the dietary control?

(d) Assessment of the practical aspects of obtaining the diet can be determined in the home: (a) Amount of money spent on food and whether the family receives Food Stamps. (b) How is food purchased: who does the purchasing, how often and where is food purchased, how do they travel to purchase food? (c) Who does the cooking? . . .

There is need for reimbursement for nutrition services in home health. The average length of time spent on my first visit to a patient is generally 1 hr. The time is broken down as: 15 min. transit time, 15 min. nutritional assessment, 25 min. for dietary instruction, and 5 min. for questions from the patient and/or family member or friend present . . .

I am the only nutritionist in a Home Health Service Provider Agency in the New Orleans area. We are now receiving calls from physicians who will order services provided nutrition consultation is available for their patients . . .

Nutritional care, including dietary counseling, should be included in all national health programs. Nutritional counseling can integrate preventive, diagnostic, curative, and restorative health services into total patient care. Decreased costs for hospitalization and home health services can be achieved when patients are taught proper normal and therapeutic nutrition as related to their physical condition and their home environment . . .

Anita Marie Hatten: Dietary counseling in ambulatory care— the nutrition consultant in home care services, J. Am. Diet. Assoc. **68:**250, 1976. Reprinted by permission. Copyright The American Dietetic Association.

---

of people. This means that nutrition education is related to the social, economic, and cultural values of food in such a way that people are motivated to make food choices which will result in their optimal nutritional well-being.

In a *Position Paper on Nutrition Education for the Public,* the American Dietetic Association defines nutrition education as the process by which beliefs, attitudes, environmental influences, and understandings about food lead to practices that are scientifically sound, practical, and consistent with individual needs and available food resources.

The American Dietetic Association takes the position that nutrition education should be available to all individuals and families. The fundamental philosophy of nutrition education is that efforts should focus on the establishment and protection of nutritional health rather than on crisis intervention. It is needed, regardless of income, location, or cultural, social, or economic practices or level of education. Nutrition education must be a continuing process through the life cycle as new research brings additional knowledge.[38]

Leverton[39] further defines nutrition education as a multidisciplinary process that involves the transfer of information, the development of motivation, and the modification of food habits where needed. It must form the bridge that carries appropriate information from the research and development laboratories to the public, the ultimate user. During this transport, nutrition educators must apply their skills and knowledge to adapt the information so it can be applied to a variety of everyday situations and then package it for distribution in a variety of

POSITION PAPER ON NUTRITION EDUCATION FOR THE PUBLIC*
Definition of nutrition education

Nutrition education is the process by which beliefs, attitudes, environmental influences, and understandings about food lead to practices that are scientifically sound, practical, and consistent with individual needs and available food resources.

The American Dietetic Association takes the position that nutrition education should be available to all individuals and families. The fundamental philosophy of nutrition education is that efforts should focus on the establishment and protection of nutritional health rather than on crisis intervention. It is needed regardless of income, location, or cultural, social, or economic practices or level of education. Nutrition education must be a continuing process through the life cycle as new research brings additional knowledge.

Planned behavioral changes

Eating behavior is psychologically motivated but is culturally and biologically determined. Any effective educational program must recognize this interaction even though it may deal actively with only one part. The solutions to nutrition problems must be diversified in approach if they are to have a significant, overall effect.

Values, attitudes, and beliefs control man's behavior; therefore, planned change is a deliberate effort to improve nutrition through intervention, and it occurs by design. The dietitian educators must understand and respect the personal meaning of these influences in others.

The process of developing planned behavioral change includes five stages:

1. Awareness—helping the individual, family, or group identify problems related to the food consumed.
2. Development of a receptive framework for learning.
   a. Establishing the credibility of the nutrition educator
   b. Becoming aware of learner's prior perceptions about food and nutrition.
   c. Helping to state desirable changes in food practices and to decide which are feasible.
3. Experimentation—testing ideas, techniques, and programs until acceptable ones are identified.

4. Reinforcement—strengthening the learning gained during the experimentation period.
5. Adoption of change—guiding the decision to accept the change and put it into practice.

The American Dietetic Association recommends that:

1. Nutrition education be identified as part of every program that educates for personal, family, and community health.
2. Consumers participate in defining their expectations and needs for nutrition information which can be met by nutrition education.
3. Persons who conduct nutrition education should be qualified by specific training in human nutrition and educational techniques.
4. Nutrition education with adequate funding be a regular part of the training of (a) teachers, (b) medical and dental professions, (c) allied health personnel.
5. The Association and members participate in the planning of emerging nutrition education programs and the coordination of existing ones.

Role of the dietitian

Knowledge of food and nutrition qualifies the dietitian as the health professional equipped to help individuals, families, and groups improve their food practices and their nutrition status. The dietitian is a translator of the science of nutrition into the skill of furnishing optimal nourishment to people. As nutrition educator and as trainer of others who conduct nutrition education, the dietitian:

1. Takes leadership in providing nutrition information.
2. Interprets nutrition facts accurately.
3. States them in terminology that people can understand and apply.
4. Aims to reduce the time lag between the discovery of nutrition knowledge and its application to food practices.
5. Recognizes and utilizes human motivation to bring about changes in food practices.

Position paper on nutrition education for the public, J. Am. Diet. Assoc. **62**:520, 1973. Reprinted by permission. Copyright The American Dietetic Association.

ways, either directly to the intended user or indirectly through intermediate agents.[39] Nutrition education as planned change is carefully discussed by Gifft, Washbon, and Harrison[40] who caution that planned change should never be undertaken lightly.

A conceptual framework for nutrition education was recommended by the panel on Nutrition Education in the Schools at the White House Conference in 1969. This framework (p. 133), or one modified to suit the situation in a community, should

WHAT IS NUTRITION EDUCATION?

Perhaps it would be helpful to review our ideas of nutrition education and in this way, arrive at some consensus of what the term means and involves, and what realistically can be expected of the process . . .

Nutrition education is a multidisciplinary process that involves the transfer of information, the development of motivation, and the modification of food habits where needed. It must form the bridge that carries appropriate information from the research and development laboratories to the public, the ultimate user.

Whether our message is general or detailed, it must be in the context that choosing food for health is not an end in itself, but a means to an end, i.e., giving us the nutritional well-being that helps us in everything we do. It is not conveyed by "eat this because it is good for you," but rather by "eating well will help you in what you want to do and to become."

There is no single approach and message that can be used in nutrition education. Each program must be tailored and related to the needs, interests, experiences, and goals of the individual or group being exposed to the subject. Probably the basic criterion for selecting what information to give is: "What will our client be receptive to?" This requires trying to discern what he thinks his problem is, which, in turn, requires our listening with a selective ear . . .

A major situation in our environment with which we must contend as we try to advance in the field of nutrition education is the prevalence of misinformation.

This, in turn, breeds a distrust by a significant portion of the public of science and technology as related to the quality of our food supply. Widespread misinformation, however, is a characteristic of any society that enjoys freedom of speech and of the press. Advanced technology in instant communication serves misinformation just as it serves accurate information.

In addition to the faddists, we have: (a) the well-meaning scientific experts with too few facts about nutrition, food composition, and human behavior related to food; (b) the self-appointed nutrition experts who qualify themselves on the basis that they eat food regularly; and (c) the eager beavers who demand a graduate course in nutrition, preferably in a 1-hr. session, even though they have never had undergraduate chemistry or physiology.

Regardless of the barriers and hurdles to be cleared, I consider that the challenge comes through loud and clear—the potential that sound, continuing nutrition education offers for health, fulfillment, and productivity is so great that it behooves us to find ways to have a consensus of the basic message and a coordination of efforts to deliver the message to all who can benefit from it. How to do it will take the thoughts and expertise of many . . .

Ruth M. Leverton: Commentary: what is nutrition education, J. Am. Diet. Assoc. **64:**17, 1974. Reprinted by permission. Copyright The American Dietetic Association.

---

be extremely useful to the nutrition educator in developing the overall concepts of nutrition information to be included in the program. In addition, it will be necessary to interpret the guidelines to obtain specific goals with defined behavioral changes for the intended target group. Further discussion of this subject appears in Chapter 6.

To reach all population groups, expanded use of the mass media and the involvement of governmental and private agencies, universities, and food industries is required. The nutrition education component of programs at the community level—in health centers, maternal and child care centers, day care centers, programs for the elderly, and Head Start—are ways to reach the citizenry with the nutrition message.

DIET COUNSELING

In dietetics, as in other health professions, the dietitian/nutritionist's interaction with clients represents a significant proportion of professional activity. More important, however, the health professional's skill in interacting with clients can affect the quality of health care and the client's health status. Although skills in interviewing and counseling are readily accepted as components of competence in the health professions, systematic techniques for assessing these skills have not been widely developed or incorporated into national examination programs.[41]

Diet counseling is the two-way process through which a nutritionist or paraprofessional guides the client or counselee in the development of a dietary plan designed to meet his nutritional requirements. Using an interviewing technique to complete a diet history in an initial orientation, the nutritionist coordinates basic information provided by the client or family members or both with the principles of diet modification

CONCEPTUAL FRAMEWORK FOR NUTRITION EDUCATION*

1. Nutrition is the process by which food and other substances eaten become part of you. The food we eat enables us to live, to grow, to keep healthy and well, and to get energy for work and play.

2. Food is made up of certain chemical substances that work together and interact with body chemicals to serve the needs of the body.
   (a) Each nutrient has specific uses in the body.
   (b) For the healthful individual the nutrients needed by the body are usually available through food.
   (c) Many kinds and combinations of food can lead to a well-balanced diet.
   (d) No natural food, by itself, has all the nutrients needed for full growth and health.

3. The way a food is treated influences the amount of nutrients in the food, its safety, appearance, taste and cost; treatment means everything that happens to food while it is being grown, processed, stored and prepared for eating.

4. All persons, throughout life, have need for the same nutrients, but in varying amounts.
   (a) The amounts needed are influenced by age, sex, size, activity, specific conditions of growth and state of health—the amounts are altered somewhat by environmental stress.
   (b) Suggestions for kinds and needed amounts of

*These concepts were recommended in the panel on Nutrition Education in Schools at the White House Conference on Food, Nutrition and Health, Washington, D.C., 1969.

nutrients are made by scientists who continuously revise the suggestions in the light of the findings of new research.
   (c) A daily food guide is helpful in translating the technical information into terms of everyday foods suitable for individuals and families.

5. Food use relates to the cultural, social, economic and psychological aspects of living as well as to the physiological.
   (a) Food is culturally defined.
   (b) Food selection is an individual act but is usually influenced by social and cultural sanctions.
   (c) Food can be chosen to fulfill physiological needs and at the same time satisfy social, cultural and psychological wants.
   (d) Attitudes toward food are a culmination of many experiences, past and present.

6. The nutrients, singly and in combinations of chemical substances, simulating natural foods, are available in the market; these may vary widely in usefulness, safety and economy.

7. Food plays an important role in the physical and psychological health of a society or a nation just as it does for the individual and the family.
   (a) The maintenance of good nutrition for the larger units of society involves many matters of public concern.
   (b) Nutrition knowledge and social consciousness enable citizens to participate intelligently in the adoption of public policy affecting the nutrition of people around the world.

COMMUNITY NUTRITION: DIAL-A-DIETITIAN

In Columbus, Ohio, anyone can Dial-a-Dietitian any Monday through Friday between 8:00 A.M. and 4:30 P.M. and ask a question about nutrition. An answering service mails each day's questions to the volunteer dietitian-of-the-day who returns all calls within 24 to 48 hr. after receiving the inquiries. Correspondence is kept to a minimum because a one-to-one telephone conversation is the basis for the Dial-a-Dietitian approach to community nutrition education. This nutrition answering service has been available continuously to the residents of Columbus and Franklin County since November 1961. It is appropriate to assess what experience and accumulated data reveal . . .

Data gathered during the decade 1962-1972 on Dial-a-Dietitian as a community service of the Columbus Dietetic Association support the usefulness of this unique experiment in community nutrition education.

The image of the dietitian as a spokesman for the science of nutrition and as a contributing member of the health team should be advanced in every way possible. Dial-a-Dietitian is a realistic vehicle which offers much needed assistance . . .

Margaret Murray Hinkle and *Edith G. Fessler:* A decade of Dial-a-Dietitian in Columbus, Ohio, J. Am. Diet. Assoc. **66**:48, 1978. Reprinted by permission. Copyright The American Dietetic Association.

required for nutritional management of the specific health condition. This counseling process combines skills in questioning, listening, probing, informing, guiding, and negotiating. Listening as an art or skill is fundamental to successful communication, and successful communication is basic to success-

ful professional practice. Some studies report that white collar workers spend approximately 40% of their day listening and that most people listen at only a 25% level of efficiency. Listening as an art is more than technical proficiency.[42]

In interviewing the client, the nutritionist seeks information about usual food intake and factors influencing food intake such as food availability, budget, life-style, work patterns, food preferences, and ethnic and religious influences on food preparation and consumption. The client should be provided with information at his own level of understanding regarding the principles involved in dietary management. Then there should be involvement in making choices and commitments to the modified dietary plan. In working with the client, the diet counselor should focus first on the most critical modification for control and survival. More details and refinements can be included in follow-up sessions where feedback can be used to assess knowledge and ability to cope with dietary change, both on short-term and long-range bases. In the continuing process of diet counseling, the nutritionist must be constantly alert to client and family needs and problems that may develop.

It is the function of the nutrition counselor to make referrals for food or financial assistance, meal programs, homemaker services, public health nursing, or other useful community services, if needed. Although the nutritionist may provide diet counseling most economically in the clinic setting or health center office, home visits for assessment of the family and food preparation facilities may be an important supportive service. Home assessment and support may be done by the nutritionist, public health nurse, trained community health worker, or nutrition aide.

A Committee of the Diet Therapy Section of The American Dietetic Association,* anticipating third-party payment for the services of dietitians in pending health care legislation, have prepared guidelines for diet counseling. These guidelines offer specifics for background knowledge and resources, the major components of diet counseling, and a procedural guide for diet counseling, which includes preparation, interview, plan

---

*Lyllis Ling, R. D., The Children's Mercy Hospital, Kansas City, Missouri; Doris Spragg, R. D., Patricia Stein, R. D., and Madge L. Myers, R. D. (Chairman), University of Kansas Medical Center, Kansas City, Kansas.

for nutritional care, follow-up, and communication.[43]

Specific terminology surfaces when reference is made to diet counseling. Definitions of terms have been presented by a Committee of The American Dietetic Association,[44] as follows:

> *Diet counseling* is ". . . providing individualized professional guidance to assist a person in adjusting his daily food consumption to meet his health needs." The process of diet counseling actually involves three activities: interviewing, counseling, and consulting.
>
> *Interviewing* is the gathering of information and/or data. Expert interviewing requires training and experience, since accurate, selective information is basic to effective counseling.
>
> *Counseling* is listening, accepting, clarifying, and helping the client to form his own conclusions and develop his own plan of action. The focus is on the client. An effective diet counselor must be able to guide the client's thinking, focus on objectives, and interpret and evaluate information accurately and effectively. The counselor translates for the patient the regimen prescribed by the physician.
>
> *Consulting* involves developing plans or proposals for a client, based on observations and evaluations. The consultant has, as a purpose, adding to and enhancing the knowledge and understanding of the person seeking help.

Diet history

Although this subject will be discussed in Chapter 8, it is important enough to mention here.

To individualize the nutritional services to the patient and to make the necessary adjustments for the home diet, a good deal of information regarding the client's food habits is essential. An interview with the client will elicit further information. A general checklist will consist of the following:

> *Dietary history*
>   Meals: where eaten, when, with whom
>   Meals skipped: which, how often
>   Food preparation: by whom, facilities
>   Meals away from home: which, how often,

GUIDELINES FOR NUTRITION COUNSELING

Although there are no hard and fast rules, the authors have found that nutritional counseling goes through the following phases:

(a) Making contact (referral system) . . .
(b) Learning "Where the person is" (assessing nutritional status and attitude).
(c) Developing rapport and mutual respect. The nutritionist must respect the value system of the individual coming for consultation if the two are to communicate freely and openly. If the individual expresses belief in crash dieting to lose weight, the counselor needs to explore his previous failures or successes with weight loss, rather than reprimand him for "wanting the easy way out." If the individual says that he is using health foods, the nutritionist will probably gain no credibility and only isolate herself from the client if she attacks the health food movement. Also, when counseling individuals who espouse macrobiotics, it is well to ferret out the details of the diet. On inquiry, it was learned that one individual who had changed from drugs and "junk" food to a modification of the macrobiotic diet, was actually eating a diet which met the Recommended Dietary Allowances for all nutrients.
(d) Introducing objective knowledge . . .
(e) Incorporating objective knowledge into the value system and setting priorities . . .
(f) Expanding nutritional consciousness . . .
(g) Achieving independence—using the nutritionist as a resource.

The growth phases discussed here are possible in any type of nutritional counseling. As the individual grows toward independent nutritional behavior, he may not fit distinctly into one phase or another, and regression is common. The quality of progress depends on the attitudes of the nutritionist and the person seeking nutritional information.

Judy Wylie and *Jeanne Singer:* Growth process in nutritional community, J. Am. Diet. Assoc. **69:**505, 1976. Reprinted by permission. Copyright The American Dietetic Association.

type of facility (lunch counter, cafeteria, school lunch, restaurant, vending machines)

Typical day's meals: 24-hour recall

Cross-check of day's meals: frequency of use of important food groups in a week, for example, milk, eggs, breakfast, cereals

Snacks: how often, types, amounts

Mineral-vitamin supplements: type, how, reasons for use

Food likes and dislikes: food intolerance, allergies

DIETARY COUNSELING

Many counselor trainers and theoreticians consider counseling to be a two-part process. The first part involves the development of rapport, empathy, and a trusting relationship; the second, the implementation of specific behavior-change strategies and techniques directed at the client's problem(s) . . . An examination of nutrition texts and journals indicates that this two-part process does exist in dietetic counseling . . .

While the dietetic counselor may be well prepared in this second phase of counseling, little or no emphasis has been placed on training in the first phase of the counseling process, that is, the development of a helping relationship. This lack is apparent despite widespread agreement that the development of empathy, rapport, and trust is an essential component of the counseling relationships.

The six relationship-building skills considered essential are:

Stage I: Understanding your needs to be a helper
Stage II: Using effective non-verbal behavior
Stage III: Using effective verbal behavior
Stage IV: Using effective self-involving behavior
Stage V: Understanding others' communication
Stage VI: Establishing effective helping relationships (Danish, S. J., and Hauer, A. L.: Helping skills: a basic training program, New York, 1973, Behavioral Publications.)

To date no studies have been done assessing the effect of training on client behavior. More specifically, the question to be asked is: do the clients of trainees change their behavior and are these changes noticeable to the clients themselves, to the clients' significant "others," and to impartial trained observers? While one would expect all training programs to be interested in such measurements, little, if any, research has been conducted along these lines. However, research is presently being done on the dietetic counseling process to answer this question.

Steven J. Danish: Developing helping relationships in dietetic counseling, J. Am. Diet. Assoc. **67:**107, 1975. Reprinted by permission. Copyright The American Dietetic Association.

Food budgeting: kinds of fruits, vegetables, meats purchased; sources of budget information; menu planning

Previous dietary restrictions: reasons for, type, how long, response to modified diet

Sources of nutrition information: use of advertising, popular publications, books

Effective dietary counseling requires a good deal of experience in communicating purposefully with people and much insight into the behavior of people. Guidelines for effectiveness in diet counseling have been outlined by the Diet Therapy Section of The American Dietetic Association.[45]

The interview will be more successful if the following data, suggested by Robinson and Lawler,[46] are gathered:

Socioeconomic history
  Occupation: hours for work, travel time to and from work
  Family relationships
  Residence: house, apartment, room
  Recreational activities: type, how often
  Ethnic background
  Religious beliefs regarding food
Medical history
  Present illness: chief complaints, especially those relating to nutrition; diagnosis
  Weight: any recent changes, comparison with desirable weight
  Appetite: any recent changes
  Digestion: ability to swallow, anorexia, vomiting, distention, cramps

Elimination: regular, constipation, diarrhea
Handicaps related to feeding: inability to chew, need for self-help devices in eating, inability to prepare food*

SUMMARY

The community health program will, in almost every situation, have a nutrition component that requires the services of a professional nutritionist as part of the health care team. Ideally, the nutritionist both should be an observer and have a knowledge of the community, its unique problems and needs, and thus be able to see to it that services are delivered and used by the community. Within a community the public service program may aim at providing care to a specific in-

---

*Robinson, C. H., and Lawler, M. R.: Normal and therapeutic nutrition. © 1977, The Macmillan Co., New York.

THE NUTRITIONIST IN COMPREHENSIVE HEALTH CARE

The Joseph C. Wilson Health Center, where I serve as a nutritionist in a team effort reimbursed through a prepayment mechanism, was opened in August 1973. This health center is part of the Genesee Valley Group Health Association, the first program of this nature developed and financed in toto by a Blue Cross and Blue Shield system—a subsidiary of Rochester Blue Cross and Blue Shield. Efforts to organize this care plan began in 1969 and, in 1971, the project was the recipient of a grant from DHEW to demonstrate the rapid development of a health maintenance organization.

Comprehensive health care services are provided to enrollees through a contractual relationship with the medical group, headquartered at the health center. The medical group was organized as a multidisciplinary health care group and has as its stated primary objective, to meet the needs of the patient . . .

The success of this multidisciplinary approach is demonstrated by statistics on physician use, enrollment, and rate of hospitalization. Members of the Genesee Valley Group Health Association currently use services at the rate of four visits per member per year. This is significantly below the 1972 national average of 5.2 visits per person per year to a physician and somewhat below the experience of a number of group practices recently sampled, which run approximately 4.5 visits per member per year . . .

In the early organizational phase of this group, the medical director made it clear that he considered nu-

trition services essential. Thus, as nutritionist, I have been part of the group since its inception. Increasingly, I have felt receptive not only toward the mutual respect and appreciation of various skills and talents in the group, but also toward a growing interdependence among our health care professionals—for example, the dependence of physicians on my services as nutritionist. My function is, essentially, to receive referrals from other primary care providers in the medical group. I maintain my own appointment book and follow patients as I see fit. I have added to my skills some simple diagnostic maneuvers, such as measuring blood pressure and ordering appropriate diagnostic studies, so as to facilitate monitoring of the on-going status of individual patients . . .

I have, over the past two years, been an integral part of a health care team and provided nutritional services in a comprehensive health care plan. We, as a team, have effectively demonstrated smooth working relationships among professionals, reduced the number of patients' visits to physicians, reduced hospitalization, and increased patient care satisfaction. The advantages of such a plan should be considered in the planning and development of national health insurance that would provide universal entitlement to the population of this country.

Lois H. Treacy: Dietary counseling in ambulatory care— the nutritionist in a comprehensive health care plan, J. Am. Diet. Assoc. **68:**253, 1976. Reprinted by permission. Copyright The American Dietetic Association.

dividual or group of the life cycle—child-bearing women, infants and children, adolescents, adults, and the elderly.

The most widespread and developed programs to date are the Maternal and Child Health Care Services provided for under Title V of the Social Security Act and the Food Assistance Programs under the auspices of the U.S. Department of Agriculture. These include the WIC Program (Supplemental Food Program for Women, Infants and Children), the Child Nutrition Programs (e.g., National School Lunch Program, Summer Food Program) and Family Food Assistance Programs (e.g., Food Stamp Program, Expanded Food and Nutrition Education Program).

Other programs too are supported by the federal government and have an important nutrition element, such as the Office of Child Development Head Start Program and the Early Periodic Screening, Diagnosis and Treatment under Medicaid. In addition, there are numerous programs that deal specifically with various problems and the relation of nutrition to them—obesity, diabetes, heart disease in adults, adolescent pregnancy, the health of migrant workers and Indian groups, and the need for counseling among certain family units.

All in all, however, the effectiveness of these programs depends on the professionals' ability and willingness to educate the public being served, to represent their interests, and to implement the operation of the program actively. The public health nutritionist employed in local health jurisdictions is urged to become a program planner and manager in a health care system that may or may not be receptive to this administrative role. Feeney presents the case well in the editorial that follows.

FUTURE DIRECTIONS FOR PUBLIC HEALTH NUTRITIONISTS EMPLOYED IN LOCAL HEALTH JURISDICTIONS

Public Health Nutritionists employed in local health jurisdictions are urged to become Program Planners/Managers in a system that does not readily ascribe to their ability to do so, or to their rationale for wanting to be so. A cyclical chain of events often prevents a Public Health Nutritionist from attaining the role of Program Manager:

1. The Public Health Nutritionist wants/should be Manager of the Nutrition Program.
2. The existing Nutrition Program in reality is often the sum of its activities.
3. Nutrition activities need to be expanded into broad-based Programs.
4. Programs require personnel and budget.
5. Many nutritionists employed by local health jurisdictions work alone without supporting staff and readily identifiable budget.
6. Hence, program management is reduced to personal time management.

The process of changing from a time manager to a Program Manager is often obstructed by traditional definitions of nutrition services many times cited in State Codes for health department services. Such codes may narrowly define nutrition services as consisting of community education and staff consultation. Another obstacle to change is the demand/need for direct service often expected by the public and sometimes assumed to be the prime function of a nutritionist even by the Health Officer. A dichotomy exists, then, between the role of a Public Health Nutritionist as perceived by nutrition professionals and that expected by the hiring agency.

Nevertheless, the trend is for nutritionists to view themselves as Program Managers participating in the planning process to assure integration of a nutrition component into preventive health services; securing grant monies to augment budget and staff; and coordinating and supervising nutrition service personnel. Discussion could be generated as to whether this is the appropriate role for a Public Health Nutritionist; assuming it is, certain forces are in effect that can hasten its development:

1. Federal funding of nutrition services that should be an extension of and monitored by an existing nutrition program.
2. Funding of project nutrition personnel who need to be functioning in coordination with the existing nutrition program.
3. Continued interest in health promotion rather than restorative diet counseling.
4. Attempts of nutritionists to identify and articulate role function of Program Manager to their superiors and peers.

Mary Jo Feeney: Future directions for public health nutritionist employed in local health jurisdictions. Presented at 60th Annual American Dietetic Association Convention, Los Angeles, Oct., 1977.

From the role of observer, interpreter of goals, communicator, and imaginator, the nutritionist will have to move with the community group into the action phase. The new role is one of advocacy and with it a new set of skills is required. Preceding the action phase, the nutritionist's role was essentially analytical and educational, clarifying the nutritional risks to a group, establishing the seriousness of consequences, and creating the belief that something can be done about the problems. Now the mission becomes one of making sure that the services are delivered. The nutritionist must be prepared to represent the interests of the groups with whom she has been working. This is social action. Put more positively, the nutritionist advocate is trying to draw the goals of her agency more closely to the population it serves.

REFERENCES

1. Association of State and Territorial Health Officials: Programs and services of state health agencies, fiscal year 1974, ASTHO-HPRS Project, 1555 Connecticut Ave., Suite 202, Washington, D.C. 20036.
2. Ad Hoc Committee, Association of Faculties of Graduate Programs: A survey of college and university undergraduate programs in community nutrition, community dietetics, and public health nutrition: final report of the results of phases I, II, and III, May, 1977.
3. Committee on Maternal Nutrition, Food and Nutrition Board: Maternal nutrition and the course of pregnancy, Washington, D.C., 1970, National Academy of Sciences.
4. Committee on Maternal Nutrition, Food and Nutrition Board: Annotated bibliography on maternal nutrition, Washington, D.C., 1970, National Academy of Sciences.
5. Bureau of Community Health Services, U.S. Department of Health, Education, and Welfare: Interim guidelines for maternal and child health services program of projects under Title V, Social Security Act, Washington, D.C., April, 1975, Government Printing Office.
6. Committee on Nutrition of the Mothers and Preschool Child, Food and Nutrition Board, National Research Council: Oral contraceptives and nutrition, Washington, D.C., 1976, National Academy of Sciences.
7. Peck, E. B.: Nutrition education specialists: time for action, J. Nutr. Ed. 8:11, 1976.
8. Ullrich, H. D.: Is this progress? J. Nutr. Ed. 7:6, 1975.
9. Poolton, M. A.: What does the nutrition education specialist need to know? J. Nutr. Ed. 9:105, 1977.
10. Weigley, E. S.: The pregnant adolescent, J. Am. Diet. Assoc. 66:588, 1975.
11. The school-age pregnant girl (editorial), J. School Health 41:347, 1971.
12. Goldstein, P. J., Zalar, M. K., Grady, E. W., and Smith, R. W.: Vocational education: an unusual approach to adolescent pregnancy, J. Reprod. Med. 10:77, 1973.
13. Backalenick, I.: A school program designed to help pregnant teenagers, N.Y. Times, p. 34, June 14, 1974.
14. Milk, J. C.: Adolescent parenthood, J. Home. Econ. 65:31, Nov., 1973.
15. Anderson, R. S.: Meeting the needs of the pregnant teenager, Ill. Teacher Home Econ. 17:14, Sept.-Oct., 1973.
16. Osofsky, H. J., Rajan, R., Wood, P. W., and Diflorio, R.: An interdisciplinary program for low income pregnant schoolgirls: a progress report, J. Reprod. Med. 5:103, 1970.
17. Hansen, C. M., Brown, M. L., and Trontell, M.: Effects on pregnant adolescents of attending a special school, J. Am. Diet. Assoc. 68:538, 1976.
18. Huyck, N. L.: Nutrition services for pregnant teenagers, J. Am. Diet. Assoc. 69:60, 1976.
19. U.S. Senate Select Committee on Nutrition and Human Needs: National nutrition policy study report and recommendations, VIII, Washington, D.C., 1974, Government Printing Office.
20. WIC Program interim regulations, Section 246.8, Nutrition Education, Washington, D.C., Jan. 8, 1976, Government Printing Office.
21. Food and Nutrition Services: Report to Congress by the Comptroller General on Evaluation of the Supplemental Food Program, Washington, D.C., Dec. 18, 1974, Government Printing Office.
22. The Urban Institute: Toward efficiency and effectiveness in the WIC delivery system, Washington, D.C., April, 1976, Government Printing Office.
23. Board of Inquiry, Citizens Crusade Against Poverty, Committee on School Lunch Participation: Their daily bread, 10 Columbus Circle, New York, 1968.

24. USDA federal feeding programs, Newsletter of the Food and Nutrition Service, Food and Nutrition, no. 45, March 8, 1976.

25. Community Nutrition Institute Weekly Report **7:**36, Sept. 15, 1977.

26. Community services administration, Federal Register, vol. 42, no. 116, June 16, 1977.

27. Dillon, H. L.: Improvement of the quality of life through a food and nutrition project, J. Am. Diet. Assoc. **67:**129, 1975.

28. Sullivan, H. J., Gere, M., Nowlin, B. J., and Kloehn, B.: Development of a nutrition education program for homemakers, J. Nutr. Ed. **8:**118, 1976.

29. Yanochik, A. V., Eichelberger, C. I., Dandoy, S. E.: The Comprehensive Nutrition Action Program in Arizona, J. Am. Diet. Assoc. **69:**37, 1976.

30. Frankle, R. T., Christakis, G.: Community nutrition teams, Hospitals **47:**56, 1973.

31. Bass, M. A.: Nutrient intake and food patterns of Indians on Standing Rock Reservation, J. Am. Diet. Assoc. **64:**34, 1974.

32. Social and Rehabilitation Service: Nutrition program for the elderly, Federal Register vol. 37, no. 162, 1972.

33. Administration on Aging: National Nutrition Program for the Elderly, Fact Sheet, DHEW publication no. (OHD) 75-20230, 1975.

34. Wells, C. E.: Nutrition programs under the Older Americans Act. In Symposium on Nutrition and Aging, Washington, D.C., 1973, Government Printing Office.

35. Facts about older Americans 1975, DHEW publication no. (OHD) 75-20007, 1975.

36. Watkin, D. M.: Nutrition for the aged: a summation. In Symposium on Nutrition and Aging, Washington, D.C., 1973, Government Printing Office.

37. National Meals-on-Wheels Program, U.S. Senate. Select Committee Hearing on Nutrition and Human Needs, April 4, 1977, Washington, D.C., Government Printing Office.

38. Position paper on nutrition education for the public, J. Am. Diet. Assoc. **62:**520, 1973.

39. Leverton, R.: What is nutrition education? J. Am. Diet. Assoc. **64:**17, 1974.

40. Gifft, H. H., Washbon, M. B., and Harrison, G. G.: Nutrition, behavior, and change, 1972, Englewood Cliffs, N.J., Prentice-Hall, Inc.

41. Andrews, B. J.: Interviewing and counseling skills, J. Am. Diet. Assoc. **66:**576, 1975.

42. Simonds, S. K.: Psychosocial determinants of dietitian's listening patterns, J. Am. Diet. Assoc. **63:**615, 1973.

43. The American Dietetic Association: Guidelines for Diet Counseling **66:**571, 1975.

44. The American Dietetic Association: Community Nutrition and Diet Therapy Section: Guidelines for developing dietary counseling services in the community, J. Am. Diet. Assoc. **55:**343, 1969.

45. The American Dietetic Association: Position paper on the nutrition component of health services delivery systems, J. Am. Diet. Assoc. **58:**538, 1971.

46. Robinson, C. H., and Lawler, M. R.: Normal and therapeutic nutrition, New York, 1977, The Macmillan Co.

GENERAL CONCEPT

The action plan is the method to achieve objectives. It involves a statement of the expected results, the systems needed to accomplish the plan, an estimate of necessary manpower and community resources, a system for training professionals, and a consideration of the audience and critics—the consumer participation (Fig. 6-1).

OUTCOMES

The student should be able to do the following:
- Design an action plan with essential components.
- Describe the four component system to deliver services.
- Provide a training curriculum to develop manpower.
- Implement a training program that includes assessment of trainees.

The action plan and behavioral change

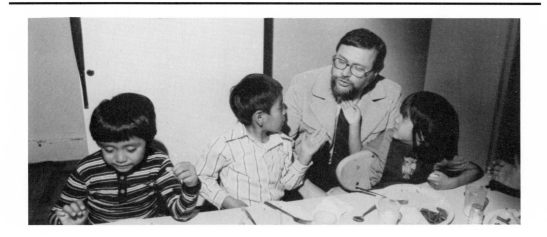

In Chapter 4, which discussed how to plan and elements in the planning process, steps 1 through 8 of the analysis required in developing a program plan were presented. To review, this includes (1) a determination of the need with the identification of the problem plus a clear description of the problem; (2) the development of an action plan concerned with what the program would accomplish, including a statement of goals and specific objectives in precise terms; and (3) a list of priorities for the plan that answer the questions: Is service needed? Is service doable? Is service affordable?

We now proceed to steps 9 through 15 (Fig. 6-1), which are concerned with an action plan to achieve the determined objectives. (See Fig. 3-3 for entire analysis of program plan.)

In Chapter 4 the planning process was discussed in terms of how to meet the needs of a community. Basically, the action plan itself will state the health problems of the community, specific objectives that will reduce those problems, the priorities for action, the methods through which objectives will be reached, and how the accomplishments will be evaluated. Previous chapters have discussed how to define the problems and how to write specific measurable objectives. This chapter will describe a specific action plan for meeting objectives, and Chapter 9 will detail how to evaluate the program's progress. The methods used to implement the action plan must lead to a measurable outcome —some specific improvement in health status. Improving health status depends on achieving desired behavioral change in individual clients and, hopefully, the community at large. This depends on systematic methods and trained personnel.

SYSTEMATIC AND REALISTIC METHODS

The methods used to implement the action plan must be systematic and realistic. Systematic implies that the steps which are

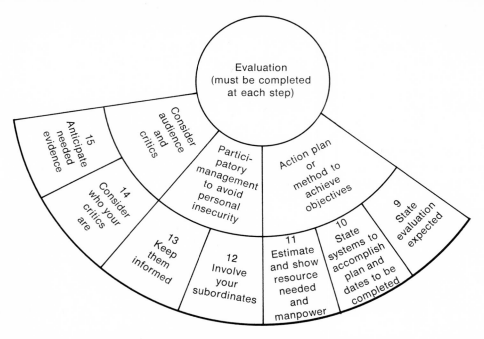

Fig. 6-1. Analyses required in developing a program plan.

taken to meet objectives should fit together as a cohesive whole. Clearly stating objectives will be a great help in making methods systematic. Too often, public health practitioners scurry from one crisis to another. A systematic plan will help personnel see the big picture so that all efforts are coordinated toward a stated outcome, such as reducing the prevalence of obesity in infants.

A systematic approach first recognizes resources. In public health the resources are usually limited. Neither the funds nor the manpower to improve the health of everyone in the community is generally available. Even the support of community leaders or legislators may be lacking. A realistic method of meeting objectives must be based on recognizing that the program cannot do everything, and so priorities must be established. For instance, it may be ideal to give one-to-one counseling on food choices to every family, but that is unrealistic.

There are three ways to make a methodology realistic. First, a priority should be established for the problems that face the community, starting with the most pressing

problems that are solvable. The nutritionist should not try to deal with all problems, large or small. For example, the hypothetical community had problems in cardiovascular disease, cancer, accidents, diabetes, anemia, and obesity, but a program should be limited to the problem that can be affected, such as obesity and/or anemia. Second, realizing that one cannot do everything for everyone, the nutritionist should identify other resources which may be able to help meet objectives. For example, the objective to reduce premature births may be shared by other groups such as the March of Dimes, the American College of Obstetricians and Gynecologists, and Health Systems Agencies. Incorporating these other agencies into a plan will make it more effective and likely to succeed. Third, the identified problem may be so extensive that it is unrealistic to tackle the entire problem. Therefore the objectives should be to demonstrate in a small subsample the potential benefits of the program. A pilot program is a more realistic approach than implementing a plan statewide when there are not statewide resources.

A systematic delivery system will be based on written procedures as to records and methods for recording and retrieving nutrition data, job descriptions, protocols for continuity of services, nutrition education plan, and an organization chart that defines responsibilities for carrying out the system, as well as an action plan. These tools should be developed early in the system because they delineate the relationships between the components of the system. They also help communicate the implementation of the plan to staff and other interested parties.

FOUR COMPONENT SYSTEM TO DELIVER SERVICES

One example of a systematic and realistic way to deliver services is through a system divided into four components: (1) screening, (2) referral, (3) follow-up, and (4) manpower development. This four component system can be applied to many public health situations where the desired outcome depends on changing clients' behavior. Client education is an integral part of this four component system.

Step 1. Screening

In the first phase of this system, various screening procedures are used to assess the needs of the population. The screening process, which includes nutrition assessment and the surveillance system that follows, is the first step in determining the need for services to clients. This important subject will be discussed in detail in Chapters 7 and 8. Another major part of the screening process should be educating individuals on what each procedure tells about health status. Screening also identifies individuals who are in need of immediate services because they demonstrate a high risk of developing health problems. For example, screening will uncover some clients with anemia, some with obesity. These may be the people who need nutrition intervention the most. Those who have normal screening values may or may not need diet counseling, but the nutritionist should remember that it is unrealistic to attempt to provide services to everyone in the community. Screening helps select those who need services the most.

If answers to the dietary screening questions suggest that habits of eating are unusual or that the diet itself is unusual or monotonous, an interview with a nutritionist should be arranged. If no evidence of dietary inadequacy is found and if the individual also "passes" the other phases of screening (physical examination, anthropometric evaluation, laboratory studies), no further evaluation will be scheduled for one or two years.

Step 2. Referral

The second component of an organized program would be the referral system, which should encompass a network that includes all services internal to the health department and all health and social services external to the health department.

The nutritionist should develop an effective system of coordination to strengthen nutrition services and prevent duplicating and conflicting information. For example, the content of educational and therapeutic guidelines for nutrition services should be agreed on so that clients are not confused and action is consistent.

The referral system has two functions, both ensuring that the client gets comprehensive services. First, a comprehensive network of services can offer solutions to clients' problems that a nutritionist's particular program does not have the resources to solve. Thus problems that already have been identified will be followed up by other agencies. Second, a two-way street, the referral system informs clients about a nutrition program by making them aware of their need for and benefits from that service. The economist would say that the referral system increases the marketability of one's product (i.e., nutrition services). Obviously, the program will not survive if the community does not demand it!

Consumer participation and community resources

At some time in the planning, preferably at an early point, thought should be given to how to organize the community. A general meeting of all community parties will be necessary to determine their interests and gain a common dedication with continuing support to develop the health program. With the passage of the National Health Planning and Resource Development Act of 1974, health councils may already be formed. Therefore it is important to determine if this mechanism already exists before proceeding with the development of another health council.

Consumer participation in health planning is a valuable principle, and, as such, it is too important to be allowed to degenerate into a slogan that can be all things to all people, with precise meaning for none. On the subject of consumer participation in health programs, Kane and Kane[1] ask the following questions: What is it? Why is it useful in health planning? Whom does it benefit? How should it be implemented? What are the potential problems? Should the goal and method of implementing consumer participation be identical across different programs and different population groups? The reader interested in answers to these question is referred to "Galloping Consumption: Consumer Participation in Health Programs."[1]

The support and involvement of community residents and agencies are essential. Health programs planned and operated without citizen participation may be ineffective, even though they offer health services that are of high quality, economical in cost, and easily accessible. A health program's success will depend on a cooperative effort by the local medical society, community groups and individuals, and institutions that are concerned with improving the health of the community. A checklist of persons and agencies who should be involved in community health programs is given in Appendix 6-1. This provides information on available community resources such as health service providers and educational institutions, influential community groups and individuals, and consumers of health services. A knowledge of these community resources will enhance the referral system.

In implementing nutrition services, cooperation, coordination, and referral between individuals, agencies, and groups in the community such as the following are important:

- Nutrition personnel of state and local health agencies and special projects. By maintaining close working relationships with one another, it will be possible to share information and coordinate goals, objectives, program plans, standards, and criteria for service.
- Nutritionists and other personnel in nonhealth agencies such as the welfare department, extension service, or homemaker service agency. Such agencies have educational or service programs that will be supportive of health care plans for individuals and families in areas such as food marketing, menu planning, food preparation, and home management.
- Nutritionists and dietitians in ambulatory health programs, treatment centers, and other group care facilities. Linkage with treatment centers is necessary for appropriate follow-up of clients on special dietary regimens who return to the home community.
- Nutritionists and other health care providers. An organized system of interdisciplinary referral for nutrition counseling is essential even in a small project, and procedures for referral between the nutritionist and the physician, nurse, and other health workers should be established.

Referral procedures are essential for continuity of care and for maximization of services available from other resources. Jointly agreed-on plans for organized procedures should be made for referral and for monitoring progress.

A nutrition referral form should include the following minimum information:

- Client identification, age, address, and telephone
- Name of referring professional or agency with address and telephone
- Diagnosis or reason for referral
- Type of service needed

Table 6-1. Problem-oriented referral system

Problem	Agency
Educational	Child day care facilities School systems Vocational training programs Department of Mental Retardation Veterans Administration Bureau of Indian Affairs Migrant opportunity program Community action programs
Economic	Employment services Vocational training program Rehabilitation programs Welfare, including food assistance programs Religious and other voluntary organizations Bureau of Indian Affairs Social Security
Medical	Hospitals Health department—state, county, and city School nurses Local physicians Crippled children's services Veterans Administration Hospital Indian Health Service Other local health services
Social	Child care facilities School systems Legal aid Local service and religious organizations Volunteer organizations Mental health services Migrant opportunity program Community action programs Welfare
Transportation	Local service and religious organizations Volunteer organizations Migrant opportunity program Community action programs
Environment	State and county health department Public service and utility companies Local government officials Agricultural extension programs
Food	Welfare, including food assistance programs Local service and religious organizations Volunteer organizations Migrant opportunities program Community action programs School lunch program Agricultural extension programs

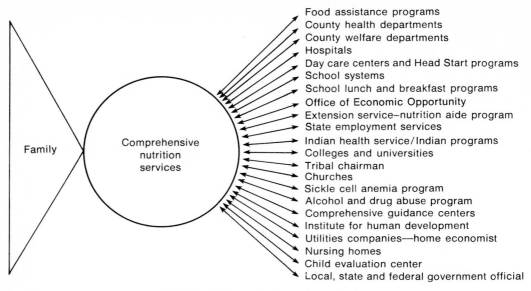

Food assistance programs
County health departments
County welfare departments
Hospitals
Day care centers and Head Start programs
School systems
School lunch and breakfast programs
Office of Economic Opportunity
Extension service–nutrition aide program
State employment services
Indian health service/Indian programs
Colleges and universities
Tribal chairman
Churches
Sickle cell anemia program
Alcohol and drug abuse program
Comprehensive guidance centers
Institute for human development
Utilities companies—home economist
Nursing homes
Child evaluation center
Local, state and federal government official

Fig. 6-2. Nutrition services referral system.

- Specific diet prescription (if applicable)
- Where nutrition services report is to be sent
- Identification of other consulting professionals presently or recently dealing with the client

A schematic diagram (Fig. 6-2) illustrates the nutrition services referral system from community to family and/or from family to community.

An example of a referral system that is problem oriented and matched to existing agencies is shown in Table 6-1.

Step 3. Follow-up

The third component of a delivery system is the actual client follow-up. If there is a suggestion of dietary inadequacy, another study (e.g., specific laboratory tests to confirm the suspicion and/or dietary counseling) should be indicated. Follow-up in a few months is generally desirable. When suggestive evidence of nutritional deficiency is detected by physical examination, appropriate laboratory studies should be undertaken to determine whether a nutritional deficiency actually exists. In some instances an interview with a nutritionist will be desirable in

BEHAVIORAL CHANGE VS. INFORMING THE CLIENT

Educators are still wrestling with their role as change agents. Some educators believe their job is complete when they have informed their client on the pros and cons of their actions. For instance, a health educator might list reasons for smoking and reasons for not smoking and then bow out to let the client make up his own mind. This laissez-faire attitude seems very democratic. After all, we cannot control people's behavior, and it is their choice whether to smoke. This is a dangerous stance for educators to take. How can an educator evaluate his effectiveness? The educator should admit that his purpose is to decrease smoking. If people stop, it is because the educator influenced them to do so. If not, he has not found the argument which will move his client to stop smoking.

Morissa White and *James Rye:* Nutrition program, Arizona State Department of Health, 1977, Phoenix.

addition to or in lieu of laboratory studies. Whenever laboratory findings confirm clinical signs of nutritional deficiency, an interview with a nutritionist should be considered essential. Once the problem has been identified at screening (e.g., anemia, obesity, cardiovascular disease risk, others), a client care plan must be developed to enable the nu-

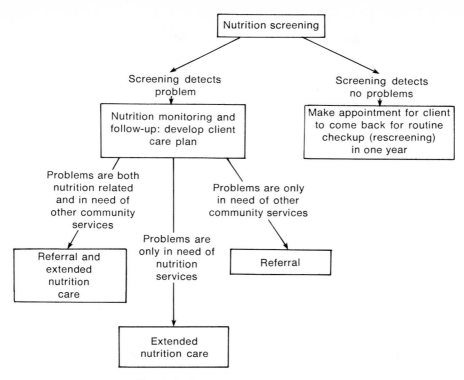

Fig. 6-3. Service delivery flow chart.

tritionist to provide follow-up care. The type of client problem will determine the design of the client care plan, which may be of three different types: a referral to another service; extended nutrition care; or a combination of referral and extended nutrition care. A Service Delivery Flow Chart (Fig. 6-3) illustrates the generation of each type of client care plan.

All of the client care plans have three common goals: (1) to increase the client's knowledge and skills in his needs area, (2) to obtain desired behavioral change, and (3) to improve health status and maintain that improvement.

Two tools are valuable aids in developing, implementing, and evaluating the client's individualized care plan:

1. *Protocols*, developed by the nutrition staff, designate what screening levels constitute risk, at what point and when to make referrals, when to evaluate for health status change, and what subject matter should be covered in client education. (See Appendixes 6-2 and 6-3.)

2. *Nutrition education plan* consists of segments devoted to each nutrition problem that requires intervention. Each segment of the plan should contain (a) behavioral objectives that state what the client needs to know and/or be able to do to help solve his health problem(s); (b) learning activities that teach the client to meet the objectives stated in each problem's protocol; and (c) an assessment or a test that enables the nutritionist, nutrition aide, or community worker to determine if the client knows or can perform what is stated in the objective. The plan can then be used with the protocols to (a) select appropriate behavioral objectives that the client needs to meet, (b) select learning activity(s) to teach the client, (c) select an assessment or test to determine if knowledge or skills have been gained, and (d) evaluate to discover whether the client's behavior and health status has changed (Appendix 6-4).

GOOD NUTRITION EDUCATION VS. THE TRADITIONAL APPROACH

There is nothing more boring than sitting down to a lecture on the nutrients from amino acids to zinc. Yet, that is how many nutritionists deliver nutrition education. How much more effective it is to let the client see an association between his own health status, the food he eats, and the nutrients the food contains. Good nutrition education should start where the client is. What are his current health problems and interests, and what are the health problems he risks in the future? Simple screening including dietary history can identify a client's nutritional status as well as his risk of future health problems. If change is necessary to improve a health problem, that change must be incorporated into the client's entire lifestyle. Changes should be small, and be made one at a time. Good nutrition education strongly considers all the variables that influence a person's food choice, including culture, economics, and taste, and of course nutritional value.

Traditionally, nutritionists have relied on pamphlets, recipes, and handouts. These are passive techniques which do not fit everyone's learning style. The client may also ignore them because they do not refer to his situation. Food intake is personal, and any attempt to change food intake should be personalized. The client should be actively involved in determining the changes necessary in his diet. Another point to keep in mind is that good nutrition education demands follow-up. The client should be praised for positive changes no matter how small, and shown his evaluation measurements as proof that the changes he made had an effect on his health status.

Morissa White and *James Rye:* Nutrition program, Arizona State Department of Health, 1977, Phoenix.

Developing the client care plan

The following suggestions are helpful in developing each of the three broad client care plans and the use of a nutrition education plan:

1. Referral plan. If a client has problems that only other services could solve, his care plan would consist of the following four steps:
   a. Identifying community services (e.g., food stamps or unemployment services) that could be of assistance (Appendix 6-5)
   b. Educating the client about why he needs the service, what the service can do for him, the eligibility requirements of the service, and where and when to make the contact

c. Referring the client through a written or verbal communication to the available service
   d. Follow-up to determine if the client made the referral contact and is receiving services
2. Extended nutrition care plan. Clients who show health problems that demand monitoring and follow-up by the nutrition program need to have an extended nutrition care plan. The plan will be individualized with respect to the client's nutrition-related health problems and must include the following:
   a. An educational component that teaches the client knowledge and skills needed to help improve his health status and maintain that improvement
   b. A component that states regular client/health worker appointments and what and when evaluation mechanisms must be carried out to monitor change in health status and reassess the client's needs
3. Referral and extended nutrition care plan. Most often a client in need of extended nutrition care will also need the attention of other community services (e.g., prenatal care, well child services, family planning clinics, special medical attention, behavioral health services, food programs). Such a plan should include the following:
   a. Educating the client about his problems and referral services that can help solve those problems
   b. Making referrals to the appropriate services while continuing to educate the client about his nutrition-related problems
   c. Regular client/health worker appointment and evaluation mechanisms to determine if referral contacts were made and to monitor the client's cognitive, behavioral, and health status change

Step 4. Manpower development

The fourth component of the entire health care delivery system will be the identification and training of individuals who will be implementing the action plan. Services may have to be delivered through existing manpower, such as public health nurses, or it may be possible to hire additional manpower. If so, it would be wise to consider hiring paraprofessionals.

The use of paraprofessionals, indigenous to a community, to provide direct services to clientele has the following advantages:

1. The paraprofessional is familiar with the community's services and economic and social structure.

2. The paraprofessional is knowledgeable about local life-styles and ethnic backgrounds and also can identify acceptable solutions to the client's problems.

3. The professional is then free to extend his or her expertise by functioning in several other ways. He or she can concentrate on promoting comprehensive health care by establishing community relations with school systems and providers of other social and health services, by analyzing program screening and evaluation data to document and report program benefits and needs, and by writing proposals and budgets to justify existing programs and documenting the need for new nutrition-related programs.

4. The same number of clients can be served effectively at a lower cost, and more clients can be seen each day with in-depth services. Both the reduced health care costs and the increase in client visits through the use of paraprofessionals have been documented in programs that use physician extenders, nurse practitioners, and community health aides.[2-6]

CURRICULUM DEVELOPMENT

Whether using existing or new personnel, the staff must be trained to deliver services. This training should not be haphazard but, instead, should follow a plan consistent with the services plan. The training plan can be called a curriculum, and it should have the following four basic components: (1) learner needs, (2) instructional objectives, (3) learning experiences, and (4) assessment (evaluation). Thus the outline of the curriculum follows the same pattern as the outline of the plan. First, a problem that needs to be solved

USE OF PARAPROFESSIONALS

The increasing demands for health services have brought to light a severe shortage of professional health manpower, especially in rural areas. The use of paraprofessionals is a potential answer to this shortage. The aide who speaks the language and knows the culture of the clients can communicate client needs to the health system.

Paraprofessionals have been shown to be effective, given the proper training and supervision. They can carry out not only routine tasks, but take on many of the functions which professionals have traditionally reserved for themselves. For this reason, many insecure professionals are not comfortable with community aides. The professionals feel their jobs may be threatened. It is short-sighted to deny the efficiency, effectiveness and practical necessity of hiring paraprofessionals. The use of paraprofessionals redefines the professional's role into that of in-service trainer, supervisor, and program planner. The professional who uses paraprofessionals effectively can extend his ability to reach people and can design and evaluate long-range, comprehensive programs rather than spend the same time counseling individuals.

Morissa White and *James Rye:* Nutrition program, Arizona State Department of Health, 1977, Phoenix.

is identified, second, objectives are stated, third, how the objectives are to be met is specified ("method" in the services plan or "learning experiences" in a training program), and fourth, the outcome is evaluated.

Once procedures for screening, referring, and following up patients are delineated, the staff must learn them. After a short initial training the staff's regular in-service training should be integrated with providing direct nutrition services to clientele. The staff ought to apply their recently acquired knowledge and skills immediately so that they both recognize the relevance of the training program to the job functions and, furthermore, develop and maintain the knowledge and skills gained in the training program.

DEVELOPING A TRAINING CURRICULUM

The concept of using a curriculum for training may be easier to understand if one first relates it to oneself. For example, right now, you are the learner and we are the trainers. We used the four basic categories of a curriculum to prepare this chapter. The *learner needs* are knowledge and skills to implement a nutrition program plan. The overall *instructional objective* is that after studying this chapter, the learner will be able to explain in writing how to implement a nutrition program plan for a model community; the learner's written explanations must meet the instructor's approval. The learning experience is, of course, this chapter as well as any other related activities and readings, and the assessment might be the successful completion of a nutrition program plan for a specific community.

The four categories of the training curriculum can be set up in the following "curriculum format."

Knowledge and/or skills learner needs for competent job performance	Instructional objectives	Learning activities	Assessment

Before we elaborate on this curriculum format, it is helpful to discuss in more detail the needs of the learner.

Learner needs

The staff should be able to deliver nutrition services through the screening, referral, monitoring, and follow-up systems. There are three levels of training needed in each system. First, staff members must know the rationale for each system and have a basic subject matter background pertaining to the offered services. Second, they have to know the mechanics of implementing that system. Third, they have to be taught how to educate clients to attain a decrease in health problems and indicate to them the risks of allowing these problems to develop. In turn, clients should be motivated to (1) increase their knowledge and skills in health care areas and (2) apply the knowledge and skills to improve their health or behavior.

Taking the systems one at a time, the knowledge and skills a trainee needs can be described. Within each system it will also be important to put in priority order each

objective, that is, which skill should be taught first, second, third, etc.

For the screening system trainees need to know *why* they are performing certain measurements, or the rationale behind them. What do height and weight measurements tell about a person's nutritional status? What does a hemoglobin test tell and what do the results or values mean? Next, the trainee needs to know *how* to screen. What is the correct way to measure height? What is the procedure for taking somebody's weight? How is blood drawn and processed for determining anemia? Finally, the trainee must develop skills to teach his client the importance of screening measurements. The trainee can use the results of screening to motivate his client if the trainee is taught educational techniques. For example, a staff member might have a client plot his own height and weight on a growth grid. If the client is obese, the screening results will show up dramatically on the growth chart and the trainee can point out that only 5% of the population is heavier than the client. This in itself may be enough to motivate the client to start a weight reduction program, but this motivation technique will not work for all clients. The training curriculum should suggest a variety of different methodologies to motivate a client from which a staff member can choose.

In the referral system a trainee should be taught the rationale for developing a referral network. As noted earlier, a referral network increases the chances that the client will receive comprehensive services and is a way of extending the effectiveness of a program. A trainee needs to know who the other agencies or people are, and this list would be the basic subject matter of the referral system. The mechanics of the referral system include how and when to make referrals. Does the agency require a form? What method of feedback would be most helpful? In addition to knowing where, why, and how to refer, the trainee must also motivate his client to follow up on referrals. The curriculum should include

Knowledge and skills learner needs for competent job performance	Instructional objectives	Learning activities	Assessment
I. SCREENING			
A. Subject matter			
1.	1.	1.	1.
2.	2.	2.	2.
3.	3.	3.	3.
B. Mechanics			
1.	1.	1.	1.
2.	2.	2.	2.
3.	3.	3.	3.
C. Educational methodology			
1.	1.	1.	1.
2.	2.	2.	2.
3.	3.	3.	3.
II. REFERRAL			
A. Subject matter			
1.	1.	1.	1.
2.	2.	2.	2.
3.	3.	3.	3.
B. Mechanics			
1.	1.	1.	1.
2.	2.	2.	2.
3.	3.	3.	3.
C. Educational methodology			
1.	1.	1.	1.
2.	2.	2.	2.
3.	3.	3.	3.
III. MONITORING AND FOLLOW-UP			
A. Subject matter			
1.	1.	1.	1.
2.	2.	2.	2.
3.	3.	3.	3.
B. Mechanics			
1.	1.	1.	1.
2.	2.	2.	2.
3.	3.	3.	3.
C. Educational methodology			
1.	1.	1.	1.
2.	2.	2.	2.
3.	3.	3.	3.

Fig. 6-4. Training curriculum format.

techniques that would enable the staff to motivate their clients. For example, a client might be motivated to follow up on the referrals if he is told that the success of the program's efforts depends on his clearing up his other problems first.

The follow-up system probably requires the most training. The basic subject matter will be the problem's specific protocols and the portion of the nutrition education plan that the staff will follow in combating nutritional problems. For this the staff must be trained in basic nutrition, nutrient needs throughout life, therapeutic diets, weight reduction, and other nutrition topics specific to the problems of one's community.

The staff also will need to be trained in the mechanics of follow-up. For example, how do they make and record appointments? How do they write a diet care plan? Where do they get the materials for teaching a client basic nutrition?

In the follow-up system the education methodology is all-important. It is not enough that the staff know basic nutrition or that they can write a client care plan which distinctly states the objectives, for example, "client will recognize when to introduce solid foods in an infant's diet." It is vitally important that the staff know techniques of motivating the client to use this knowledge to change his behavior. The thrust of the program is to encourage clients to change their behavior to improve their nutritional status. Thus one of the greatest training needs will be to teach the staff how to motivate clients to change their behavior. Having established training needs, the staff now can state objectives precisely, specify learning activities, and assess achievements.

A more elaborate form of the training curriculum format is shown in Fig. 6-4.

The other three categories of the training curriculum are the *instructional objectives, learning experiences,* and *assessment.*

Instructional objectives

Once the learner needs that are necessary to perform in the nutrition delivery system are identified, instruction must be provided to the learner. The important thing to do now is to decide what the outcome of this instruction should be. In other words, what should the learner be able to do as a result of instruction given in a certain area? Well-written instructional objectives state the desired result or outcome of instruction. A set of well-written instructional objectives for the instructor is analogous to a well-drafted blueprint for an architect that defines direction and outcome. The objectives will identify both to the instructor and the student, or trainee, exactly what the trainee is supposed to know or be able to do. The instructional objectives will make it easy for the instructor to do the following:

1. Develop pretest items to evaluate whether the trainee already knows or can perform what the objective requires (i.e., meet the objective).
2. Select appropriate subject matter and instructional techniques to teach the trainee to meet the objective.
3. Develop posttest items to assess or evaluate the outcome of instruction.

Both Mager[7] and Lynch and Holloway[8] provide excellent guidance in writing instructional objectives, and they may be referred to for further detail.

However, adapted from their example is the following well-written instructional objective. It has been developed from a need that the learner must satisfy to function competently in the referral system. The need can be stated as follows: "How does one correctly fill out a referral form?" The instructional objective can be stated as follows: "Given a case study that describes a client in need of three other community health services and a Z-21 referral form, the trainee will correctly fill out the referral form for one of these services. The form must be filled out with the appropriate information for all four items on the form." This instructional objective, like all others, has four main components. It can be broken down into its components as follows:

1. Condition—Given a case study that describes a client in need of three other

community health services and a Z-21 referral form.

2. Learner—the trainee.
3. Behavior or performance—will correctly fill out the referral form for one of these services.
4. Criterion—The form must be filled out with the appropriate information for all four items on the form.

The *condition* describes the conditions under which the trainee must perform. The *learner* tells who it is that is required to perform. The *behavior or performance* contains an action verb and states what you want the learner to be able to do (as a result of instruction). (Refer to objectives below.) The *criterion* states

---

THE VERB IN INSTRUCTIONAL OBJECTIVES

It is critical to use a verb in the instructional objective that states an observable behavior. Verbs such as "understand," "realize," "recognize," "appreciate," and "see" do not state a readily observable behavior, and therefore it is difficult for both the learner and instructor to determine if the instructional objective was achieved. There are many action verbs that do state a measurable behavior, and therefore are useful in the objective-writing process. Additionally, these action verbs can be categorized under six levels of behavior, ranging from simple to the more complex. These levels of behavior are more properly called "cognitive outcomes." This list contains some action verbs that have been categorized according to function. The list contains some action verbs that do the following:

Knowledge	Comprehension	Application
define	translate	interpret
repeat	restate	apply
record	discuss	employ
list	describe	demonstrate
recall	identify	use
name	locate	dramatize
underline	report	schedule

Analysis	Synthesis	Evaluation
distinguish	plan	judge
analyze	propose	evaluate
differentiate	design	rate
appraise	formulate	compare
calculate	arrange	revise
experiment	assemble	score
test	collect	select
compare	construct	

Arizona Department of Health and Nutrition Bureau.

---

the degree of accuracy with which the learner must perform, that is, how accurate the learner must be to "meet" the objective.

These instructional objectives state a behavior that is an important job function. We could further specify this behavior as the "terminal" behavior. The trainee can readily understand the purpose of mastering an instructional objective that states a job performance, and the trainer will be able to assess the trainee through an on-the-job or job-related performance. However, oftentimes background knowledge and skills must be learned to master an objective that states as its behavior a job performance. Frequently, the instructor attempts to state all the knowledge and skills as well as the "terminal behavior" in one instructional objective. It is less frustrating to state "enabling behaviors" separately from the "terminal behavior." For example, in the case of the referral system, it would be ideal for trainees to demonstrate that they have acquired certain knowledge and skills dealing with the referral system prior to demonstrating the ability to complete a referral form correctly. These prior knowledge and skills demonstrations would give trainees a background in the referral system and also enable them to demonstrate the ability to complete a referral form correctly. Some examples of enabling behaviors that may be desirable to have the trainee demonstrate prior to completing the referral forms are as follows:

1. Explaining what is meant by comprehensive health care
2. Identifying a certain number of other health and social services in the community
3. Interviewing other health and social services regarding their function and eligibility requirements
4. Constructing a referral list of health and social services
5. Identifying clients in need of services on the referral list and explaining why

Learning experiences

In developing any learning experience, the developer's principal focus should be to provide experience that will enable the learner to perform as stated in the instructional objective. Ideally, the final part of a learning experience should have the trainee practicing the behavior stated in the objective. In other words, the experience should enable the learner to meet the objective. In developing a learning experience, two factors must be considered: (1) what the *content*, or subject matter, will be and (2) how to teach the subject matter (the process or technique to be used). The learning experience should have as its principal *content* the subject matter most directly related to the knowledge and/or skill needed.

The technique one chooses will depend on the following six factors: (1) the size of the learner group; (2) the learner's style of learning; (3) the relevance of the technique to the job situation for which the trainee is being trained; (4) the desire to maximize trainee participation; (5) the resources available to the trainer; and (6) the comfort, confidence, and competence of both trainee and trainer.

Many techniques for teaching the subject matter have been identified[9-11] and can be put into four categories as follows: (1) presentation techniques, (2) participation techniques, (3) simulation techniques, and (4) human relations techniques.

Presentation techniques are employable in both large and small groups and include lecture, television videotape, debate, interview panel, demonstration, motion picture, slides, and programed and self-instructional learning materials, which include learning modules.

Participation techniques are also employable in large and small groups. Those most usable in a large group include question and answer period, forum, buzz groups, and audience role playing. Six small group participation techniques have been demonstrated to be most useful: brainstorming, interviewing, case discussion, book-based discussion, problem-solving discussion, and guided discussion.

Simulation techniques are most beneficial in teaching small groups and include role playing, case study method, in-basket exer-

cises, and a variety of simulation games.

Human relations techniques are also most adaptable to small groups. T-groups, laboratory training, sensitivity training, nonverbal exercises, and value clarification exercises are all human relations techniques.

To recapitulate, in choosing the appropriate technique or techniques, the trainer should weigh strongly the benefits to the trainee that are gained from his being actively involved in the learning experience and the possibilities of making that learning experience job related. Obviously, many of the presentation techniques just mentioned naturally lend themselves to trainee participation. The content, or subject matter, with which the public health nutritionist, as a trainer, must be concerned is reflected in the knowledge and skill of the "learner needs." In other words, the subject matter of the staff training curriculum must be directly related to the following three areas: (1) basic background and rationale for screening, referral, and monitoring and following up clients; (2) the mechanics of screening, referring, monitoring, and following up clients; and (3) the educational methodology required to teach clients during the screening, referral, monitoring, and follow-up process.

The technique selection factors should relate to the needs of the community. For example, using the hypothetical community presented in Chapter 4, Everywheresville, U.S.A., the following would be pertinent considerations:

1. The size of the group is small, consisting of health worker trainees. Therefore the trainer (nutritionist) can pretty much rule out those large group presentation techniques.

2. The learning style of the health workers may vary, but it is likely that they will learn best from concrete experiences and active experimentation, both of which maximize trainee participation. Small group participation and simulation techniques may be ideal here.

3. Since the health workers are being trained to deliver nutrition services in a public health setting, learning techniques especially relevant to the job situation would in-

clude brainstorming, case discussions, problem-solving discussions, role playing, and case studies.

4. Since most trainees learn best from being actively involved, the trainer should try to formulate a personalized system of instruction and a program that utilizes learning modules and requires a great deal of learner participation. These should provide immediate and direct feedback. Additionally, the learning module makes the trainee more independent of the trainer because learning modules usually are self-instructional and contain all the subject matter and self-tests necessary to develop the knowledge and skill needed. The time available for training while setting up the nutrition program may be less than desired, and the learning module can be a viable solution to a time problem. The trainer then becomes more of a resource person, developing and helping the trainee by suggesting activities relevant to the learning module's subject matter and administering a formal assessment after completion of various parts of a module. The construction of a curriculum that employs learning modules is described by Keller and Sherman.[12] The modular system is currently being used in various settings to train health care paraprofessionals and professionals in the areas of nutrition and nursing.

5. Resources existing in the community should be considered in planning for the learning experiences of the health workers, including (a) all other health department personnel; (b) other health and social services, both internal and external to the health department; (c) the limitations on screening equipment; and (d) the educational settings, including high schools, junior college, and vocational school. Other health department personnel also may have useful training materials and expertise. They can be helpful in training paraprofessionals on the background needed to deliver services through the referral system. Other health and social services, such as well-baby clinics, family planning clinics, and prenatal clinics may provide a laboratory for teaching health worker trainees screening, monitoring, and follow-up

skills that they will need. Finally, the educational settings may be advantageous for two reasons: they could offer classes that would provide needed background and skills for the trainees, and they offer a library and often have informative audiovisual materials, such as films and projectors.

6. The comfort, confidence, and competence of the trainee will be directly affected by the nutritionist's self-confidence and competence in training techniques and subject matter content. The trainer may already feel confident and comfortable doing lectures and demonstrations because of practical experience, but skill in using other techniques (role playing, small group discussions, gaming, values voting, etc.) can come through reading about them, observing them, and integrating them with training sessions. Trainees are more likely to develop their needed skills when allowed to learn through a variety of practice activity techniques. The community's educational resources as well as other health care professionals may be able to help structure learning experiences that maximize learning without being particularly risky to either the trainee or trainer.

An instructional objective that could be included in the training curriculum for the two paraprofessionals was stated earlier: "Given a case study that describes a client in need of three other community health services and a Z-21 referral form, the trainee will correctly fill out the referral form for one of these services. The form must be filled out with the appropriate information for all four items on the form." Keeping in mind how the two trainees and the hypothetical community influence the selection of training techniques, a good learning experience to enable the trainees to meet the instructional objective is described below in a planned sequence of steps.

1. Each trainee uses a questionnaire to gather data about the different health services that are available, obtaining information on each service's function, location, time offered, and eligibility criteria.

2. The trainer guides a discussion with the

trainees as they share their question-naire results and make up a referral list of the interviewed health services.

3. The trainees examine four health work-er/client case studies and identify other health services on their referral list that could help the clients.

4. The trainer demonstrates to the train-ees how to fill out a Z-21 referral form for two of the clients.

5. Based on the health service needs of the other two clients, the trainees fill out Z-21 referral forms and the trainer conducts a discussion about the accu-racy with which the referral forms were completed.

Assessment

To determine both the trainee's level of knowledge at the start and base skill and to evaluate the effectiveness of the learning ex-perience, a training curriculum must have an assessment category. The assessment cate-gory should include an assessment, or what is commonly called an assessment tool or test, for every instructional objective. The learn-ing experience is to enable the trainee to gain the knowledge, skills, and/or practice, that is required to perform the instructional objec-tive. The assessment tool or test enables both the trainer and trainee to determine if the trainee can do precisely what the instruction-al objective states, whether it be demonstrat-ing knowledge, skills, job-related perfor-mance, or a combination of these. The pre-cision with which such determinations can be made will depend on how well the instruc-tional objective was originally stated. In oth-er words, was the terminal behavior that was stated in the instructional objective measur-able, and did the objective state criteria or the degree of accuracy that terminal behav-ior must display?

In writing the assessment for each instruc-tional objective, it is critical that it directly measure that behavior stated in the instruc-tional objective. For example, if one's objec-tive states that "the trainee will identify the proper forms to use for screening, referring, and evaluating a client," one might write an

assessment requiring the trainee to read case studies of three different client/health worker situations in which the client needed to be screened, referred, or evaluated. The trainee would then be given a number of forms and asked to select the form needed by the health worker in each case study.

If the trainer's assessment measures the behavior stated in the instructional objective, three people will benefit in various ways: (1) the trainee will be able to determine what progress he or she has made; (2) the trainer will be able to ascertain if the trainee has de-veloped the desired knowledge and/or skill and so gain insight into the effectiveness of the planned learning experience; and (3) the person(s) paying for the training will be able to assess their investment.

Many forms of assessment tools are avail-able to the trainer, including (1) the objective test; (2) the matching test; (3) the perfor-mance test (e.g., taking a 24-hour recall, measuring height, weight, and head circum-ference, taking blood, using the colorimeter and centrifuge to process hemoglobin and hematocrit tests); (4) the essay; and (5) the oral test. Of these forms, the performance test is often the most beneficial in determin-ing if a person can perform competently in a job situation. Through a job-related perfor-mance assessment the trainer can see wheth-er or not the trainee can actually perform a desired job function. Such an assessment measures the application of knowledge and skills in the job environment.

An example is given using the instructional objective stated earlier: "Given a case study that describes a client in need of three other community health services and a Z-21 refer-ral form, the trainee will correctly fill out the referral form for one of these services. The form must be filled out with the appropriate information for all four items on the form." The following is an example of a job-related, performance-based assessment, as addressed to the trainer:

Provide the trainee with a Z-21 referral form and a case study of a client with which he or she is familiar. The case study should indicate a need to refer this client to three other health-related services. Have the trainee read the case study and fill out the Z-21 referral form for one health-related service to which he or she wishes to refer the client. Then use a correctly filled out Z-21 referral form to check to see if all four parts of the form are completed correctly.

The assessment tools described in the training curriculum are short term. They do not allow the trainer to ascertain if the trainee maintains an acceptable level of job performance over a period of time. Therefore, for those instructional objectives stating a terminal behavior that is a performance critical to the trainee's job, it is vital that the trainer also develop and implement a long-term assessment. A long-term assessment is accomplished through purposeful on-the-job observations over the trainee's period of employment.

An example of a long-term assessment for the instructional objective just discussed could include setting up a feedback system with the referral sources so that the trainer could note the number of correctly written, correctly designated referrals out of all the referrals made.

Using the training curriculum

The use of a training curriculum in a training program has at least two major benefits in that it (1) provides a structured sequence of objectives which the learner needs to achieve and (2) enables the trainer and learner to make optimal use of training time by assisting the job-related knowledge and skills the learner already possesses. The steps to follow in using the curriculum are as follows:

1. *Administer assessment* for each objective first to determine if the learner already has the ability to do what is stated in the instructional objective.
2. Identify those *instructional objectives* in the curriculum for which the learner does not pass assessment. These are the objectives the learner did not "meet."
3. Provide *learning experiences* to teach the learner to be able to perform according to what is stated in each unmet instructional objective.

4. Administer assessment for each unmet objective again to determine if the learner has gained the ability to do what is stated in each instructional objective.

This set of steps is a cyclic process and can be depicted in a circular illustration:

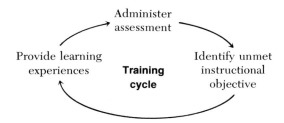

Often the learning experience that enables the learner to meet a given instructional objective will involve more than one activity, and it is then useful to develop an action plan for such an instructional objective. Action planning is part of the "management by objective" (MBO) process,[13] but it can be used at the training level too. In the action plan the various activities comprising a learning experience can be sequenced in steps by date and listed under the category "steps to complete to meet instructional objective."

Each step may require the input of more than one person, as well as a variety of resources. The last step in the action plan should always be the assessment for the instructional objective. The learning experience for the given instructional objective that has been used as an example has been sequenced in several steps. Table 6-2 demonstrates the use of the action plan format for this instructional objective, its learning experience, and assessment.

Participating in the planning and action process

Throughout this chapter strategies were developed for the trainee to meet the needs of the consumer. The unique roles of the trainer and trainee were stressed. The relationship is even more crucial when a total program plan is being developed. Every employee, whether a nutritionist or a communi-

Table 6-2. Action plan for objective 12

Objective 12: Given a case study that describes a client in need of 3 other community health services and a Z-21 referral form, the trainee will correctly fill out the referral form for one of these services. The form must be filled out with the appropriate information for all 4 items on the form.

Date step is to be completed	Steps to complete to meet instructional objective	Person(s) responsible	Resources required	Progress notes
6/1/78	1. Learner receives questionnaire and interviews other health-related services that are both internal and external to the county health department.	Trainer Sanitarian Nurses Health educator Maternal and Child Health Director Social worker Health director Clinic physician Learner	Question-naire Transporta-tion	
6/2/78	2. Learner participates in guided discussion in which interview results are shared and a referral list is constructed.	Trainer Learner	Complete question-naire Butcher paper	
6/3/78	3. Learner examines health worker/client case studies and identifies other health services on referral list that could help clients.	Trainer Learner	Case studies Referral list	
6/4/78	4. Trainer demonstrates mechanics in completing a Z-21 referral form for several clients from the case studies in step 3.	Trainer	Z-21 referral form Overhead projector	
6/5/78	5. Learners fill out Z-21 referral forms for several clients from the case studies in step 3, and trainer critiques the completed form and guides a discussion on the accuracy with which the form was completed.	Trainer Learner	Z-21 referral form completed and blank Overhead projector	
6/6/78	6. Learner takes the assessment for the instructional objective. If the learner passes assessment, he or she is directed back to appropriate activities in the learning experience.	Trainer Learner	Assessment tool	

ty worker, must be included in the planning process at every stage. By including the staff in the planning process from the initial stages, each team member will feel a part of meeting the planned objectives. If participatory management is not a part of the administrator's or planner's style, then personal insecurities may come to the surface. Involving employees and keeping them informed at every stage of the development of the plan is a vital step that is often overlooked. (See Fig. 6-1.)

Documenting results of the action plan

One major step in developing the action plan is to consider the audience and potential critics. The consumer of services may be pleased with the results, but the administrator may be skeptical about the time and money being spent on a specific effort. Both these elements must be considered. Therefore always anticipate the needed evidence and document results at every stage of the plan. (See Fig. 6-1.)

SUMMARY

The four components of a system to deliver services have been discussed. An important part of putting a plan into action is the design and implementation of a training curriculum for the staff. It should be emphasized to health worker trainees that the process used for training them will be the same process they use to educate clients. This process includes the following steps: (1) identifying knowledge and skill needs, (2) stating instructional objectives, (3) participating in learning activities, and (4) successfully completing assessments. Whereas the *learner needs* identify knowledge and skills required to perform various job functions, the *instructional* objectives state how and to what level the learner will demonstrate that he or she has gained the knowledge and skills needed to perform competently. The *learning experiences* teach the learner, through appropriate techniques, the subject matter and skills he or she needs to perform as stated in the instructional objective. The *assessments* enable the trainer to measure whether the learner can perform as stated in the instructional objective. Tests that utilize a checklist to assess a job-related performance are especially beneficial in a training program. Once the short-term assessment for specific objectives has been successfully completed by the learner, effective long-range assessment that measures retention of skills, knowledge, and application in job performance needs to be carried out.

It is through such a four-step process that clients, too, will achieve the desired behavioral change which will lead to an improvement in their health status. The plan is implemented when the nutritionist designs systematic methods for delivering services, trains the staff, supervises the staff to effect behavioral change in the clients, and designs an evaluation mechanism to measure improvement in health status as a result of the changes in client behavior.

Application of the available health knowledge is the weakest link in the chain of health protection. It is in the "public" part of public health that health professionals are weak. The behavioral scientists have shared their concepts, tools, and methodology to help health professionals bring about behavioral change in their clients.

The social scientists and epidemiologists have also guided health professionals. It is a team effort. As Rosen[14] has written: "A knowledge of the community and its people . . . is just as important for successful public health work as is knowledge of epidemiology or medicine . . . The first principle in community organization is to start with people as they are and with the community as it is."

REFERENCES

1. Kane, R. A., and Kane, R. L.: Galloping consumption: consumer participation in health programs. In Kane, R. L., editor: Challenges of community medicine, New York, 1974, Springer Publishing Co., Inc.
2. Gilladay, A.: Allied health manpower strategies: estimates from the potential gains from efficient task delegation, Med. Care **6:**457, 1973.
3. Spitzer, W. D., et al.: The Burlington randomized trials of nurse practitioners, N. Engl. J. Med. **290:**251, 1974.
4. Egeberg, R. O.: Allied health workers now and tomorrow, Manpower **2:**Oct., 1970.
5. Yanochik, A.: Community nutrition workers—their effectiveness in a nutrition delivery system, Public Health Currents, Oct., 1973.
6. Wingert, W. A., et al.: Effectiveness and efficiency of indigenous health aides in a pediatric outpatient department, Am. J. Public Health **65:**849, 1975.
7. Mager, R. F.: Preparing instructional objectives, Belmont, Calif., 1975, Fearon Publishers, Inc.
8. Lynch, B. L., and Holloway, L. D.: Writing objectives for health instruction: an introductory manual, Gainesville, Fla., 1974, University of Florida.
9. Family Planning Manpower Development Project: Training paraprofessional family planning workers,

Books I and II, New York, 1972, Planned Parent-hood-World Population.

10. Hyman, R.: Ways of teaching, Philadelphia, 1970, J. B. Lippincott Co.

11. Margolis, F. H.: Training by objectives: a partici-pant oriented approach, Cambridge, Mass., 1970, McBer & Co.

12. Keller, F. and Sherman, S. G.: PSI: The Keller Plan, Menlo Park, Calif., 1974, W. A. Benjamin, Inc.

13. Raice, A. P.: Managing by objectives, Glenview, Ill., 1974, Scott Foresman & Co.

14. Rosen, G.: The community and health offices—a working team, Am. J. Public Health **44:**14, 1954.

Appendix 6-1*

CHECKLIST OF PERSONS WHO SHOULD BE INVOLVED IN COMMUNITY HEALTH PROGRAMS

Health service providers and educational institutions

- Health professionals: physicians, dentists, nurses, veterinarians, pharmacists, and other allied health professionals
- Health institutions and professional training programs

  Hospitals and other patient care facilities, including ambulatory care centers

  Medical schools, universities, colleges, junior colleges

  Medical laboratories

- Government health and welfare agencies
- Voluntary health and welfare agencies (e.g., Red Cross, Community Chest)
- Health planning organization (e.g., Regional Medical Programs, State and Areawide Comprehensive Health Planning Agencies, Health Services Agencies)

Influential community groups and individuals. Those reputable individuals or organizations who are actually involved or have the potential for productive involvement in community decisions. Individuals reputed to play a critical role in non-health community issues may or may not exert the same influence on health matters.

- Industry (owners and employees at all levels)
- Business—local merchants
- Non-health professionals (e.g., lawyers, engineers, etc.)

- Farm organizations—the Farm Bureau, the Grange, 4-H, etc.
- Civic groups—PTA, Chamber of Commerce, women's and men's clubs, Urban League, etc.
- Student organizations
- Management and employee organizations
- Religious leaders
- Educational leaders
- Local government officials
- Local medical auxiliaries and other professional auxiliaries
- Cooperative Extension Service

Consumers of health services. Individuals not previously mentioned, residents of the area to be served by a community health program. Inclusion of these individuals should not be optional to the planning body. When encouraged to accept a meaningful role, their involvement will provide valuable input in developing programs to meet the area's health needs.

- Criteria to assure broad representation

  Representative of all educational levels

  Representative of all family income levels

  Representative of ethnic groups

  Representative of age groups

  Vocational representation of the community (i.e., industry, commerce, agriculture, etc.)

- Criteria to assure individual competence

  Basic knowledge of and concern for health problems of the community

  Ability to represent the interests of the group from which an individual is chosen

*From American Medical Association: Guidelines for community health programs, Chicago, Ill., The Association.

Appendix 6-2

ARIZONA NUTRITION SERVICES
Obesity follow-up protocol

A. Obese clients for the Weight Reduction Program may be selected from the following:
   1. Screening-in clinics, Head Start centers, or schools
   2. Screening and follow-up in homes
   3. Referrals from community agencies
   4. Self-referral

B. Complete screening on clients includes the following:

   Hemoglobin   Heart disease risk factors
   Hematocrit   Height
   Serum cholesterol   Weight
   Blood pressure   Socioeconomic data as appropriate

C. Have the client determine his ideal weight from "Four Steps to Weight Control."

D. Administer the questionnaire on factors affecting weight.

E. Explain the Behavior Modification Weight Reduction Program to the client (including what to expect). Discuss the causes, effects, and disadvantages of being obese.

   Behavior modification means just that: The client must change his eating habits to lose weight and keep it off. The client became overweight because he is eating too many calories and not exercising enough. If he examines his behavior, he will find that other things besides hunger cause him to overeat. This plan will require that he be honest, consistent, and responsible. Through this program the client *can* lose weight. Many people have. It means that he has to find out what things around him cause him to overeat and underexercise and what things he *must* change to lose weight; he must change them and receive *immediate* rewards for these changes (being 50 pounds lighter in 6 months is not enough to keep going on a daily basis).

1. Only *he* can do the work, although a family member or friend *must* help.

2. He will be expected to keep records of his eating behavior.

3. He will be expected to assist you, the nutrition aide, in working out a plan for his weight reduction. His plan will be based around the following:
   a. Eliminating eating behavior in situations where it is inappropriate
   b. Following a well-balanced meal pattern modified from what and how he now eats
   c. Increased exercise based on what physical activity he now likes
   d. Following a reward system that he designs
   e. Regular monitoring of his progress by the nutrition team
   f. Involving a family member (parent or spouse) to support, encourage, and reward

4. He will be expected to follow his plan for 24 hours a day, 7 days a week.

5. He will sign a contract with you in which he pledges that he will do everything in his power to lose weight.

6. He will make appointments with you to check weight, discuss problems, etc.

7. He will accept nutrition counseling for his total dietary intake (including any other problems that may have been detected in screening).

8. He will understand that weight reduction will be slow but if he teaches himself new habits through this program, he will solve his weight problem permanently.

F. If the client understands, client agrees to follow a plan and signs a contract. A copy is given to the client.

G. The client is given food records, which he is to complete (one for each day) for 1 week.

Explain the mechanics of completing. Ask the client to calculate calories each day using the "Four Steps to Weight Control."

H. If the client is more than 30% overweight, the physician should be notified that he is involved in a weight reduction program.

I. Make an appointment for a clinic or home visit in 1 to 3 weeks.

J. Analyze the client's eating behavior. When records are received in the mail, do the following:

1. Analyze for calories and other nutrients as appropriate. (See blood levels on screening slip.) Most obese women lose weight well (1 to 2 pounds a week) on a diet of 1,000 to 1,200 calories a day (a decrease of about 1,000 calories a day). Consult with the nutritionist before recommending a calorie level for children.

2. Analyze for eating behavior problems, time, place, mood, and other activities while eating. Circle problem areas; for example, eats problem foods every afternoon while watching TV.

K. Devise a nutrition care plan consisting of the following:

1. Calorie level needed for a 1- to 2-pound weight loss weekly.

2. Diet plan is based on the present diet (modifications as few as necessary) *or* exchange diet.

3. Behavior control changes, including a list of modifications and individual changes as necessary.

4. Regular daily exercise—one activity the client enjoys—to be filled in when you visit (using information from questionnaire). Write out the information.

5. Rewards to be worked out on second visit with the client's spouse, parent, or friend present.

Rewards for adhering to the diet and exercise plan can be made daily, biweekly, or weekly (the more often the better). All kinds of material things can be used as rewards, including, for an adult, tokens to be cashed in for things or the thing itself, that is, conversation, evening out, sex, trips, babysitter for an afternoon, toys for children, clothes, new hairdo.

If the client is a female child, every day that she follows her diet and takes a 20-minute walk, her mother gives her 25 cents. When she has enough, she can purchase her toy. If she wants to spend her 25 cents daily, she is entitled to do so. An additional reward is praise. Members of families should be encouraged to offer praise when weight loss is achieved. No punishment, chiding, or criticism should be made by family or nutrition aides.

L. If the client has been taking a "fad" diet, review its fallacies and dangers. Also consult "The Way to Quick Weight Loss."

M. If the client would like more variety in the diet, provide one or two recipes each home visit and, if necessary, demonstrate the preparation. Aides should keep a recipe file of low-calorie recipes.

N. Monitoring of progress. Arrangements should be made for the client to be weighed regularly (and any other appropriate screening indices). The client should keep a progress chart of weekly weight gains and losses and daily food records for several weeks of his weight control plan. If the client's weight begins to plateau or increase, reevaluate the plan. Provide nutrition information so that wise dietary choices can be made.

When the ideal weight or goal has been achieved, the client should be instructed in a weight maintenance diet (may increase the calories gradually until the weight is stabilized) and should be seen at 3-month intervals to evaluate weight maintenance. Exercise should be continued.

Appendix 6-3

ARIZONA NUTRITION SERVICES
Anemia follow-up protocol

A. Clients for anemia follow-up may be identified at the following:
1. Screening-in clinics, Head Start centers, schools
2. Screening and follow-up in homes
3. Referrals from community agencies
4. Self-referral

B. Complete screening on clients includes the following:

Hemoglobin   Height
Hematocrit   Weight
Mean corpuscular hemoglobin Dietary intake
  concentration (MCHC)*

C. Standard criteria for follow-up†

Age	Sex	Hemo-globin (9/dl)	Hema-tocrit	MCHC (gm/dl RBC)
6-23 mo	Both	10.0	31.0	30
2-5 yr	Both	11.0	34.0	30
6-14 yr	Both	12.0	37.0	30
<14 yr	Male	13.0	40.0	30
<14 yr	Female	12.0	37.0	30
Pregnant	Second tri-mester	11.0	35.0	30
	Third tri-mester	10.5	33.0	30

D. Vitamin-mineral supplementation
1. Referrals to the physician for vitamin supplementation will be made when the hemoglobin is greater than 1 gm below cutoff given above; the hematocrit is greater than 4%; and/or there are other medical problems suspected.
2. Routine prescription of vitamin and mineral supplements is of uncertain value and should not be relied on for correcting inadequate food intakes or faulty food habits.
3. When a vitamin and/or mineral supplement is indicated, the prescription should take into consideration the Recommended Dietary Allowance for specific age, sex, condition, and usual food intake.
4. A physician's order is required for the prescription of vitamin/mineral supplementation.

E. Suggestions for scheduling follow-up
1. Visit within 2 weeks of screening for dietary evaluation—24-hour recall and discussion of feeding practices and eating habits. Make an appointment for next visit.
2. Schedule a second visit within 1 or 2 weeks to reinforce information given at the first visit.
3. If the information has been well accepted and change can be noted, visits may be decreased to one a month until rescreening.
4. Make a home visit and take 24-hour recall 1 week before rescreening is scheduled.
5. After rescreening make one last visit to close the case and to answer any questions even if values are normal—*praise improvement*. Suggest rescreening in 1 year and advise that the client can call if any problems or questions arise.
6. If values have not improved, schedule weekly visits for a month and a case conference.
7. Do a second rescreening in 3 months.

F. Guidelines for consultation and patient education
1. Causes
  a. Insufficient dietary intake of iron, protein, folic acid, and other vitamins
  b. Malabsorption of iron (probable effect in pica)

---

*Ratio between hemoglobin and hematocrit; amount of hemoglobin per red blood cell.
† From Center for Disease Control, Atlanta.

c. Blood loss due to trauma, gastrointestinal bleeding, menstruation
d. Rapid growth especially during infancy
2. Symptoms
   a. Weakness and fatigue
   b. Pallor
   c. Irritability with decreased attention span
3. Consequences
   a. Decrease in growth and development potential
   b. Increased susceptibility to infection
   c. Decrease in receptiveness to learning opportunities
4. Explanations of the meaning of hemoglobin, hematocrit, function of iron, and food high in iron
   a. Hemoglobin is a measurement of the iron in the blood.
   b. Hematocrit is a measurement of the number of red blood cells in the body.
   c. Iron is essential for the blood to carry oxygen all over the body. If iron in blood is low or less than normal, a person is said to have anemia.
   d. Foods high in iron include liver, meats, dark green vegetables (turnip, mustard or collard greens, spinach, verde lagas), beans, enriched or whole grain breads and cereals, eggs, peanut butter, and raisins.
   e. Vitamin C helps the body utilize the iron in foods; therefore high-iron foods should be eaten with foods high in vitamin C, that is, oranges, grapefruit, tomatoes, chili peppers, cabbage, cantaloupe, and strawberries.
   f. Young children are often anemic because of excessive intakes of milk, usually from a bottle. Milk is a good food, but it contains very little iron. By the time a child is 1 year old, he should be off the bottle, eating a variety of solid foods, and drinking at most 4 cups of milk a day.
   g. For the initiation of breastfeeding, mothers are well advised to have an adequate diet during pregnancy. The nutritional goals for lactation will highlight increased calorie and protein needs along with added vitamins and minerals as directed by the RDAs. To meet her nutrient needs without exceeding her energy needs, a lactating mother must select a diet of higher nutrient density than at any other time in her life.

Appendix 6-4

NUTRITION EDUCATION PLAN
Behavioral objectives: Coding and Abbreviation for Tickler Card

Code	Abbreviation	Behavioral objectives
1.A.1.	Ideal weight	Parent will identify *ideal weight* for his/her infant.
1.A.2.	Weight and height	Parent will see the *relationship between weight/height and health.*
1.B.1.	Weight gain	Parent will explain *factors affecting weight gain* during infancy.
1.B.2.	Key nutrients	Parent will identify the *key nutrients and their functions* during early growth.
1.B.3.	Eating problems	Parent will identify *eating problems* occurring during infancy leading to obesity.
1.B.4.	Modify behavior	Parent will identify *modifications in eating behavior to reach ideal weight* for his/her infant.
1.B.5.	Eating habits	Parent will explain the *relationship of infant eating habits* to the development of *adult eating habits.*
1.C.1.	WIC foods	Participant will identify acceptable *WIC foods as sources of nutrients* and energy.
1.C.2.	Other foods	Participant will identify *other* economical and culturally *acceptable sources of nutrients and energy.*
1.C.3.	Plan diet	Participant will *plan* an economic and culturally acceptable *diet to meet* the *nutrient and energy needs* for age, sex, activity, nutrition, and health status, etc., and to be incorporated into her usual family dietary pattern.
1.C.4.	Home economics	Participant will identify (1) economic *shopping practices*, (2) safe methods for *preparing and serving* foods, and (3) safe methods for storing foods.
1.D.1.	Referral services	Parent will identify the *sources, functions, and eligibility criteria for services* to which they have been referred.
1.D.2.	Supplements	Parent will identify *reasons for vitamin/mineral supplement* prescribed by physician.
1.D.3.	WIC tasks	Parent will explain the *reasons and required tasks for participation in the WIC program.*
2.A.1.	Pregnancy risk	Participant will explain the *risk factors for poor pregnancy* outcome.
2.A.2.	Limited nutrition	Participant will discuss *factors that limit or prevent adequate nutrition during pregnancy and lactation* (cultural, economic, social, religious, psychological).
2.A.3.	Plot weight gain	Participant will plot and *interpret* her *weight gain* during *pregnancy.*
2.B.1.	Increased needs	Participant will identify the *reason for increased nutrient and energy needs* during pregnancy and lactation.
2.B.2.	Weight gain	Participant will explain a *normal weight gain* pattern and the *components of total weight gain* during pregnancy.

Code	Abbreviation	Behavioral objectives
2.B.3.	Reduce risk	Participant will identify *methods to reduce the risk of anemia, toxemia, and prematurity.*
2.B.4.	Breast feeding	Participant will identify reasons to *breast feed or bottle feed* an infant.
2.B.5.	Use services	Participant will identify *reasons for early use of prenatal services and the relationship to outcome of pregnancy.*
2.B.6.	Pregnancy outcome	Participant will explain the *role of nutrition* in the maintenance of *health in pregnancy* and *successful outcome.*
2.C.1-4		See 1.C.1-4.
2.D.1-3		See 1.D.1-3.
3.A.1.	Hemoglobin or hematocrit	Parent/participant will identify *reasons for completing hemoglobin and hematocrit* and indices to determine nutritional status.
3.B.1.	Anemia	Parent/participant will identify *causes, symptoms, and consequences* of anemia.
3.B.2.	Blood production	Parent/participant will *identify and explain the function of iron, vitamin C, folic acid, and protein in blood production.*
3.B.3.	Nutrition and health	Parent/participant will explain the *role of nutrition in maintenance of health.*
3.C.1-4		See 1.C.1-4.
3.D.1-3		See 1.D.1-3.
4.A.1.	Height and weight	Parent will identify *reasons for completing height, weight, and head circumference measurements* and indices to determine nutritional status.
4.A.2.	Feeding skills	Parent will identify *appropriate feeding skills* for the infant or child.
4.A.3.	Plot height and weight	Parent will *plot and interpret screening values for height, weight, and head circumference* on growth grids.
4.B.1.	Growth risk	Parent will explain the *risk factors* for physical and mental retardation *associated with poor or inadequate gain* in weight, height, and head circumference.
4.B.2.	Nutrients and growth	Parent will identify and explain *functions of key nutrients during early growth.*
4.B.3.	Nutrition and health	Parent will explain the *role of nutrition in the maintenance of health.*
4.C.1-4.		See 1.C.1-4.
4.D.1-3.		See 1.D.1-3.

Appendix 6-5

RESOURCES FOR FOOD ASSISTANCE

A. Nutrition (food assistance) programs supported by the U.S. Department of Agriculture include the following:

1. *School Food Programs*
   School Feeding Program provides lunches and breakfast to schoolchildren. Low-income children can receive meals at free or reduced prices. Funds are made available to the states for purchase of food, maintenance, operation, and expansion of nonprofit school lunch programs.
   Special Milk Program allows any school or nonprofit child care institution to provide needy children with free milk.

2. *Child Care Food Programs* provide for nutritious meals to preschool and school-aged children in child care facilities. Through grants and/or other means, states can initiate, maintain, or expand nonprofit food service programs for children in institutions providing child care, for example, day care centers, family day care program, Head Start centers, and institutions providing day care service for handicapped children.

3. *Summer Food Programs* help get nutritious meals to needy preschool and school-aged children in recreation centers, summer camps, or during vacations in areas operating under a continuous school calendar. Any nonresidential public or private nonprofit institution or residential public or private nonprofit summer camp is eligible if it develops a summer food program for children from low-income areas. Federal funds are given to eligible institutions for the costs involved in obtaining, preparing, and serving food under this program (including administrative costs and rental of office space and equipment).

4. *Supplemental Food Program for Women, Infants and Children (WIC)* is operated on a project basis and administered through the state health agency. It provides for selected foods to infants, children up to 5 years of age, and pregnant and lactating women who are eligible on a health/nutritional and economic need basis.

5. *The Food Stamp Program* enables eligible low-income households to buy more food of greater variety to improve their diets. The program is usually administered by the local welfare department. To qualify for food stamps, households must meet certain nationwide eligibility standards.

B. *Nutrition Programs for the Elderly*, administered by the state Agency on Aging unless another agency is designated, provide meals for older Americans, primarily from low-income groups, from within the project area. In addition to serving nutritionally sound meals, the program provides supportive services such as nutrition education, shopping assistance, recreational activities, transportation to the center site, health services, and information referral.

C. *Community Food and Nutrition Programs* administered by the Community Services Administration (formerly OEO Emergency Food and Medical Services Programs) may be available in some communities. Such programs are usually administered by local community action agencies.

D. *Home-delivered meals, or Meals on Wheels*, a nonprofit program of home-delivered meals, is a community service administered by an official or voluntary or welfare agency. The service is provided to ill, disabled, and elderly persons whose physical, emotional, mental, or social conditions handicap their ability to obtain or prepare meals for themselves. Such services often make it possible for individuals to remain in their own homes, reducing institutional care, or to obtain special diets they could not prepare. Support is usually from local sponsorship and income generated from the meals.

E. Many church missions and community organizations keep an emergency food pantry, which is an excellent resource for individuals and families in need of food on a short-term basis.

GENERAL CONCEPT

To proceed with an action plan, nutritional assessment and subsequent surveillance are necessary. Assessment and surveillance provide information on nutritional status and allow an ongoing documentation for program needs and the effectiveness of implementation.

OUTCOMES

The student should be able to do the following:

- Define the needs and objectives of a nutrition survey: the needs and objectives of a nutrition surveillance system.
- Review in general terms the significance and findings of the Ten State Nutrition Survey, the Preschool Nutrition Survey, and the first Health and Nutrition Examination Survey.
- Discuss the methodology for developing a nutrition surveillance system.
- Review the functions and accomplishments of the Center for Disease Control Nutrition Surveillance System.

Nutritional assessment and surveillance

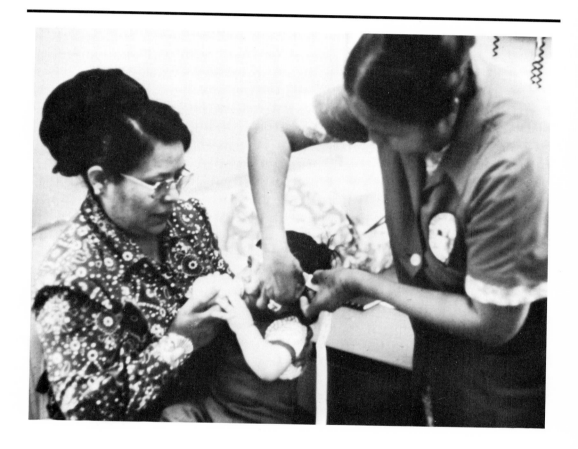

In the preceding chapters several of the analyses required to develop a program plan have been presented. These include (1) the determination of need, (2) the development of a precise plan that encompasses establishing goals and developing specific objectives, (3) the listing of priorities to be tackled, and (4) the development of an action plan to achieve the determined objectives. See discussion on analysis required in developing a program plan (pp. 65 to 67). Steps 1 to 8 are covered in Chapter 4; steps 9 to 15 in Chapter 6; steps 16 to 19 in Chapters 7, 9, and 10.

Despite the fact that nutritional assessment and surveillance would seem to be basic to planning, implementing, and evaluating program activity, they have not been a major focus of public health nutrition programs thus far. A surveillance program, specifically planned for a particular state or locale is the

NUTRITION ASSESSMENT—WHY?

Public health is in a very different situation today. For practical purposes, no patients in the United States have purely nutritional diseases; perhaps we should even drop the word "disease" from our vocabulary when discussing public health nutrition. An occasional psychotic or mentally defective mother has a marasmic baby, and an occasional alcoholic gets beriberi, but these are exceptions. Instead, society is composed of individuals whose nutritional status places them in one of a variety of risk categories for developing ill health at some future date. Everyone, 100 percent of the population, falls into some risk category for morbidity and mortality for chronic diseases. Everyone, 100 percent of us, could benefit from further nutrition education and modification of our diets. Since we simply don't have resources to approach 100 percent of the population with serious nutritional counselling and personal nutrition education, we must develop screening techniques to identify that portion of the population most in need of nutritional services.

J. Michael Lane and *Morissa White:* Personal communication, 1977.

only way to identify the nutritional needs unique to that geographic area. Nichaman and Collins[1] indicate that national surveys may suggest problem areas and high-risk population groups, but only a continuing or planned periodic surveillance within the community can provide data basic to a well-founded program. (See Fig. 7-1.)

To operate a surveillance program, specific tools must be utilized that will determine the nutritional status and the needs of the community.

Owen and Lippman[2] point out that the nutritional status of a population group or of a community is best evaluated by correlating results of dietary, clinical, and biochemical studies. An individual's nutritional status, according to Christakis,[3] is his condition of health as it is influenced by his intake and utilization of nutrients. These can be determined from the analysis of information obtained from (1) dietary intake studies, (2) clinical findings, (3) biochemical data, and (4) anthropometric measurements.

Such definitions of nutritional status indicate the necessity of baseline data—dietary, clinical, biochemical, and anthropometric—in making judgments about the need and out-

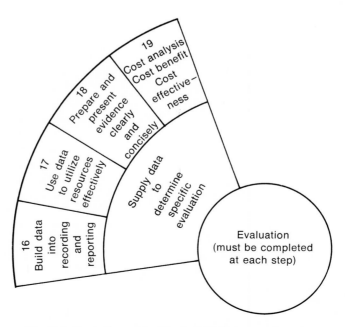

Fig. 7-1. Analysis required in developing a program plan.

NUTRITIONAL ASSESSMENT—A VEHICLE FOR GOOD MEDICAL CARE

Successful nutritional care of individuals and population groups can only be based on adequate and valid data . . . Nutritional assessment and awareness should be an integral part of any medical care system, and a nutritional surveillance system can be the vehicle to develop this nutritional awareness.

Milton Z. Nichaman: Developing a nutritional surveillance system, J. Am. Diet. Assoc. **65:**15, 1974.

comes of surveillance and nutrition programs. Without nutritional assessment one cannot determine where the effort began and what results occurred, if any. To proceed effectively with the action plan, nutritional assessment must be an integral part of the planning and implementation processes. The nutritional assessment system should be able to identify the facts and determine the action that will improve the nutritional status of the population or community.

BACKGROUND ON DEVELOPMENT OF NUTRITIONAL ASSESSMENT

The first conference to discuss the physical, clinical, and physiological aspects of nutritional assessment to detect malnutrition was held in Berlin in 1932 by the Health Organization of the League of Nations. Work on nutritional assessment proceeded through 1937 when the Technical Commission on Nutrition of the Health Organization published a monograph indicating standard procedures for conducting nutrition surveys.

In 1949 the first Joint Food and Agriculture Organization/World Health Organization (FAO/WHO) Expert Committee on Nutrition met. This committee recommended that national nutrition policies should be designed once information about the following could be determined: (1) knowledge of the nutritional status and dietary patterns of the population, (2) food supplies, and (3) economic conditions. A guide discussing the assessment of nutritional status was prepared in 1951 by the Joint Expert Committee of WHO. This guide did not recommend standard procedures for nutritional assessment

but described in general terms the application of anthropometric, clinical, and dietary methods.

The Interdepartmental Committee on Nutrition for National Defense (ICNND) was organized in 1955 with the major objectives of giving developing countries technical assistance in assessing their nutritional status, defining problems of malnutrition, and developing action plans to alleviate critical nutrition problems by using resources locally available. Technical advice was obtained by a group of consultants from universities and research institutions with expertise in nutritional science and international work. Harold R. Sandstead, one of the founders of the ICNND, was the first Executive Director of the committee.

In 1951 the ICNND published the first edition of the *Manual for Nutrition Surveys,*[4] which was intended for conducting nutrition surveys of military personnel in the Near and Far East.

In 1963 the second edition of the manual[5] was published with additional emphasis on the following:

1. Establishing uniformity in methods, techniques, procedures, and guidelines for conducting surveys to make meaningful comparisons of results within and between countries
2. Outlining and defining the responsibilities and duties of team members
3. Providing a guide to interpretation of the dietary, biochemical, and clinical data collected
4. Being a working reference of major facts essential to proper appraisal of nutritional status and aiding in the interpretation of findings to draft practical, effective recommendations for alleviating nutritional problems
5. Assisting in training personnel in nutritional appraisal techniques and stimulating continued nutrition work

Then the WHO Expert Committee on Medical Assessment of Nutritional Status recommended that a standard guide be published, giving detailed instruction about planning and conducting nutrition surveys and reporting results. Following this recommendation, *The Assessment of the Nutritional Status of the Community*[6] was published in 1966.

Although nutrition surveys were being conducted throughout the world with the initial survey commencing in Pakistan in 1956, it was not until the late 1960s that the United States began to address its own nutrition problems. Two surveys were undertaken almost simultaneously to determine the extent of malnutrition in the United States, the Ten State Nutrition Survey, 1968-1970, the Preschool Nutrition Survey, 1968-1970. In 1971 a third survey, the first Health and Nutrition Examination Survey (HANES), was begun, which was completed in 1974.

In addition, a Nutrition Surveillance System was developed by the Center for Disease Control (CDC). In 1974 through 1975 the five states, Arizona, Kentucky, Louisiana, Tennessee, and Washington, were the first to submit data to CDC on selected indices of nutritional status. This system will be elaborated on later in this chapter.

NUTRITIONAL ASSESSMENT: SURVEYS
Definition of surveys

Nichaman[7] describes a nutritional survey as the most traditional data gathering method. It is the examination of a population group at a particular point in time and thus is considered a cross-sectional examination. The "cross-sectional" survey provides information on the prevalence or magnitude of a condition or characteristic in a population at a specific time; it does not provide data on the number of individuals who may be expected to develop a condition during a period of time.

Jelliffe[6] defines a nutritional survey as both a prevalence and incidence study that requires epidemiologic investigations into the nutritional status of a population by various direct and indirect methods, taking into account an evaluation of the determinant ecologic factors in the environment.

Goals and objectives of a survey

The ultimate goal of a nutrition survey is to develop measures to control and eradicate malnutrition, including undernutrition and overnutrition in a population. To accomplish this goal, there are several objectives that must be fulfilled, as follows:

1. The magnitude and geographic distribution of undernutrition and overnutrition at a given point in time must be determined.
2. The ecology of the population that is directly or indirectly involved in the nutrition problem must be recognized and understood.
3. The dietary needs and appropriate corrective measures to alleviate the problems must be ascertained.
4. The community must be motivated to take action that will achieve better health through improved diet.
5. The policy makers and administrators who are responsible for the development of applied nutrition programs must be informed about the extent of overnutrition and undernutrition in the population.
6. The value of methods proposed for specific programs must be tested.
7. Information on the most effective measures used to determine nutritional status should be gained.
8. Information on the effect of nutrition as a factor in improving socioeconomic and health conditions in a community should be provided.
9. The survey should be utilized as a teaching device for both professional and paraprofessional health personnel and also for helping students to understand the importance of nutrition as a public health problem.
10. The standardization of laboratory methods for more definitive interpretation of the data should be encouraged.
11. Laboratory methods applicable to public health workers involved in field studies, and the opportunity to test these methods in an applied situation, should be developed.
12. The impact of the food industry on public buying and eating habits, family

budgets, and changes in dietary patterns should be recognized.

13. Ethical advertising and production policies of the food industry should be promoted.

14. The need for legislation regarding health care, agriculture policy, needs of vulnerable groups, and feeding programs throughout the life cycle should be recognized and encouraged.

Examples of national surveys
Ten State Nutrition Survey

The Ten State Nutrition Survey has been the largest and most comprehensive nutritional health survey of the United States population to date. It was conducted from 1968 through 1970 as a result of an amendment to the Partnership for Health Act in 1967. Congress ordered the Secretary of Health, Education, and Welfare to make a comprehensive survey of the incidence and location of serious hunger, malnutrition, and health problems in the United States and to report back with findings and recommendations for dealing with these conditions within 6 months from date of enactment of the law.

The bill was signed on December 5, 1967. By February 1, 1968, the Nutrition Program of Health Services and Mental Health Administration (formerly the Interdepartmental Committee on Nutrition for National Defense—ICNND) was selected by The Department of Health, Education, and Welfare to be responsible for organizing and directing the Ten State Nutrition Survey.

The first subject was examined in May, 1968, and the last subject in May, 1970. The plan of operation, selection of states random sample, methodology, and guidelines for interpretation of the findings were reviewed and discussed before the Select Committee on Nutrition and Human Needs, of the U.S. Senate—Testimony Part 3, January 22-29, 1969.

Thus the objective of the survey was to make appropriate recommendations after determining the prevalence and location of serious hunger, malnutrition, and resultant health problems that occurred in low-income populations. These populations were selected from ten states located in different geographic regions of the United States.

In response to legislative mandate, the states included were New York, Massachusetts, Michigan, California, Washington, Kentucky, West Virginia, Louisiana, Texas, and South Carolina.

Family selection was determined according to the 1960 census, which listed the families that made up the lowest economic quartiles of their respective states at that time. Approximately 5% of the families selected had incomes more than three times that of the poverty level, thereby allowing for some comparison of results according to economic considerations.

Thirty thousand families were identified in the selection process; 23,846 of these participated in the survey. Data regarding more than 80,000 individuals were obtained through interview; of these individuals,

---

BIOCHEMICAL DATA FROM THE TEN STATE NUTRITIONAL SURVEY
Vitamin A

The high prevalence of "unacceptable" serum vitamin A levels in children 0-16 years of age in seven of the ten states and especially in pre-school children should be of vital concern. The pre-clinical period, that is where blood concentration is being depleted and prior to appearance of overt physical lesions, of vitamin A deficiency is usually prolonged due to liver storage. However, the subsequent stage, ("deficient") of continued depletion can lead to overt disease in a short time and proceed with disastrous rapidity leading to xerophthalmia and blindness in children. Fortunately, no child was diagnosed as having severe eye lesions. In the first five states studied, Texas, Louisiana, Kentucky, Massachusetts and New York, clinical physical lesions associated with vitamin A deficiency were noted, follicular hyperkeratosis in 1 per cent of children under six years of age. Bitot's spots, an eye lesion, associated with but not always specifically due to vitamin A deficiency, was seen in 23 subjects. Twenty of these were found in Texas where a high prevalence of "unacceptable" vitamin A values was noted.

Arnold E. Schaefer: Nutrition in the United States. In McLaren, D. S.: Nutrition in the community, New York, 1976, John Wiley & Sons, Inc., p. 375. Reproduced with permission. Copyright © 1976, John Wiley & Sons Limited.

40,847 were examined. There was a large representation of children in the sample. More than 50% of the persons examined were 16 years of age or less; 30% were from 17 to 44 years, and 17% were above 44 years.

The study design of the survey included the following data:

1. Extensive demographic information on each of the families
2. Clinical evaluation, which included a medical history, physical examinations, anthropometric measurements, x-ray examinations of the wrist
3. Dental examination
4. Biochemical assessment including hemoglobin, hematocrit, total serum protein, serum albumin, serum vitamin A and carotene, and serum vitamin C
5. For those with a hemoglobin of 10 gm/dl or less: blood smears, total serum iron and iron-binding capacity, and serum folic acid and vitamin B_{12}
6. Urinary analysis—creatinine, thiamin, riboflavin index
7. Dietary food intake data

Findings. The results of the Ten State Nutrition Survey[8] revealed that a significant number of the population surveyed was malnourished or at high risk of developing nutritional problems. The results also demonstrated that the elements of malnutrition vary from one locality to another and in different populations within the locality. In developing solutions for these problems, the social, cultural, and economic characteristics must be considered, since each problem is unique to each population.

The survey showed that malnutrition was found most commonly among blacks, less commonly among Spanish Americans, and least among whites. In general, there was increasing evidence of malnutrition in those persons with the lowest incomes. Although income is a major determinant of nutritional status, other factors such as cultural, social, and geographic differences play a significant role in the nutrition level of a population.

Biochemical determinations. Specific findings of certain nutrients in the survey included the following.

IRON. Iron-deficiency anemia, as evidenced by a high prevalence of low levels of hemoglobin, was a widespread problem. In those individuals who were found to have hemoglobin concentrations below selected values, determinations of serum iron and iron-binding capacity were also made to document the extent of iron deficiency. A surprising finding was that many adolescent and adult males had low hemoglobin levels.

VITAMIN A. A major finding was that Mexican Americans living in the Southwest had lower levels of plasma vitamin A than did the black or white populations. From 1 year of age through adolescence, 50% of the Mexican-American children living in the Southwest had plasma vitamin A values below 20 $\mu g/dl$.

There was a general increase in plasma vitamin A concentrations with increasing age. In states with the highest income levels (California, Massachusetts, Michigan, New York, and Washington), mean values showed a progressive increase. In the five states representing the lowest economic levels of the sample, the mean vitamin A levels for all age groups were generally lower. Thus it appeared that slightly higher levels of plasma vitamin A were associated with higher family incomes.

VITAMIN C. Generally, more men had lower vitamin C levels than did women, although vitamin C nutriture was not a major problem among any of the groups selected. There was an apparent relation between vitamin C levels in serum and reported dietary intakes of the vitamin—a relation unique for vitamin C.

PROTEIN. In general, dietary protein intakes were well above levels considered to be adequate. However, a relatively large proportion of pregnant and lactating women demonstrated low serum albumin levels. A question has been raised as to the adequacy of standards for protein levels of pregnant women, since the optimum level of protein required during pregnancy has not been satisfactorily determined.

RIBOFLAVIN AND THIAMIN. Riboflavin status was poor among blacks and among young people of all ethnic groups. Thiamin levels in the population surveyed appeared to be adequate.

IODINE. No evidence of iodine deficiency was found. The data showed no evidence between the prevalence of goiter and iodine status, suggesting that goiters which were seen in the study did not result from iodine deficiency

Anthropometry

GROWTH. Height, weight, and other body measurements are some of the tools used to identify populations in which nutritional inadequacies are reflected by retarded growth and development. An excess of underweight and undersized children and adolescents were found in all population groups studied when compared with the standards commonly used in the United States. A greater per capita income was associated with greater height, greater body weight, greater thickness of subcutaneous fat, advanced skeletal development, advanced dental development, earlier maturation, and earlier attainment of maximum stature. The data from the Ten State Nutrition Survey provided a clear indication of the magnitude of the economic impact on dimensional, skeletal, dental, and sexual development.[9]

Despite lower income levels, black children generally were taller than white children and were more advanced in skeletal and dental development, indicating that racially based differences as well as nutrition factors affect growth.

FATNESS AND OBESITY. Obesity was found to be most prevalent in adult women, particularly black women. In some age groups more than 50% of the adult women were found to be obese. White men in both the adolescent and the adult age groups had a relatively higher prevalence of obesity compared with black men. The wide range of caloric intakes seen in the dietary data was consistent with the findings of underweight and overweight children and adolescents, as well as with the adults.

DENTAL HEALTH. Poor dental health was encountered in many segments of the population. One of the significant factors was the consumption of refined carbohydrates between meals. In adolescent children of all races, the caries index progressively rose as dietary components increased. When only those adolescents who consumed no refined carbohydrates between meals were considered, Spanish-Americans living in higher income areas had the lowest caries index, and whites and blacks living in low-income areas, the highest. Considering all racial groups together, family income was not related to the prevalence of caries.

DIETARY RESULTS. The educational attainment of the person usually responsible for buying and preparing the family food most naturally had an effect on the nutrition of the children under the age of 17 years. As the homemaker's educational level increased, the evidence of nutritional problems in the children decreased. The caloric content of the diets and the intakes of all nutrients studied were lowest for blacks and Mexican-Americans living in the Southwest.

Although the diets of individuals living in low-income families did not differ from middle-income groups, in the concentration of essential nutrients (units/calories), the amount of calories provided by the food available was directly related to family income. The total food intake of children in low-income families was limited, and this was reflected in growth performance. There were also distinct differences related to family income level in the nutrient intake of pregnant women. However, on the average, pregnant women in all economic and ethnic groups had insufficient dietary iron.

The Preschool Nutrition Survey

In the mid-1960s it became apparent that little was known about the nutritional status of the population of the United States. Some information was available on young children, but the studies were often limited in scope and sample size. Only selected nutritional indices such as anthropometric measurements and dietary information were available. In 1966 a proposal was submitted to the Research Division of the Children's Bureau by George M. Owen, Department of

Pediatrics, at the Ohio State University College of Medicine.[10] The proposal included a description of pilot studies to be completed in 2 years, with a national study being initiated at the end of the second year.[11-13] Funds were granted for the project, and the Preschool Nutrition Survey was conducted between November, 1968, and December, 1970. In the preliminary discussions on developing the survey, decisions were made to collect substantial information about socioeconomic status to characterize families in study. This included information on eating habits, current dietary intake, medical history, physical examination, and biochemical determinations.

Objectives of the study and sample. The primary objective of the Preschool Nutrition Survey was to provide an overview of descriptive data on nutritional status of a cross-sectional sample of preschool children throughout the United States. This contrasted with the Ten State Nutrition Survey, which focused on the population presumed to be most at risk because of poverty; the Preschool Nutrition Survey was not designed to determine the prevalence or severity of malnutrition in poor children or in children of any particular racial or ethnic group. The data collected would provide realistic bases for comparisons with other data from present and future studies.

GREATER ATTENTION NEEDED TO NUTRITIONAL WELL-BEING OF INFANTS AND YOUNG CHILDREN

With increasing use of processed, highly refined and manufactured foods, the practitioner must pay greater attention to the nutritional well-being of infants and young children who because of rapid growth and increased needs are at particular risk of developing subclinical malnutrition. The relatively frequent occurrence of intercurrent illness during childhood and the common use of chemotherapeutic agents represent additional important factors influencing nutritional status.

George M. Owen, et al.: Evaluation of the individual child's nutritional status. In Kelley, V., editor: Practice of pediatrics, New York, 1975, Harper & Row, Publishers, vol. 1.

In a 2-year period some 3,400 children between 1 and 6 years of age were studied in thirty-six states and the District of Columbia; 14.5% of these children were black, whereas Spanish-Americans and American Indians accounted for 5.8% of the study population.

Study design

Clinical examination and anthropometry. A team of nurses and pediatricians was responsible for locating, scheduling, staffing, and operating clinics in which, initially, medical histories and the mother's obstetric history were reviewed. Complete data on the child's birth weight and other pertinent information were obtained. The children were then weighed and height measured, head circumference and skinfold thickness were obtained, radiographs of the left hand and wrist were taken, and venipunctures were performed for blood samples. Abnormal clinical findings were reported to physicians, the health department, or clinics that had been designated by the family for follow-up.

Laboratory examination. Samples of urine and blood (venipuncture) were taken from each child who came to the clinic.

Laboratory examinations performed on blood samples included hemoglobins and hematocrits, tests for transferrin saturation, iron and iron-binding capacity, total protein, albumin, vitamin A, vitamin C, cholesterol, and triglyceride content of plasma. Urine samples were analyzed for glucose and protein (qualitative) and urea nitrogen, riboflavin, thiamin, creatinine, and iodine.

Dental examination. Dental caries were expressed in a modification of a DEF (decayed, extracted, or filled) index.

Dietary interviewing. Detailed information concerning the composition of each family with preschool children was obtained by trained dietary interviewers, including dietitians, nutritionists, and home economists. Estimates of energy and nutrient intakes were computed from 2-day records of food intake kept in the home. Interviewers obtained exact descriptions of foods consumed, including brand names of commercial products and identifying information on the label.

Information on vitamin and mineral supplementation was also collected.

Findings. The Preschool Nutrition Survey indicated that evidence of "nutritional risk," that is, lower dietary intakes, lower biochemical indices, and smaller physical size for age, were clustered among preschool children of lower socioeconomic status. A large segment of the population surveyed were regularly taking vitamin supplements.

It was also evident from the survey that racial, genetic, and socioeconomic factors are important determinants of growth, nutrition, and health.

The findings may be summed up as follows.

Clinical findings. There was a paucity of the classic clinical signs of malnutrition for which the physician has traditionally been taught to search. Thus it is necessary for the physician to consider demographic and socioeconomic variables and dietary and medical histories and to make appropriate laboratory examinations before a valid diagnosis can be made.

Medical history. There was a greater prevalence of low birth weight infants among Warner Rank I children. (According to this classification, Rank I equals the lowest socioeconomic rank.) These children may have reflected the fact that 40% of their mothers reported being younger than 17 years of age when first pregnant. In Warner Rank I children there seemed to be less increase in birth weight associated with birth order than was noted for children in higher socioeconomic status (Warner Ranks III and IV, lower middle and upper middle rank).[4]

Physical examination. Relatively few children were noted to have signs suggestive of specific nutritional disorders. Some clinical signs suggestive of malnutrition are short height for age, lower intakes of calories and some nutrients, and lower levels of some biochemical factors. Such characteristics were found mostly in Warner Rank I, in contrast to Warner Ranks III (lower middle socioeconomic level) and IV (upper middle socioeconomic level) (Table 7-1).

Anthropometry. Black children were found to be heavier and taller than white children. In contrast, for every age and sex group white children had greater skinfold thickness. Head circumferences showed slight and inconsistent differences between black and white children. It was also noted that black and white differences in stature were greater among boys than among girls, whereas the differences in weight were greater among girls.

There were also significant correlations between height, weight, head circumference, and skinfold measurements of preschool children. Taller and heavier children were more advanced in skeletal maturity and dental development.

Radiograph of hand-wrist. Within ethnic and age groups, black children have greater numbers of ossification centers than do white children. Thus at any age black children were found to have greater bone-equivalent ages than white children.

Biochemical determinations

HEMOGLOBIN. Mean hemoglobin values were lower in Warner Rank I and increased progressively in each rank. Mean levels of hemoglobins were higher in whites than in blacks for each age group, but whereas vitamin-supplemented white children as a group

Table 7-1. Mean Z scores of selected anthropometric and biochemical variables according to socioeconomic status (Warner Rank)*

Variables	Warner Rank†			
	I	II	III	IV
Height	−0.24	−0.04	0.05	0.16
Weight	−0.10	−0.02	0.00	0.14
Head circumference	−0.28	−0.04	0.06	0.15
Hemoglobin	−0.14	−0.02	0.00	0.16
Iron	−0.17	−0.03	0.03	0.13
Vitamin C	−0.16	−0.14	0.15	0.41
Vitamin A	−0.36	−0.06	0.09	0.18

*Owen, G. M., Kram, K. M., Garry, P. J., et al.: A study of nutritional status of preschool children in the United States, 1968-1970, Pediatrics 53 (suppl.):597, 1974.
†Warner Rank I comprised families with median annual income of $3,500, while families in Warner Rank IV had median annual incomes of $13,000. Warner Ranks II and III were intermediate.

consistently had higher mean hemoglobin values than nonsupplemented white children, the same pattern did not apply in blacks, among whom the converse was sometimes true.

TRANSFERRIN SATURATION. Differences in transferrin saturation among the children were more apparent among supplemented children than among those not taking supplements. However, when mean values were compared by age and Warner rank for supplemented and unsupplemented children, the differences were inconsistent. Furthermore, there was no significant or consistent sex-related difference in transferrin saturation values.

TOTAL PROTEIN. The overall mean for the population was 6.8 gm/dl, with 95% of values between 6.0 and 7.6 gm/dl. The mean values remained essentially constant with age, but there was a trend toward a decrease in total protein with increasing socioeconomic status, reflecting a decreased concentration of globulins. In every age group, total protein levels tended to be higher in black children than in white children. This can be accounted for by globulins that probably reflect greater exposure to infections and contagious diseases.

ALBUMIN. The level of albumin remained essentially constant throughout all age groups, with mean values of 3.9 or 4.0 gm/dl, although children in Warner Ranks III or IV had a greater percentage of higher albumin levels.

CHOLESTEROL. A mean cholesterol value of 161 mg/dl was found for all children examined and did not change significantly with age. In the youngest age group (12 to 23 months) mean values increased somewhat in higher Warner ranks.

TRIGLYCERIDE. Generally, triglyceride values decreased with increasing age and related positively to dietary intake of total energy, carbohydrates, fat, and protein, all of which decreased significantly with age. There was also a trend for the values to rise with socioeconomic status. As with cholesterol, vitamin/mineral supplementation seemed to have no appreciable effect on tri-glyceride levels. Also, there was no statistically significant correlation between plasma triglyceride and dietary intakes of carbohydrates, fats, protein, or total energy.

VITAMIN A. There was poor correlation between current dietary intake of vitamin A and plasma levels of retinol in individual children. Supplemented children did have higher levels than unsupplemented children. In comparing plasma retinol concentrations in children who had relatively low intakes of vitamin A with those of children who had relatively high intakes, the difference between the children's mean plasma retinol value was significant.[15]

VITAMIN C. When plasma vitamin C values were evaluated, there was a significant difference between blacks and whites in every age group. The magnitude of difference seemed consistent, whether or not children received vitamin/mineral supplements. Again, increasing values with increasing Warner ranks were noted.

UREA NITROGEN. Plasma urea nitrogen value fluctuated little for most age, sex, ethnic, and socioeconomic stratifications. Children with vitamin/mineral supplementation had slightly higher levels than unsupplemented children. This corresponded to the slightly higher protein intake in the supplemented group. There were no sex differences, but mean values for whites were significantly higher at every age interval than mean values for blacks and reflected somewhat higher protein intakes of whites than of blacks.

Urinary urea nitrogen concentration decreased with age, reflecting lower protein intake and the fact that creatinine excretion increases with age. It may also indicate a more efficient utilization of nitrogen-containing nutrients by the body as it ages.

THIAMIN. Urinary thiamin levels decreased with age, although not markedly, and probably reflected increased creatinine excretion, since thiamin intakes generally increased with age. Average values for supplemented children are almost twice those of unsupplemented children.

RIBOFLAVIN. Essentially the same observations made for thiamin are true for riboflavin.

Values decreased with age; no sex difference was observed; levels in supplemented children were almost twice those in unsupplemented children.

IODINE. There was no obvious trend of fluctuation of iodine levels according to Warner rank, sex, or the use of supplements.

Dental health. Children in the lower socioeconomic groups, and particularly black youngsters, had the highest caries attack rate. Data for a subsample of white children (12 to 36 months of age) were analyzed to determine if deciduous tooth eruption was related to height, weight, and head circumference.[16] The coefficient of association was positive for all comparisons. Statistical analyses demonstrated significant associations between tooth eruption and height, weight, and head circumference in boys; the associations in girls were significant for teeth as opposed to height. These findings indicate that the timing of deciduous tooth eruption is related to general somatic growth and perhaps also to nutritional status.

Dietary status. It is possible to look at dietary intake data according to distributions of values in various subsets of the population, but then no conclusions are warranted with respect to usual intakes of individual children. Suggested guidelines for evaluating

energy and nutrient intakes of individual children have been designed by Owen and co-workers (Table 7-2).

Inspection of the dietary intake data showed fairly consistent and expected changes according to the age of children irrespective of socioeconomic status. It was apparent that supplements contributed substantial amounts of vitamins to the total intakes of preschool children, with percentage increases greatest for children of lower socioeconomic status.

Food sources of energy and nutrients. Age, race, and socioeconomic status are important variables that influence eating patterns. There was a progressive decrease in the use of dairy foods with increasing age in all socioeconomic groups. This was most evident among Warner Rank I children and particularly among black children. Total consumption of meat and poultry varied little by socioeconomic status. Despite reduced money available for food, poor families did not scrimp on meat in children's diets.

Cereal grains were major contributors of iron and of calories to children's diets. As socioeconomic levels increased, breads, rolls, biscuits, cereals, pastas, and grain mixtures contributed progressively less energy. In the higher socioeconomic groups, cakes, cookies, pies, and sweet rolls contributed more energy for children. More children in the upper socioeconomic families consumed heavily iron-fortified breakfast cereals, primarily the ready-to-eat variety.

Fruits contributed progressively more energy and nutrients, whereas vegetables generally contributed less as socioeconomic level increased. Contrary to popular belief, poor children did not substitute soft drinks for more nutritious fruit juices or vitamin-fortified beverages. Vegetables were most frequently mentioned as being least preferred by older children.

Health and Nutrition Examination Survey (HANES)

The first Health and Nutrition Examination Survey (HANES) was begun in 1971 and completed in 1974.[17] The purpose of the sur-

Table 7-2. Suggested guidelines for evaluating energy and nutrient intakes of individual child*†

	Age (yr)	
	1-2	**4-6**
Energy (kcal)	1,000	1,300
Protein (gm)	15	22
Protein (gm/kg)	1.5	1.5
Calcium (mg)	450	450
Iron (mg)	5	5
Vitamin A (IU)	800	1,000
Thiamin (mg)	0.3	0.5
Riboflavin (mg)	0.5	0.7
Vitamin C (mg)	20	20

*From Owen, G. M., Kram, K. M., Garry, P. J., et al.: A study of nutritional status of preschool children in the United States, 1968-1970, Pediatrics 53 (suppl.):597, 1974.
†Intakes of nutrients below these levels may be unacceptably low for most children.

vey was to establish a continuing national nutrition surveillance system by measuring the nutritional status of the population and monitoring changes in status over time.

The HANES survey was actually a part of the National Health Survey and represented the first time a nutrition component had been incorporated into the health survey. Funding for these activities emanated from the National Health Survey Act of 1956, which provided for the establishment and continuation of a National Health Survey to obtain information about the health status of the population in the United States, including the services received for or because of health conditions. Responsibility for this program was placed with the National Center for Health Statistics (NCHS), a research-oriented statistical organization within the U.S. Department of Health, Education, and Welfare.

Prompted by the preliminary results of the Ten State Nutrition Survey and various programs being carried out by a number of federal, state, and local agencies to combat nutrition problems, the need for data on the magnitude and distribution of these problems in the United States became more evident. The Department of Health, Education, and Welfare in 1969 then established HANES, a continuing national nutrition surveillance system under the authority of the 1956 National Health Survey Act.

Objectives of study. The objectives for HANES were based on the recommendations made by the National Center for Health Statistics (NCHS) Task Force, which was the body selected to formulate a scientifically sound plan for the collection, analysis, and dissemination of the data required by the Department of Health, Education, and Welfare.

Some of the major objectives were the following:

1. Each cycle of HANES would cover approximately a 2-year period based on a sample of about 30,000 persons, 1 through 74 years of age.

2. All sample persons would receive a specifically designed nutrition examination, with a one-fifth subsample of those 25 to 74 years of age also receiving a more detailed examination based on the Health Examination Survey (HES) component.

3. The sample would be more heavily weighted with low-income groups, older age groups, preschool children, and women of childbearing age.

4. The nutrition aspect would consist of a general physical examination; dermatologic, ophthalmologic, and dental examination; body measurements; biochemical assessment; and dietary intake measures.

5. Demographic data, health history, health care needs, dietary information, and data on participation in food programs would be obtained through the use of questionnaires.

Sample design. There were four major nutrition components in HANES:

1. Dietary intake based on a 24-hour recall and a food-frequency questionnaire
2. Biochemical levels of various nutrients based on assessments of blood and urine samples
3. Clinical signs of possible nutritional deficiencies
4. Anthropometric measurements

Dietary component. Most of the dietary interviews were conducted in clinic settings, with a small number completed on home visits. The 24-hour dietary recall questionnaire was administered for the total day before the day of examination. After the 24-hour recall a second questionnaire on dietary frequency was answered, which obtained information about how often certain foods had been eaten during the preceding 3 months. Household questionnaires and food program questionnaires were also administered.

Biochemical levels. Samples of blood and urine were obtained by a laboratory technician. Laboratory determinations with blood or serum included hemoglobin, hematocrit, erythrocyte count, and indices (MCV, MCH, MCHC), white cell count, sedimentation rate, iron, iron-binding capacity, folates, cholesterol, vitamin A, vitamin C, magnesium, total protein, and albumin. Examination of urinary constituents included qualitative tests for glucose, albumin, and occult blood; quantitative determinations were made of creatinine, thiamin, riboflavin, and iodine.

Clinical signs and medical history. The physicians' examinations were oriented toward gathering data on physical conditions pertinent to nutrition habits and on certain chronic diseases. Medical history questionnaires were administered and reviewed by the physicians.

The ophthalmology examination included an ocular history regarding previously known eye disease or previous surgery and a detailed examination of the eyes.

A dermatology examination, historic review, and detailed clinical examination of the skin and its appendages were all included.

Dental examination. A complete dental examination was done by dentists. The teeth were classified as sound, filled, decayed, filled-defective, and nonfunctional.

Anthropometry. Height and weight measurements were completed on all subjects. In addition, all examinees received a determination of handedness and six other measurements: elbow breadth, upper arm girth, triceps and subscapular skinfolds, bitrochanteric breadth, and sitting height. Children 1 to 7 years of age were also measured for head and chest circumferences. Those receiving a more detailed examination had chest circumference measurements made of full inspiration and expiration.

Also, for the detailed examination the range of motion of certain joints, including the hip and knee, was measured goniometrically. Finally, hand-wrist radiographs were completed in those aged 1 to 17 years only.

Findings

Dietary data. The mean nutritive content of diets consumed by different age, sex, race, and income groups was compared, using indices of iron, calcium, and vitamin A and C intakes. Only the major findings obtained from the first Health and Nutrition Examination Survey have been published.[18]

Some of the major findings include the following:

1. Iron was the nutrient most often found below the standard in population groups. This was shown in three age groups: children 1 to 5 years, for whom the mean measurements were 31% to 40% below the standard; adolescents 12 to 17 years who were 23% to 33% below the standard, and women 18 to 44 years who were 41% to 51% below the standard.

2. Black children 6 to 11 years and adults, regardless of race, 45 to 59 years in the lower income groups also consumed amounts of iron that were below the standards.

3. Most age groups, regardless of both race and income levels, had calcium and vitamin A and C intakes that either approached (90% to 100% of the standard) or were above the standards. The exceptions were black women 18 to 44 years, regardless of income levels, who had inadequate mean calcium intakes that were 20% to 23% below the standard; and white women of the same age group in the lower income level, who had mean vitamin A intakes 18% below the standard.

4. A higher percentage of white children 1 to 5 years and white women 18 to 44 years in the lower income group tended to have vitamin A and C intakes that were less than the standards when compared with black individuals of similar age-sex-income groups. Corresponding percentages in the upper income group were higher for blacks than for whites.

Biochemical data. Major findings from the biochemical tests include the following:

1. Black adults 60 years of age and over in the lower income group had the highest prevalence of low hemoglobin and low hematocrit values. Of this group 29.6% had low hemoglobin values and 41.7% had low hematocrit values.

2. The percentage of blacks with low hemoglobin values was more than four times that of whites in the age groups 6 to 11 and 12 to 17 years at each income level.

3. The highest prevalence of low percent transferrin saturation values occurred in the age groups 1 to 5, 6 to 11, and 12 to 17 years.

4. In the age group 1 to 5 years the prevalence of low transferrin saturation value greatly exceeded that of low serum iron, hemoglobin, and hematocrit values.

5. Black children in the age group 1 to 5 years showed the highest prevalence of low serum vitamin A values.

6. There were no observed low serum albumin values in the age groups 1 to 5, 6 to 11, and 12 to 17 years.

7. Whites had a higher prevalence of low serum protein value for all age groups regardless of income level.

Clinical findings. Evidence of clinical signs suggesting possible nutrient deficiencies was generally slight, particularly high-risk signs.[19,20] This confirmed similar findings from previous surveys such as the Ten State Nutrition Survey and the Preschool Nutrition Survey. Two generalizations can be made about the clinical findings: First, the prevalence of most clinical signs increases with age, a finding that coincides with previous investigations in highly developed countries. Many of the nutritional deficiencies in the older age groups are secondary to underlying diseases and abnormalities (e.g., alcoholism). Second, it seems that blacks show higher prevalences for most signs than whites of the same age, sex, and income groups.

Clinical protein deficiency does not appear to be a problem and particularly not in young children. There appears to be some vitamin B complex deficiency in certain older age groups. A similar situation exists in regard to vitamin C. Some dietary deficiency may have a role in the prevalence of bleeding and swollen gums in adolescents. Vitamin A deficiency may exist among young children and women of childbearing age and more so among whites than blacks.

The prevalence of Chvostek's sign, which indicates increased neuromuscular irritability associated with relative calcium deficiency, was generally higher in blacks of all ages regardless of income.

The prevalence of goiter was relatively low in most age-sex-income groups except in black adolescents from groups just above poverty level income and in young black women in the same income group. Here it reached public health significance, which is greater than 10%.

Anthropometry. Anthropometric findings in the age groups 1 to 18 years showed that blacks generally were slightly taller and heavier but whites had greater median skin-

REFINING THE TOOLS FOR NUTRITIONAL ASSESSMENT

In medical centers and regions where infants and children are referred or followed because of failure to thrive or because of conditions known to be associated with altered gastrointestinal function or metabolic disorders and among whom clinical findings might be expected, it is interesting how infrequently they are reported. This may mean either they have not occurred or the physician has failed to recognize them. It does seem likely that when clinical signs of nutritional disease are manifest, the deficiency is severe. Alternatively, one may conclude there are no subtle clinical signs of nutritional disorders. Further research is needed to improve biochemical methodologies to allow early detection of subclinical nutritional disorders and to monitor nutritional status.

George M. Owen, Kathryn M. Kram, Philip J. Garry, et al.: A study of nutritional status of preschool children in the United States, 1968-1970, Part II, Pediatrics **53** (suppl.):597, 1974.

folds. Dietary findings are compatible with the latter but do not explain the former.

In adults 20 to 74 years the prevalence of both leanness and obesity was observed. There were more lean blacks, especially men, than whites and more obesity among white men than blacks. However, the percentage of obese black women was as high as leanness among black men.

Children and adolescents in the income groups just above poverty level were usually fatter, heavier, and had greater median skinfolds than those in other income groups.

Black women were identified as the highest risk group regarding the contraction and mortality from certain diseases such as hypertension, heart disease, and diabetes. Both control and preventive programs need to be implemented for these high-risk groups. Further research is needed to improve methodologies to allow for earlier detection of certain diseases that have a nutritional component.

Regional and local surveys

In addition to the three major studies just outlined, many investigators have undertaken dietary and nutritional status surveys among various population groups in the United States, summarized in Table 7-3.

Table 7-3. Selected regional and local studies with children*

Sample	Location	Findings and comments
170 Mexican-American 0-66 months of age	San Ysidro, California	Some children with low intakes of energy, vitamin C, niacin, and iron. Vitamin A intakes good and plasma vitamin A concentrations normal. Iron deficiency prevalent. Some youngsters had low plasma vitamin C.
41 black inner city preschoolers	Philadelphia	Comparable intakes of iron by day-care (0.7 mg/kg/day) and by non-day-care (0.5 mg/kg/day). Anemia more prevalent among non-day-care than among day-care children.
50 blacks of low income	Nashville	Approximately 10% of children were anemic and 15% had low plasma vitamin A.
281 mixed racial 2-3 years of age	Honolulu	Intakes of calcium, vitamin A, ascorbic acid, and riboflavin low for some groups (inversely related to income). Between 5% and 10% were anemic.
168 Mexican-American 6-9 years of age	Coachella Valley, California	52% had hemoglobin less than 10 gm/dl.
178 black pre-schoolers	South Carolina	25% anemic (hemoglobin < 10 gm/dl); 50% iron deficient (serum iron < 40 μg/dl).
300 Mexican-American migrant workers' pre-school children	Colorado	10%-20% of children had clinical signs (skin and eye) suggestive of vitamin A deficiency. 20% had low plasma vitamin A. 5% had skeletal findings (ribs and wrists) suggestive of rickets.
642 Puerto Ricans, Chinese, blacks, and whites 10-13 years of age	New York City	5% with anemia. Nutrient intakes followed ethnic and cultural patterns (24 hour recall of intake by the children).
115 whites 2-6 years of age	Minnesota	Dietary survey only. Some low intakes of iron and vitamin C.
7800 children less than 10 years old, blacks and whites	Three National surveys (see text)	Systematic difference of approximately 1.0 gm/dl of hemoglobin between blacks and whites.
109 blacks and whites 4 months-5 years of age	Michigan	10% with severe iron deficiency anemia; mild iron deficiency anemia 13%; and 23% with nonanemic iron deficiency.
250 Mexican-American and whites 0-17 years of age	Denver	Evidence of low zinc stores among 45% of children under 4 years of age (based on hair zinc determinations).
843 Eskimos 2-6 years of age	Alaska	Low levels of intake of calories, calcium, and vitamin C among some children. Protein intakes were generally high.
70 whites 0-18 months of age	Seattle	More than half of the nonanemic (hemoglobin ≥ 11 gm/dl) infants studied had iron deficiency (transferrin saturation < 15%).
36 blacks 4-10 months of age	South Carolina	Approximately 10% of infants had low levels of albumin and plasma vitamin C.
60 families	Iowa and North Carolina	Dietary survey only. Adequate intakes of protein, calcium, vitamins C, B_1, and B_2 as well as iron.
113 Indian families	Fort Belknap, Montana	Some children with low intakes of vitamins A and C as well as of calcium. Approximately one-third of children had low levels of hemoglobin, plasma vitamin A, and erythrocyte riboflavin.
40 whites	Nebraska	Urinary thiamin and riboflavin excretion varied with income. Approximately 10% of children had low levels of hemoglobin.

*From Owen, G. M., and Lippman, G.: Nutritional status of infants and young children: U.S.A., Pediatr. Clin. North Am. **24:**214, 1977.

Continued.

Table 7-3. Selected regional and local studies with children—cont'd

Sample	Location	Findings and comments
160 Mexican-Americans 0-9 years of age	Lower Rio Grande Valley, Texas	Clinical signs of vitamin A and vitamin D deficiencies. One-third of children with low level of vitamin A in plasma. 10% were anemic.
100 low income 0-14 years of age	New York City	No clinical signs of riboflavin deficiency, although 10% had biochemical evidence of deficiency.
386 whites 3-10 years of age	Tennessee	Many children had low intakes of iron (6%-18%), vitamin C (20%), energy (30%), and vitamin A (50%).
465 Apache Indians 1-6 years of age	Arizona	20% of children with low levels of hemoglobin, vitamin A, and vitamin C. Iron deficiency and anemia were prevalent.
100 black pre-schoolers	Tennessee	15% iron-deficient; 95% with low levels of vitamin A.
129 Eskimos 0-12 years of age	Alaska	40% of children under 5 years of age had hemoglobin < 10 gm/dl.
200 newborns, 60 percent blacks	Kentucky	No correlation between maternal and infant hematological values (iron, total iron-binding capacity, hemoglobin, packed cell volume).
300 blacks 0-6 years of age	Tennessee	25% with "low" hemoglobin, 40% with low plasma vitamin A levels. Average height (stature) at 25th percentile of reference chart.

These studies have focused on either specific geographic locale or segments of society that deserved special attention. By means of dietary survey or biochemical assessment or both, these studies provide insight into those special areas and indicate particular needs.

NUTRITIONAL ASSESSMENT: SURVEILLANCE

To the public health practitioner the idea of a nutrition survey in the traditional sense implies rigorous sampling procedures, costly biochemical determinations, and a large budget for providing the necessary tools and information that make the survey data meaningful. However, even this kind of detailed survey only can provide information about the prevalence of a condition in a population at a given point in time. Such data do not give insight into the number of individuals who may be expected to develop a nutritional problem over time. Two additional problems are unresolved with survey data alone: (1) Neither specific locations nor the relative magnitudes of problems in different localities are identified. (2) Little or no local information is provided that is necessary to de-

velop a sound program based on rational program planning.

On the other hand, if nutrition surveys are conducted in the same population at two or more points in time, utilizing similar sampling methods and methodologies, useful information regarding changes that occur over time can be discovered. The Health and Nutrition Examination Survey can provide this type of information through its "monitoring" or "surveillance" aspects.

The importance of a surveillance system becomes clear when one considers that once the nutrition practitioner finally has access to funds for developing a state survey, a question arises: Is it wise to spend these funds on a survey that will identify problems but has no mechanism to begin correcting the problems?

The need for a "watching over" plan at state and local levels that would be a start in implementing positive action was recognized by Nichaman and Lane at the Center for Disease Control, Atlanta, who devised a pragmatic system utilizing selected nutritional indices. It is known as the Nutrition Surveillance System.[21]

PURPOSE OF SURVEILLANCE

As opposed to assessment and monitoring, surveillance implies an ongoing system intimately linked to an active health program. Thus, surveillance should not be a separate enterprise in and of itself. Rather surveillance data should be produced by the ongoing health programs themselves . . . Another hazard in developing surveillance systems is the temptation to turn them into research projects. It is, for example, inappropriate to attempt to define the clinical or health importance of such things as zinc or chromium in the context of a surveillance system.

Jean-Pierre Habicht, Michael Lane, and Arthur McDowell: Nutrition surveillance. Presented at the Symposium on National Nutrition Surveillance, American Institute of Nutrition Meeting, Chicago, April, 1977. Reprinted from Federation Proceedings **37**:1181, 1978.

Definition of surveillance

Surveillance, as contrasted to survey, implies continuity—"a frequent and continuous watching over." As Nichaman stated, "Repeated surveys do not accomplish this, particularly if the period of time between population sampling is protracted. Therefore, an activity that monitors individual groups, particularly high-risk groups, on a continuous, uninterrupted basis, is desirable. . . ."[7] One highly desirable feature of the surveillance system is that a "sample of convenience," that is, data available from any source that accurately describes the sample, can be utilized effectively.

Examples of "ready-made" data sources include Medicaid, Early Periodic Screening, Diagnosis, and Treatment program (EPSDT) information, Maternal and Infant Care projects; children and youth projects; public health well-baby clinics, maternal and family planning clinics: Head Start data; and the school system. These are just a few sources that can be tapped and retrieved at little cost.

Major components

The major components of a competent surveillance system are (1) nutritional assessment, (2) nutritional monitoring, and (3) nutritional surveillance in its specialized sense.[22]

Nutritional assessment includes the measurement and description of the nutritional status of a population in relation to those economic, sociodemographic, and physiologic variables which can affect the nutrition of that population.

Nutritional monitoring is the measurement of changes over time in the nutritional status of a population or of a specific group of individuals. Monitoring thus requires repeated comparable assessments at regular intervals.

Nutritional surveillance indicates a frequent and continuous watching over. It gives direction to the early detection of community nutritional problems so that they then can be corrected. A good surveillance system not only gathers and analyzes data but also quickly presents the data to those who make administrative decisions that will affect the health and nutrition of the community.

These components are in accord with the objectives presented by the United Nations Expert Committee Report on Methodology of Nutritional Surveillance for such a system.[23]

1. To describe the nutritional status of the population, with particular reference to defined subgroups who are identified as being at risk. This will permit description of the character and magnitude of the nutrition problem and changes in the features.

2. To provide information that will contribute to the analysis of causes and associated factors and so permit a selection of preventive measures which may or may not be nutritional.

3. To promote decisions by governments concerning priorities and the dispersal of resources to meet the needs of both normal development and emergencies.

4. To enable predictions to be made on the basis of current trends in order to indicate the probable evolution of nutritional problems. Considered in conjunction with existing and potential measures and resources, these will assist in the formulation of policy.

5. To monitor nutritional programs and to evaluate their effectiveness.

Developing a nutrition surveillance system for a program

In developing any program plan, a *needs assessment* must be determined before a problem can be identified. As was discussed in Chapter 4 on program planning, a need is described as a lack of something required or desired. In looking at the need, the public health practitioner must answer the following questions: In what population groups do nutritional problems exist? What is the geographic location of these populations? What is the ethnic mix, economic status, and age of these populations? What is the extent of the problem? How can a program be implemented to alleviate these problems? What resources of manpower and money are already available and what additional resources are needed?

The information from the three national surveys (Ten State, Preschool Nutritional Survey, and HANES), described earlier, indicate similar findings—that anemia is a problem and that people in low-income populations are at greater nutritional risk. It is noteworthy that although these three surveys used different approaches to assess the nutrition problems, their results coincide in almost all instances. Reviewing these survey data should give the practitioner an indication of the "universal" problems.

Developing the nutritional assessment profile

To further delineate the local problems and to assist in initiating a nutritional surveillance system, one must determine what is to be measured and how the data will be collected. Such information is called the "nutritional assessment profile." The tools of nutritional assessment, both for individuals and population groups are "(1) *biochemical* measurement of nutrients in body fluids and tissues; (2) *clinical* examinations, including assessment of growth by utilizing body measurements; and (3) collection of *dietary* information."[7]

Anthropometric and biochemical measurements constitute the major objective data used in determining nutritional status, yet dietary intake data are useful in determining avenues for intervention. Dietary information should be confirmed by the presence or absence of clinical signs, by biochemical data, and by body measurements. Since the collection of dietary information is extremely difficult and fraught with many inconsistencies such as problems concerning analysis of food composition data, nutritional losses during handling and cooking of food, and difficulty with clients' memories, to mention only a few, this information must be substantiated with more objective data such as biochemical values and anthropometric measurements. If in the hypothetical community dietary data reveal that a population is below the Recommended Dietary Allowance for iron intake, information on hemoglobin and hematocrit of the populations should be obtained before diagnosis of "iron deficiency" can be made.

Guide to nutritional assessment and the surveillance system

To assist with the development of nutritional assessment, an excellent guide, *Nutritional Assessment in Health Programs*, edited by Christakis,[3] was published by the American Public Health Association under the auspices of the Nutrition Program, Center for Disease Control (CDC). It was aimed primarily at community public health workers. The guide is one of the most important tools in practicing public health today and should be a part of every practitioner's library. It is the tool to be used in evaluating the nutritional status of a target population, and thus it is effective in defining the "need" and ultimately reducing this need in a community.

Data collection for continuity

The procedure for developing a program plan, presented in Chapter 6, states the importance of supplying data to determine the specific evaluation. The scheme indicates that a built-in method for recording and reporting data is vital if one is to present evidence of change clearly and concisely. Selecting which data to report is the key to sound evaluation results; frequently one collects entirely too much data of the wrong kind. Determining results from this mass of information is difficult, if not impossible.

Once the data-gathering forms and mechanisms have been determined by the staff, several further steps are necessary as follows:

1. The data should be analyzed at a central point or location.
2. The data should also be compared with reference populations so that comparisons can be made between reporting sets.
3. A mechanism for assessing and improving the quality of the data must be built into the data collection system.

Consideration also should be given to monitoring the quality of both anthropometric and biochemical measurements. Because of inadequate equipment and lack of training among personnel, measurements such as height and weight can be inaccurately made, and such data can lead to unsound program planning. Inappropriate field equipment used to complete hemoglobin and hematocrit determinations can lead to the same situation —an unrealistic view of the problem being identified.

Uses for nutrition surveillance data

The usefulness of surveillance information cannot be overemphasized in public health practice. Nichaman,[21] in the Center for Disease Control report, cites six ways in which data from a nutrition surveillance system can be utilized:

(a) To define the prevalence of particular nutritional problems in target populations. One may start with a simple beginning such as recording heights and weights, then add hemoglobin and hematocrits. Flexibility should be built into the system in order to accommodate the addition of more indices. An example of this is the Arizona Surveillance System where serum cholesterol determinations were added to the assessment profile.

(b) To facilitate medical care by providing a basis for identifying individuals in need of follow-up treatment.

(c) To provide "before" and "after" information so that the value of intervention and preventative programs, both for individuals and population groups, can be measured. The opportunity to provide data on the result of the program is one of the most important aspects of the surveillance system.

(d) To provide data to establish priorities for the allocation of funds and personnel resources.

(e) To provide information about the local situation that will enable effective targeting of federal, state and local feeding programs.

(f) To provide a research base for investigating the relationship between various levels of nutritional status and health consequences.

Nutrition surveillance in the United States: state of the art

The list of federal agencies involved in nutritional surveillance is formidable. They include the Department of Agriculture, Department of Defense, Veterans Administration, Department of Health, Education, and Welfare, National Center for Health Statistics, Food and Drug Administration, Com-

---

IDENTIFY HIGH-RISK GROUPS AND THEN DESIGN PROGRAMS TO REDUCE RISK

In general, it is clear that nutritional deficiency must develop in the following manner: first, there is an inadequate intake of the nutrient; second, the tissue reserves of the nutrient fall; third, after the tissues are depleted, clinically evident disease develops. The objective of any adequate nutrition program must be to *prevent* the disease from developing—not to cure the disease after it develops. Thus, if there is any appreciable amount of clinically evident disease in a population, the surveillance system has failed. Clearly, a system that relies largely on counting the numbers of malnourished persons is inadequate. The system must identify "high-risk groups" and call for programs that will reduce the risk. This is an extremely important point and one that is usually not appreciated.

D. Mark Hegsted: A national surveillance system. In Mayer, J., editor: U.S. nutrition policies in the seventies, San Francisco, 1973, W. H. Freeman & Co., Publishers. © 1973.

NUTRITION SURVEILLANCE IN ARIZONA

Approaching public health nutrition through a health care delivery system enables planners to assess the status of the population first before trying to intervene. Changes in program planning and setting of priorities have occurred because of what the surveillance data showed. With the serum cholesterol data before us, we were encouraged to reevaluate our assumption about the Mexican-American diet.

Anita Yanochik-Owen and *Morissa White:* Nutrition surveillance in Arizona: selected anthropometric and laboratory observations among Mexican-American children, Am. J. Public Health **67**:151, 1977.

municable Disease Center, and Environmental Protection Agency, among others.

The types of assessment studies that have been completed are equally widespread. They range from assessment and monitoring of food supply to food production costs and to household food consumption. Many of these have been implemented by the Department of Agriculture.

Other data sources are studies of the nutritional value of foods and ingestion of contaminants carried out by the National Center for Health Statistics, Food and Drug Administration, and Environmental Protection Agency. The Communicable Disease Center and National Center for Health Statistics have also made studies of nutritional status and health-related variables. In addition, the Departments of Labor and Agriculture have investigated costs of food purchased and price indices related to food.

A report published in March, 1976, by the Congressional Research Service for the Senate Select Committee on Nutrition and Human Needs indicates various kinds of research studies in agencies such as the Department of Agriculture, Department of Health, Education, and Welfare, Depart-

ment of Defense, and Veterans Administration.[24]

This rather unorganized system of nutritional surveillance presents some problems for the practitioner, such as the following: Where is a total listing of completed studies that can be useful for field experiences? How readily available are reports of these studies?

Most of the data collected to date have been regarding undernutrition. Few data are available on the areas of overnutrition such as obesity, a number one public health problem. An attempt to address these concerns was made in May, 1977, when the National Center for Health Statistics convened a standing panel of experts and ad hoc consultants to evaluate HANES and extend its studies into overnutrition problems.

A nutrition surveillance system of the Center for Disease Control (CDC): a model

The Center for Disease Control (CDC) has been operating a nutrition surveillance system that can serve as an excellent model for a statewide system. It shows the public health nutrition practitioner the practical application of a surveillance system.

Realizing that information on nutritional status has been collected in a variety of medical care settings and that there was no concurrent system to analyze these data, Nicha-

---

NUTRITIONAL STATUS MONITORING SYSTEM

During a June 29, 1977 discussion of the HEW appropriations bill on the Senate floor, concern was expressed by Senator Chiles (D. Fla.) with the lack of knowledge and federal effort in the area of nutrition. With his urging, the Appropriations Committee has directed the HEW Assistant Secretary of Health to submit within 90 days a proposal for a comprehensive nutritional status monitoring system. This will include an assessment system to determine the extent of nutrition-related health problems in the United States, a surveillance system to identify nutrition-related health problems in individuals or local areas, and program evaluations to determine the adequacy, effectiveness and efficiency of Federal nutrition programs in reducing health risks. He hopes that appropriations will be authorized next year to undertake a comprehensive effort on nutrition.

Nutrition Notes, American Institute of Nutrition Newsletter **13**:3, Sept., 1977.

OBESITY: A SERIOUS PUBLIC HEALTH PROBLEM

The public health importance of obesity is considerable, both because of its prevalence in the United States and because of its detrimental effects on performance, health and survival. Unfortunately, there are less than a dozen well designed studies investigating the relationships between energy intake, the ills of obesity, and exercise. . . . must be followed up by better measures of energy intake and exercise before they can be considered conclusive these results illustrate the usefulness of a national nutrition assessment survey in identifying new areas of public concern.

Jean-Pierre Habicht, Michael Lane, and *Arthur McDowell:* Nutrition surveillance. Presented at the Symposium on National Nutritional Surveillance, American Institute of Nutrition Meeting, Chicago, April, 1977. Reprinted from Federation Proceedings **37**:1181, 1978.

man and staff at CDC initiated the development of a nutrition surveillance system in 1974. They utilized data from five states, Arizona, Kentucky, Louisiana, Texas, and Washington, as the pilot for the system.

The nutrition surveillance system at CDC has four major components:

1. A data collection system
2. A mechanism for analyzing the data
3. A mechanism for returning the results to the originating clinic or activity for their use
4. The development of a nutrition surveillance report on a quarterly basis to be distributed nationwide with data on the nutrition indices given state by state

The ultimate goal of the CDC surveillance program is to develop a simple computer system that can be presented to individual states, which will then be able to handle their own data. As well as systematically providing data for program planning, an additional benefit of the CDC system is that it is an educational tool for nutrition staff and health department personnel. It makes the staff cognizant of the kind of data with which they will be dealing and the importance of collecting accurate information, and it helps improve the quality of their services.

Method of operation

A format was developed for gathering and submitting data from several different sources in a standardized, computer-compatible manner. The format was devised with recommendations from federal and state health agencies and subcommittees representing the American Academy of Pediatrics and the Food and Nutrition Board of the National Academy of Sciences–National Research Council (NAS–NRC).

The basic data collected by these states include measurements of height, weight, hemoglobin, or hematocrit. The results of data from January through March, 1975, and April through June, 1975, are shown in Tables 7-4 and 7-5. Although these indices are limited in scope, they do reflect the major nutritional problems that have been identified in the United States, such as growth deficit, obesity, and iron-deficiency anemia.

The Center for Disease Control is performing the analyses of the data at present. Monthly tabulations are provided to clinics and programs at the state level. They consist of listings of individuals requiring nutrition follow-up, together with clinic summaries— the number and percentage of children who require follow-up because of deficiencies in one or more of the indices. Quarterly and annual summary tabulations are also made to enable geographic comparisons, as well as selected agency and program comparisons.

The basic data handling system can be modified to permit future incorporation of additional nutritional indices into the basic

Table 7-4. Nutrition indices of persons less than 18 years of age by state, January-March, 1975*

State	Hemoglobin[2]		Hematocrit[2]		Height for age[1]		Weight for age[1]		Weight for height[1]		
	No. exam.	% low	No. exam.	% low	No. exam.	% low	No. exam.	% low	No. exam.	% low	% high
Arizona	2,088	14.5	3,245	14.7	5,210	19.1	5,242	9.1	5,120	5.3	16.2
Kentucky	993	15.0	1,207	17.3	2,909	14.7	2,917	8.6	2,870	6.0	14.1
Louisiana	5,399	21.4	1,470	15.0	7,053	9.9	7,111	7.3	6,925	5.1	6.9
Tennessee	526	5.5	5,256	18.9	5,806	10.1	5,913	5.6	5,745	5.2	9.5
Washington	390	11.0	2,912	10.5	3,798	13.0	3,807	6.3	3,779	2.8	11.5
Total	9,396	17.9	14,090	15.7	24,776	12.9	24,990	7.3	24,439	4.9	11.0

*From Center for Disease Control: Nutrition surveillance report, Washington, D.C., 1975, HEW publication no. 77-8295, Government Printing Office.
[1]Children <1 month of age excluded.
[2]Children <6 months of age excluded.

Table 7-5. Nutrition indices of persons less than 18 years of age by state, April-June, 1975*

State	Hemoglobin		Hematocrit		Height for age		Weight for age		Weight for height		
	No. exam.	% low	No. exam.	% low	No. exam.	% low	No. exam.	% low	No. exam.	% low	% high
Arizona	1,874	13.4	2,067	11.9	3,690	15.2	3,721	7.2	3,638	4.0	13.2
Kentucky	824	20.0	1,109	17.1	2,550	13.6	2,553	7.2	2,512	5.1	11.7
Louisiana	930	18.8	215	16.7	1,198	9.9	1,208	6.5	1,185	3.3	7.8
Tennessee	374	6.7	6,411	21.5	7,197	10.2	7,358	5.9	7,111	4.2	9.9
Washington	386	3.9	1,915	10.3	2,799	12.0	2,799	6.2	2,777	2.9	11.6
Total	4,388	14.4	11,717	17.5	17,434	12.0	17,639	6.4	17,223	4.0	11.0

*From Center for Disease Control: Nutrition surveillance report, Washington, D.C., 1975, HEW publication no. 77-8295, Government Printing Office.

format on a routine basis. One example, mentioned previously, is information regarding serum cholesterol determination that was submitted by Arizona.

Guidelines for interpretation and reference data in the CDC nutrition surveillance system*

Comparisons must be made with known values derived from appropriate reference populations to make meaningful interpretations of data. In this system the indices were physical growth of children and anemia.

Height and weight. The reference populations utilized for the height-weight data were as follows:

Age	Reference population data
Birth to 24 months	Fels Research Institute Growth Study
25 to 59 months	Preschool Nutrition Survey
60 to 143 months	National Health Exam Survey Cycle II
144 to 215 months	National Health Exam Survey Cycle III

These data are reasonably representative of the total population of the United States. Until recently, reference values for a randomly selected sample, representative of the general population, were not available. The most commonly utilized values were the "Harvard and Iowa standards" of Stuart and

Meredith, which were drawn from special studies conducted several decades ago on small numbers of relatively well-nourished children.[25] Although the Stuart-Meredith work has proved to be useful as baseline data, these standards cannot be considered to be normative values for children in the United States today.

Methods of comparison for heights and weights. The system employs three commonly utilized relationships expressing height or weight: height for age, weight for height, and weight for age.

HEIGHT FOR AGE (MEASURE OF SHORTNESS AND TALLNESS). A low height for age is indicated when height for age is less than the 5th percentile of a person at the same sex and age in the reference population. Height for age is the best indication of long-term undernutrition if it has been of sufficient severity and duration to have caused stunting of growth. It is a most helpful measure in detecting the short stature that may result from chronic undernutrition in children and their mothers.

WEIGHT FOR HEIGHT (MEASURE OF THINNESS AND FATNESS). To determine low weight for height, the weight for height would be less than the 5th percentile of a person at the same sex and height in the reference population. To determine height-weight for height, the weight for height would be greater than the 95th percentile of a person of the same sex and height in the reference population. Weight for height is an excellent indicator of recent undernutrition or of overnutrition and overweight.

*Modified from Center for Disease Control: Nutrition surveillance, Washington, D.C., Jan., 1975, HEW Report 27, Government Printing Office.

WEIGHT FOR AGE (RATIO OF HEIGHT OBSERVED TO HEIGHT EXPECTED, FOR THAT AGE AND SEX). To determine low weight for age, the weight for age would be less than the 5th percentile of a person of the same sex and age in the reference population. Although weight for age was used extensively in the past, it is of limited use, since it may be misleading as an index by itself.

Hemoglobin and hematocrit. In the CDC surveillance system the reference values are adapted from the World Health Organization study on nutritional anemias and the Ten State Nutrition Survey. Individuals below these measures are considered to be anemic.

Methods of comparison for hemoglobin and hematocrits. It is most useful to array the data as percentage distributions at successive 0.5 gm/dl intervals for hemoglobin and at 1.0% intervals for hematocrit.

These data are also analyzed according to the percentage of the population at various age intervals that fall below the following specified levels:

	Hemo-globin (gm/dl)	Hemat-ocrit %
6 to 23 months (both sexes)	10.0	31.0
2 to 5 years (both sexes)	11.0	34.0
6 to 14 years (both sexes)	12.0	37.0
15 years and over (males)	13.0	40.0
15 years and over (females), nonpregnant	12.0	37.0
15 years and over (females), pregnant	11.0	34.0

These cutoff points that are used to define groups with potential nutrition problems have been derived from consultation with many individuals and professional groups.[21]

Results of nutrition surveillance programs in states

Two state nutrition programs have published information on their nutrition surveillance systems. In 1973 the Nutrition Section of the Louisiana Health and Social and Rehabilitation Service Administration developed one of the most comprehensive nutrition surveillance programs in the United States. The first findings and implications of

ASSESSMENT: WHY?

Having assessed the problem, the nutritionist and community health worker together develop a patient care plan for each client found by screening to be at unusual nutritional risk. The client is seen at home, and other family members are encouraged to undergo screening. The plan includes intensive diet counseling in the family setting. The meaning of the screening values is explained and behavior changes (simple modifications one at a time) are suggested within the person's ethnic and cultural framework. Reevaluation of the anthropometric and biochemical values as well as the patient's diet and food practices is scheduled. The patient care plan also includes the necessary referrals, utilizing community resources according to the patient's unique problems, e.g. legal aid, service, day care facility, extension program, etc.

Anita Yanochik-Owen and *Morissa White:* Nutrition surveillance in Arizona: selected anthropometric and laboratory observations among Mexican-American children, Am. J. Public Health **67:**151, 1977.

the Louisiana assessment are well described by Langham.[26] The program is based on data collected from the states Early Periodic Screening, Diagnosis, and Treatment Program (EPSDT). The data from the surveillance system in Louisiana are used to plan intervention programs and bring marginal nutritional defects to the attention of the families of the affected children and to the medical care authorities that control the clinical aspects of the Medicaid program.[27]

Arizona's Nutrition Program at the Department of Health Services has been collecting nutritional data on the state's population since 1970. The nutrition surveillance system functioning in public health clinics is providing data for patient care and program planning. Through this system, Arizona's Mexican-American population has been shown to differ from other ethnic groups that are seen in clinics. Anemia and low height for age are significant problems in the Mexican-American population. Overnutrition in the form of overweight and high cholesterol are also problems in this population. Changes in program planning and setting of priorities have occurred because of the results of the surveillance data.[28-30]

SUMMARY

It has become increasingly clear that the art of nutrition program planning, implementation, and evaluation requires the initial step of a nutritional assessment and then a follow-up by means of a nutritional surveillance system. This is true whether activity is directed toward an individual, a community group, or a special population or is on the national level.

To discover nutritional status, which may be defined as the condition of health as it is influenced by the intake and utilization of nutrients, nutritionists analyze baseline data that are gleaned from clinical (or medical), dietary, and biochemical (laboratory) studies.

It is only recently that nutritional studies have proceeded on a large scale. Among the most important national surveys, for which the ultimate purpose was to locate, determine, and make recommendations regarding malnutrition, have been the Ten State Nutrition Survey, the Preschool Nutrition Survey, and the Health and Nutrition Examination Survey (HANES). Each of these surveys relied on information from a variety of sources, using various tools, including anthropometric measurements, clinical examination, dental examination, medical history, dietary recalls, and biochemical determinations. The results of these findings, including socioeconomic or cultural considerations, were then correlated to make the most accurate conclusions. Each tool or methodology alone, of course, has limitations, and conclusions based on uncorrelated data can be misleading.

REFERENCES

1. Nichaman, M. Z., and Collins, G. E.: Nutrition programs in state health agencies, Nutr. Rev. **32**:65, March, 1974.
2. Owen, G. M., and Lippman, G.: Nutritional status of infants and young children: U.S.A., Pediatr. Clin. North Am. **24**:211, 1977.
3. Christakis, G., editor: Nutritional assessment in health problems, Am. J. Public Health, **63** (suppl.): 1, 1973.
4. Interdepartmental Committee on Nutrition for National Defense: Manual for nutrition surveys, Washington, D.C., 1957, Government Printing Office.
5. Interdepartmental Committee on Nutrition for National Defense: Manual for nutrition surveys, ed. 2, Washington, D. C., 1963, Government Printing Office.
6. Jelliffe, D. B.: The assessment of the nutritional status of the community, Geneva, 1966, World Health Organization.
7. Nichaman, M. Z.: Developing a nutritional surveillance system, J. Am. Diet. Assoc. **65**:15, 1974.
8. U.S. Department of Health, Education, and Welfare: Ten State Nutrition Survey in the United States 1968-1970, Washington, D.C., 1972, publication no. (HSM) 72-8134, Government Printing Office.
9. American Academy of Pediatrics Committee Statement: The Ten State Nutrition Survey: a pediatric perspective, Pediatrics **51**:6, 1973.
10. Owen, G. M., Kram, K. M., Garry, P. J., et al.: A study of nutritional status of preschool children in the United States, 1968-1970, Pediatrics **53** (suppl.): 597, 1974.
11. Owen, G. M., Kram, K. M., Garry, P. J., et al.: Nutritional status of Mississippi preschool children: a pilot study, Am. J. Clin. Nutr. **22**:1444, 1969.
12. Owen, G. M., and Kram, K. M.: Nutritional status of preschool children in Mississippi: food sources of nutrients in the diet, J. Am. Diet. Assoc. **54**:490, 1969.
13. Owen, G. M., Nelson, C. E., Kram, K. M., and Garry, P. J.: Nutritional status of preschool children in two counties in southern Ohio: pilot study in August and September, 1968, Ohio Med. J. **65**: 809, 1969.
14. Warner, W. L.: Social class in America: a manual of procedure for the measurement of social status, New York, 1960, Harper & Row, Publishers.
15. Owen, G. M., Garry, P. J., Lubin, H., and Kram, K. M.: Nutritional status of preschool children: plasma vitamin A, J. Pediatr. **78**:1042, 1971.
16. Infante, P. F., and Owen, G. M.: Relation of chronology of deciduous tooth eruption emergence to height, weight and head circumference in children, Arch. Oral Biol. **18**:1411, 1973.
17. U.S. Department of Health, Education, and Welfare: Plan and operation of the Health and Nutrition Examination Survey, U.S. 1971-1973, Washington,

D.C., 1975, HEW publication no. (HSM) 73-1310, Government Printing Office.

18. USPHS–Health Resources Administration, National Center for Health Statistics: dietary intake and biochemical findings, Preliminary findings of the first Health and Nutrition Examination Survey, U.S., 1971-1972, Jan., 1974, Rockville, Md.

19. USPHS–Health Resources Administration, National Center for Health Statistics: Anthropometric and clinical findings, preliminary findings of the first Health Nutrition Examination Survey, U.S., 1971-1972, Rockville, Md., April, 1975.

20. Lowenstein, F. W.: Preliminary clinical and anthropometric findings from the first Health and Nutrition Examination Survey, U.S., 1971-1972, Am. J. Clin. Nutr. **29:**918, 1976.

21. Center for Disease Control: U.S. Department of Health, Education, and Welfare: Nutrition surveillance, Washington, D.C., Jan., 1975, HEW publication no. 77-8295, Government Printing Office.

22. Habicht, J. P., Lane, M., and McDowell, A.: Nutrition surveillance. Presented at the Symposium on National Nutritional Surveillance, American Institute of Nutrition Meeting, Chicago, April, 1977.

23. United Nations Expert Committee: Report of methodology of nutritional surveillance, FAO/UNICEF/WHO Technical Report Series no. 593, 1976.

24. U.S. Senate Select Committee on Nutrition and Human Needs: Research in nutrition, report prepared by Congressional Research Service, Washington, D.C., March, 1976, publication no. (67-532), Government Printing Office.

25. Vaughn, B. C., III: Growth and development textbook of pediatrics, ed. 9, Philadelphia, 1969, W. B. Saunders Co.

26. Langham, R.: CDC surveillance report: nutrition surveillance in Louisiana, a review of the first year's experience, Washington, D.C., 1975, U.S. Department of Health, Education, and Welfare.

27. Langham, R.: A state health department assesses undernutrition, J. Am. Diet. Assoc. **65:**18, 1974.

28. Owen, A., and White, M.: Nutrition surveillance in Arizona: selected anthropometric and laboratory observations among Mexican-American children, Am. J. Public Health **67:**151, 1977.

29. Center for Disease Control, U.S. Department of Health, Education, and Welfare: Nutritional surveillance report, Washington, D.C., April, 1975, Government Printing Office.

30. Yanochik, A., Eichelberger, C., and Dandoy, S.: The comprehensive nutrition program in Arizona, J. Am. Diet. Assoc. **69:**37, 1976.

SOURCES: NUTRITIONAL STATUS IN THE UNITED STATES

Christakis, G., editor: Nutritional assessment in health programs. Proceedings of a conference, Oct. 18-20, 1972, Washington, D.C., 1973, American Public Health Association, 82 pp. ($4.00).

Owen, G. M., Kram, K. M., Garry, P. J., Lowe, J. E., and Lubin, A. H.: A study of nutritional status of preschool children in the United States, 1968-1970. Part 2, Pediatrics **53** (suppl.):597-646, 1974, American Academy of Pediatrics, Evanston, Ill.

Somogyi, J. C., Assessment of nutritional status and food consumption surveys, Basel, 1974, S. Karger.

Consumer and Food Economics Research Division, U.S. Department of Agriculture, Washington, D.C., Government Printing Office

*Dietary levels of households in the United States, spring 1965: Household Food Consumption Survey 1965-66, Report no. 6, 1969, 117 pp.

Food and nutrient intake of individuals in the United States, spring 1965: Household Food Consumption Survey 1965-66, Report no. 11. 1972, publication no. S/N 001-000-01599-1 ($5.15).

U.S. Department of Health, Education, and Welfare, Washington, D.C., Government Printing Office

Body dimensions and proportions, white and Negro children 6-11 years, United States, Vital and Health Statistics, Series 11, no. 143, 1974, HEW publication no. (HRA) 75-1625, S/N 017-022-00361-9, 66 pp. ($1.30).

Chase, H. C.: Trend in low birth weight ratios—United States and each state, 1950-1968, publication no. S/N 017-022-00281-7 ($0.90).

Height and weight of children: socioeconomic status, United States, Vital and Health Statistics, Series 11, no. 119, 1972, HEW publication no. (HSM) 73-1601, S/N 017-022-00146-2, 87 pp., ($1.10).

Height and weight of youths 12-17 years, United States. Vital and Health Statistics, Series 11, no. 124, 1973, HEW publication no. (HSM) 73-1606, S/N 017-022-00249-3, 81 pp. ($1.25).

Moore, W. M., Silverstein, M. J., and Read, M. S., editors: Nutrition, growth and development of North American Indian children, publication no. S/N 017-046-00013-6, 246 pp. ($2.40).

Plan and operation of the Health and Nutrition Examination Survey, United States 1971-1973, Vital and Health Statistics, Series 1, no. 10b, 1973, HEW publication no. (HSM) 73-1310, S/N 017-022-00254-0, 46 pp. ($1.00).

Preliminary findings of the first Health and Nutrition Examination Survey, United States 1971-1972: Dietary Intake and Biochemical Findings, 1974, HEW publication no. (HRA) 74-1219-1, S/N 017-021-00013-3, 183 pp. ($2.15).

Skeletal maturity of children 6-11 years, United States, Vital and Health Statistics, Series 11, no. 140, 1974, HEW publication no. (HRA) 75-1622, S/N 017-022-00404-6, 62 pp. ($1.45).

Ten-State Nutrition Survey, 1968-1970 (in 5 parts), Center for Disease Control, 1972, HEW publication no. (HSM) 72-1830, -1831, -1832, -1833, -1834, S/N 017-023-00056-0 ($10.55).

---

*Out of print.

GENERAL CONCEPT

Community assessment provides a picture of the
health of the community utilizing demographic,
cultural, and geographic data. The major tools
for nutritional assessment include dietary studies,
clinical and anthropometric studies, and laboratory studies.

OUTCOMES

The student should be able to do the following:
- Identify the specific areas for inquiry in community assessment programs.
- Discuss the objectives, methodologies, and
  limitations of dietary studies.
- List the considerations of the clinical and anthropometric assessments.
- List the biochemical tests applicable to nutrition surveys.

Tools of nutritional assessment

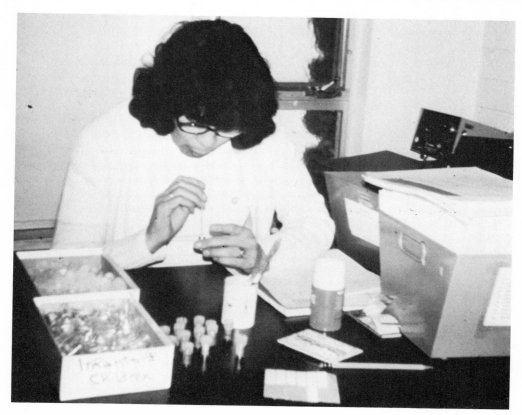

As stated earlier, the assessment of a community is best determined by correlating results of dietary, clinical, biochemical, and anthropometric studies. In the descriptions of the national nutrition surveys (Ten State Nutrition Survey, Preschool Nutrition Survey, and Health and Nutrition Examination Survey) and of the nutrition surveillance system, the major tools and methods required for assessment have been mentioned. These include a community diagnosis or assessment, dietary assessment, clinical and an-

thropometric assessment, and laboratory or biochemical assessment. Data collected from these assessments are part of the analysis required in developing a program plan. (See Fig. 7-1.) Table 8-1 summarizes the information needed for the assessment of nutrition status.

CHAPTER 8

COMMUNITY ASSESSMENT: DIAGNOSING THE COMMUNITY'S NEEDS

Nutrition problems originate from complex interrelationships between environmental

Table 8-1. Information needed for assessment of nutritional status*

Sources of information	Nature of information obtained	Nutritional implications
1. Agricultural data Food balance sheets	Gross estimates of agricultural production Agricultural methods Soil fertility Predominance of cash crops Overproduction of staples Food imports and exports	Approximate availability of food supplies to a population
2. Socioeconomic data Information on marketing, distribution and storage	Purchasing power Distribution and storage of foodstuffs	Unequal distribution of available foods between the socioeconomic groups in community and within family
3. Food consumption patterns Cultural—anthropological data	Lack of knowledge, erroneous beliefs and prejudices, indifference	
4. Dietary surveys	Food consumption	Low, excessive or unbalanced nutrient intake
5. Special studies on foods	Biological value of diets Presence of interfering factors (e.g., goitrogens) Effects of food processing	Special problems related to nutrient utilization
6. Vital and health statistics	Morbidity and mortality data	Extent of risk to community Identification of high risk groups
7. Anthropometric studies	Physical development	Effect of nutrition on physical development
8. Clinical nutritional surveys	Physical signs	Deviation from health due to malnutrition
9. Biochemical studies	Levels of nutrients, metabolites and other components of body tissues and fluids	Nutrient supplies in body Impairment of biochemical function
10. Additional medical information	Prevalent disease patterns including infections and infestations	Interrelationships of state of nutrition and disease

*From WHO Expert Committee: Medical assessment of nutritional status, Geneva, 1963, WHO Technical Report Series no. 258, World Health Organization.

and social factors and the individuals in a community. Therefore, to look at a community only in terms of medical assessment of nutritional status (clinical, dietary, and biochemical), is of limited practical value if the different factors from which problems result are ignored.

Community assessment is one of the most practical methods of obtaining an overview of the nutritional status of a given community. Assessing a community actually means diagnosing a community. As stated in Chapter 4, community diagnosis is defined as an attempt to identify, as fully as possible, which are health problems with nutritional implications and what resources are currently available that will enable the practitioner of community nutrition to implement solutions. In

effect, community assessment paints a picture of the health of the community, its ecology, and the factors influencing the way that people live. To do this, epidemiologic, demographic, cultural, and geographic data must be utilized.

Community assessment relies primarily on existing sources of information. It is a relatively simple technique for which cost and manpower requirements are relatively small. Some existing sources of information may include statistics from United States census studies, vital statistics, hospital records, public assistance records, private and public health agencies, and social welfare agencies. One readily available source of data is the Health Planning Agencies in each state. Since 1966 health planning has been a viable component of the health care scene. One major thrust of federal legislation in 1966 was to collect data on existing health problems in a state. Since the National Health Planning and Resources Development Act was passed in 1974, additional information should be available in the Health Systems Agencies (HSAs).

Christakis[1] specifically lists areas of information that pertain to community assessment and describes each of these areas of inquiry as follows:

1. Demographic information
2. Socioeconomic stratification
3. Health statistics resources: morbidity and mortality
4. Local health resources
5. Dental health
6. Cultural factors
7. Community political organizations
8. Housing
9. Food supply—food costs, food standards, nutrition resources
10. School nutrition programs
11. Social welfare programs—population receiving assistance
12. Transportation
13. Education
14. Occupational data
15. Geography and environment

Demographic information

Webster defines demography as the statistical study of human populations, especially with reference to size and density, distribution, and vital statistics. Age, ethnicity, sex, population density, birth rates, and death rates are all important aspects of demographic data. The United States census tabulations are good source documents for such data, but there are some inherent limitations in using census material—for instance, the infrequency of census enumerations (every ten years) and the lack of detail for geographic areas smaller than a census tract. Places to obtain information for small areas where problems exist include the local Health Systems Agency; local city planning; health, welfare and social service agencies; school boards; chambers of commerce; local banks; and local newspapers.

Socioeconomic stratification

One of the fundamental tools of community nutrition analyses is determining socioeconomic stratification. The two main devices for social stratification include (a) socioeconomic profile of geographic areas, which is useful to define and locate poverty pockets, and (2) evaluation of individuals, for which levels of income are relevant because income may be directly related to the adequacy of nutritional status.

Census data are useful in stratifying areas, since they contain information on socioeconomic indicators such as crowding, racial composition, housing characteristics, etc.

Housing adequacy and the health environment correlate closely with socioeconomic status and are indicators of potential nutritional problems. Local health departments usually have these data.

In dealing with an individual's or family's socioeconomic status, two of the best known tools are the Hollingshead and the Orshansky indexes.[2,3] The Hollingshead Index considers the individual's education, occupation, and income and comes up with a single numerical value that can be used for comparative purposes. The Orshansky Index is a ratio between income and the official figures for the cost of an adequate diet as issued by the U.S. Department of Agriculture.

Health statistics resources: morbidity and mortality

The vital statistics department of any health agency has a wealth of information derived from local and state data on the health problems in the community. The vital statistics department usually has actual numbers of births and crude birth rates. This information is especially important if comparisons are made over periods of years. Additional data that are significant in nutritional assessment are the numbers of illegitimate births, births of less than 1½ pounds (2,500 grams), the number of home births, and births to mothers under 18 or over 40 years of age. These may indicate community health problems. High neonatal, postnatal, and infant mortality is a gross indicator of the need for better health and nutrition services.

For the community as a whole, compiling the causes of deaths and the number of deaths attributed to each cause can be useful. However, the common practice of examining the ten leading causes of death provides inadequate information for community nutritional assessment. Nutritional factors are often a highly important component of the morbidity and mortality due to coronary heart disease, hypertension, diabetes, and alcoholism. These disease indices should all be looked at in terms of their nutritional implications.

Statistics on the prevalence or incidence of diseases that may be poverty related, for example, tuberculosis or other nutritionally related diseases, such as coronary heart disease, hypertension, diabetes, and alcoholism, are often available from public health sources or voluntary health organizations that are concerned with these specific diseases. Family planning clinics also have data on diet histories that can be made available to the assessment team.

Data available in the EPSDT portion of the Medicaid program are also a valuable source of health information, particularly for children from birth to 18 years of age. The WIC Program, the supplemental feeding program for pregnant and lactating women, infants, and children, is another source of data for specific indices such as height, weight, hemoglobin, or hematocrit.

Local health resources

Some of the questions that might be asked of agencies working in the area of community health and nutrition services include the following:
- Are nutritionists available to agencies' staff?
- Is a health educator available?
- Are effective well-child programs in operation? Do these have adequate nutrition evaluation? Is parent education adequate?
- Are maternity clinics adequate, and do they have credible nutrition programs?

- Is nutrition a significant part of local health units or public education programs?
- Are public programs available for coronary heart disease, diabetes, and hypertension? Is the nutrition component an effective and significant one?
- Does an effective alcoholism program exist? Does it have an effective nutrition component?
- Do drug addiction and rehabilitation programs have a nutrition component?
- Do child feeding and school lunch programs exist and under whose supervision? Are there qualified people to run them?

Hospitals, extended care facilities, and nursing homes also should be identified and their bed capacity and occupancy rates evaluated in terms of the community's health needs. Within these institutions the number of qualified dietitians employed and adequacy of food service facilities should be measured. Also, public health care agencies should be viewed in terms of their nutrition component.

In a particular area the number of available health personnel such as physicians, dentists, public health nutritionists, public health nurses, school nurses, health educators, social service workers, nurse practitioners, and other health workers should be determined, including osteopaths and other licensed practitioners. This information can be obtained from local licensing agencies, professional societies, and social service agencies. It may be wise to explore other influences on community health, such as the extent to which a population utilizes faith and spiritual healers or other quasi-medical practitioners. In an Indian population, for example, the number of healers is a particularly important consideration.

Dental health

The availability of dental care for all members of the community regardless of income or age should be investigated, since nutrition is an important factor in dental health. If dental health programs do exist, the amount and number of patients being seen in various economic categories should be determined.

The existence of dental screening studies and community dental education programs also should be assessed. Information concerning these topics can be obtained from the local dental society and health agencies. It is worth while to discover if dentistry programs including preventive dentistry are available in schools, health agencies, and other publicly funded efforts. The existence of community fluoridation programs is another important consideration.

Cultural factors

Knowledge of cultural factors in a community such as differences in life-style and ethnic eating patterns are crucial to any community nutritional assessment. Although some of these cultural factors are difficult to define and isolate, community assessment should summarize the identifiable cultural traditions and the goals of the community and its subgroups, particularly with reference to food preferences and eating habits. An evaluation should be made of the shopping area where produce and meat are purchased and of shopping patterns as well.

These data may only be available from local nutritionists, dietitians, home economists, school lunch supervisors, public health nurses, and social service workers, who are generally a good source of information.

Community political organizations

A program for a given community should never be conceived exclusively by health professionals without any input from the community. This type of approach can ensure failure from the very beginning. Thus it is necessary to determine who the community leaders are and where the power structure lies. Interviews with various government officials, community coordinators, and people in administrative positions can provide clues as to who is in charge. Health Systems Agencies should also be able to provide information as to the sources of funds for health programs, the major contributors,

and recipients of these funds. Interviews can be made of the public officials and community leaders in the following way:

1. Determine whether nutritional problems exist in the community. Is the community aware of them?
2. Determine whether an educational program is necessary to increase awareness of the local government and community groups to the need for health action programs.
3. Determine how to locate and utilize available resources for developing programs in this area.

The need to know about the community's political organization is depicted by a recent story about a neighborhood health center where a team of professionals began to work with the community leaders. The team of professionals conceived a highly sophisticated cardiovascular program with major output for costly approaches to assist patients who had already experienced a coronary occlusion. However, in meeting with community leaders, it was discovered that their main concern was how to feed their babies "to make them intelligent and healthy." This was a learning experience for the professionals, since the community leaders' approach to health care had an entirely different emphasis.

Housing

Housing data are important in community and nutrition assessment for two reasons: (1) they are an excellent indicator of the social and environmental deprivation, and (2) the family's ability to utilize foodstuffs is directly related to the adequacy of kitchen facilities.

Since these data again can be a useful source of selected housing characteristics, they can be used to measure crowding, that is, the number of persons per room, and the sanitation facilities.

Data on kitchen facilities might be supplemented by information from local utility companies, which may have records of household appliances such as stoves, refrigerators, freezers, and dishwashers. If a direct household survey has been completed in the area, this certainly is even more informative.

Specific information on housing may be obtained from local housing authorities, the local health department, and urban planning groups.

Food supply

Assessments of the local marketplaces, supermarket, small grocery stores, food cooperatives, delicatessens, health food stores, organic food stores, and other food outlets are necessary for a complete community diagnosis. The number of small corner vendors, snack stands, and other popular chains and the extent to which they are utilized by the population are also relevant.

Food consumption studies on a national basis are available from the U.S. Department of Agriculture in their regional and national offices. There are other factors such as the following to consider.

Food costs. The determination of relative food costs for a community, indicating if an adequate food supply can be purchased, is important. Local departments of welfare, market departments, community service agencies, and consumer groups often compile food costs on a weekly and monthly basis. Department of Agriculture publications, issued on a regular basis, indicate costs of food in various part of the United States. A yearly survey is done on food costs and is often reported in local newspapers. Another consideration is credit purchases as opposed to cash purchases of food. This may also indicate variances in cost.

Food standards. It is desirable to determine the presence or absence of compliance with local or state food standards, including fortification requirements, and also if the state has an enrichment law for breads and cereals. It should be ascertained whether a consumer protection agency is available and how strong its role is in local government.

Nutrition resources. A survey of the numbers of nutritionists, dietitians, home economists, and nutrition aides within the community, their level of training and certification, their functions, and a definition and assessment of the population they serve is desirable. The amount of inservice training of these various personnel groups should be known, as well as the kinds of institutions and universities that provide their training. It is important to see if a nutrition council, where cooperation and coordination between various agencies working toward the alleviation of nutrition problems, is available. Such a council is often necessary so that duplication of services among agencies is not a problem.

School nutrition programs

The number of school breakfast and school lunch programs and the presence or absence of vending machines for pastries, snacks, and soft drinks require evaluation. The amount of federal funds compared with local funds for school lunch and school breakfast programs is also a consideration.

The extent of nutrition education in the school systems and also at the preschool level should be defined. If at all possible, the quality of these curricula should be evaluated. Further possibilities for nutrition education programs for teachers in the primary and secondary schools, their students, and food service personnel has become a reality with the passage of the Child Nutrition Act (H.R. 1139 Amendments to the National School Lunch Act and Child Nutrition Act of 1966), which includes nutrition education for these groups and a funding allowance of 50 cents per child. Feeding programs such as the WIC Program, which has a strong medical component, should be identified if they are available.

Social welfare programs

National figures and percentages of the population receiving public assistance may be discovered from local welfare departments and social service agency records. Eligibility standards may need careful review, particularly since many barriers stand in the way of people obtaining social services. It is useful to find out about the extent of the commodity program in the community and the eligibility standards for Medicaid. The use of food stamps, donated foods, and supplemental food programs all require documentation as well as description and evaluation of the quality of the diets provided by these programs. The accessibility of these feeding programs for the client should be investigated.

Food and social services for senior citizens (Title VII programs) and children should be explored. For example, are there day care programs for senior citizens? Does the program provide nutrition education and meal services? In children's programs, such as Head Start, are the meals adequately prepared and is there an adequate nutrition component including food service and nutrition education?

Transportation

Transportation facilities are important to nutritional patterns for the following reasons:
1. They provide accessibility to food supplies.
2. Mobility of individuals has a direct bearing on their ability to obtain nutritional counseling, to visit health and educational facilities, and to obtain food.
3. Freeways and other barriers may present problems that limit social or commercial contacts between segments of the community.

Usually communities have a transportation department that can provide information on the transportation patterns of a given area. If not, bus companies and highway departments and city planning agencies should have this information.

Education

An understanding of the literacy and the extent to which the English language is understood and spoken must be considered in the evaluation of health and nutrition programs. If the program is to be oriented toward an English-speaking population and the nutritionist is dealing with a primarily Spanish-speaking population, obviously the program is doomed to failure. Unfortunately, detailed data in this area are difficult to acquire, but public and parochial schools can often provide useful facts concerning education levels, illiteracy, and whether or not English is understood. Frequently, community leaders also can give this kind of information.

Occupational data

Data on occupations, unemployment, and industrial health practices may not be essential to a nutritional assessment but may be helpful in providing a profile of the whole community. Industrial populations are already a known group of adults in a controlled environment; however, they are excellent areas for health and nutrition screening.

Geography and environment

In rural and underdeveloped areas, particular attention should be given to soil type and other factors related to agricultural production. Maps may be obtained from city and county engineers' offices and from highway departments. The level of food supply can be a direct function of whether and in what conditions the crops affect production.

Man-induced environmental changes are significant considerations as well. Polluted feeding areas, creation of land subsidies, and crop or livestock loss from the air or water contamination are all factors in determining food availability and, consequently, nutritional status.

Standards relating to adequate community levels of nutrition and the social indicators known to correlate with malnutrition have not yet been agreed on universally. However, knowledge about the preceding fifteen factors from Christakis[1] can provide enough information to make sound judgments on community assessment. A word of caution is necessary in doing community assessment: Specific cutoff points on the collection of data must be made. It is self-defeating if the gathering of data becomes the main objective and the true purpose of alleviating the nutrition problems in a given area is lost.

DIETARY METHODOLOGIES: A TOOL OF NUTRITIONAL ASSESSMENT
Objectives of dietary studies

Dietary studies constitute an important part of any complete nutrition survey in that they provide essential information on nutrient intake levels, sources of nutrients, food habits, preparation practices, and attitudes. They cannot be taken as absolute indications of adequate nutrition, but they are widely used to obtain presumptive evidence of dietary inadequacies or excesses in individuals, specific population groups, institutions, or other community agencies.

Christakis[1] cites some of the overall objectives of dietary studies:

1. To assess the need for appropriate intervention programs by determining dietary or nutrient intake of one or more individuals.
2. To determine the need for community nutrition programs among various population groups, e.g. maternal, child, adolescent, or elderly programs.
3. To evaluate ongoing programs and compare dietary status of groups within a given geographic area or with similar groups from the area.

Considerations in planning dietary studies

There are several methods employed in nutritional surveys to determine dietary studies, from very simple to very detailed. They range from relatively simple studies describing a rough estimate of food consumption to detailed histories of individual dietary intake. The objectives of the entire study must be well in place before the selection of the most appropriate dietary method can be made. One should allow no more detail or expense than is necessary in doing dietary studies. Other considerations that would apply to selecting the appropriate type of study include the following:

1. The number of persons to be surveyed, their degree of understanding, cooperativeness, and available time
2. Methods of data collection analysis and interpretation necessary to achieve the predetermined objective
3. The training and availability of personnel to conduct the study
4. How the dietary information is to be related to the clinical and biochemical findings in a survey

There are two categories of dietary data collection: data that record food intake of families or larger groups and data on the intakes of individuals. Both of these offer information that may be translated to give an appropriate estimate of nutrient intake. The primary value may be used for comparative studies, to suggest a need for further and more precise measurements, or to provide the basis for program planning.

Individual dietary intake

Dietary data on individuals may be collected to obtain more precise measurements for determining the average nutrient intake of groups to be used in comparison with other similar groups and then for finding out if there are dietary inadequacies in the study group. Another purpose for assembling data on the nutrient intake of a given individual is to correlate it with clinical and biochemical measurements also obtained from that individual.

Unless an individual's dietary measurements cover an extended period, there is no point in correlating them with individual biochemical or clinical nutrient determinations, since the latter reflect the long-term results of adequate or inadequate nutrition. Short-term dietary intake data of groups, however, have shown positive correlations with biochemical and clinical observations.

Food intake surveys of individuals range from a qualitative type of food habit inquiry to those having a more quantitative nature. These may include the following:

1. The parent or child's recall of food intake during the previous 24 hours or longer.
2. Records of foods eaten by an individual according to weight, household measures, or estimated quantities over a stated period of time.
3. A questionnaire or interview to obtain general dietary data or information on specific foods if the study is focused on one or more nutrients.
4. A diet history usually obtained by a trained interviewer that will indicate the amounts of food eaten over a relatively long period of time.

5. Laboratory studies in which nutritive values are determined by careful laboratory weighing and analysis of duplicate samples of all food portions. This method is generally used only by research groups with special facilities for collection and analyses, such as metabolic research wards.

6. Food frequencies measured in combination with 24-hour recall. Frequency indicates the use of selective food groups over a period of time in a given household.

Family or group dietary intake methods

Family food accounts, food records, and food lists are the means through which food usage of families or groups having the same food supply may be studied.

1. Family food accounts are usually simple descriptions of food purchased and produced for household use. They are not precise and are rarely used today.

2. Food records constitute an inventory of foods on hand at the beginning and close of the study with a day-to-day accounting of the food brought into the home. Kitchen and plate waste (refuse) may sometimes be recorded.

3. Food lists comprise an estimate of the quantities of food used during a given period of time, which is obtained through an interview with the person responsible for buying the food.

One difficulty with the food record and food list occurs in estimating food wastes, that is, food fed to animals, discarded, or

Text continued on p. 209.

Record No.			Date Record Started	
			MEALS EATEN THIS WEEK	
Person	Sex	Age	Number of meals eaten at home or lunches carried	Number of meals eaten out, not using home food supply

---

ON THE FOLLOWING PAGES, WE WOULD LIKE A RECORD OF THE FOODS AND DRINKS USED IN YOUR HOME FOR ONE WEEK.

1. When you start the record, write down the amounts of the foods *on hand* which you may use during the week.
2. As food is brought into the house from store, farm or elsewhere during the week, write it down.
3. At the end of the week, write down the amounts of food left from those you have put on your record.

HOW TO KEEP THE RECORD:

Under *amount* put down the numbers, weights, measure, or sizes.
Under *kind of food* write the exact name of the food, for example, "cornflakes," not cereal. Write whether foods are fresh, canned, dried, or frozen.
Under *price for amount bought*, put down price.
Under *source*, write whether foods are from store, own farm, bought from farm, dairy, bakery, gift, etc. If food is home-canned or home-frozen, record this, and tell the original source of the fresh food.

AMOUNT	KIND OF FOOD	PRICE FOR AMOUNT BOUGHT	SOURCE

END OF WEEK:
Amounts of food left over from those listed above:

AMOUNT	KIND OF FOOD

Fig. 8-1. Household record of food used for 1 week. (From Christakis, G., editor: Nutritional assessment in health programs, Am. J. Public Health **63**[suppl.]:1-82, 1973.)

HOUSEHOLD DIETARY QUESTIONNAIRE*

Name _____ Address _____ Date _____

1. Persons fed: (give sex and age for each)

   _____
   _____
   _____

2. Grade of school completed
   by homemaker _____

3. Occupation of head
   of household _____

4. Income level $ _____

   Sources of income _____

5. Where do you usually get your food supplies?
   If purchased:

   Kind of store? _____ Cash or credit? _____

   Distance to store? _____ Transportation? _____

   How often shop for food? _____ Why? _____

   If home produced, what? _____

   _____
   _____
   _____

   Do you home preserve? _____ What? How much? _____

   _____
   _____

   Other sources? _____

   _____
   _____

   Are food stamps available? _____ Do you purchase? _____

   How much do you pay? $ _____ Value get? _____

   Are donated or surplus foods available? _____ Do you use? _____

   _____

6. How much did you spend for food last week? _____

   Is this the usual amount? _____

7. Do you feel you have adequate storage facilities for food? _____

8. Do you feel you have adequate cooking facilities? _____

   Kind? _____ Working oven? _____

9. Do you feel you have adequate refrigeration? _____

   Kind? _____

---

*Adapted from National Nutrition Survey, Nutrition Program; Division of Chronic Disease Program, DHEW, Atlanta, Ga. Rev. 3/69.
VIII A-Dietary—Household—General Information. NCCD-3-8a (DC).

Fig. 8-2. Household dietary questionnaire. (From Christakis, G., editor: Nutritional assessment in health programs, Am. J. Public Health **63**[suppl.]:1-82, 1973.)

24-HOUR RECALL

Name _____

Date and time of interview _____

Length of interview _____

Date of recall _____

Day of the week of recall _____

1-M 2-T 3-W 4-Th 5-F 6-Sat 7-Sun

"I would like you to tell me everything you (your child) ate and drank from the time you (he) got up in the morning until you (he) went to bed at night and what you (he) ate during the night. Be sure to mention everything you (he) ate or drank at home, at work (school), and away from home. Include snacks and drinks of all kinds and everything else you (he) put in your (his) mouth and swallowed. I also need to know where you (he) ate the food, and now let us begin."

What time did you (he) get up yesterday? _____

Was it the usual time? _____

What was the first time you (he) ate or had anything to drink yesterday morning? (list on the form that follows)

Where did you (he) eat? (list on form that follows)

Now tell me what you (he) had to eat and how much?

(Occasionally the interviewer will need to ask:)

    When did you (he) eat again? Or, is there anything else?

    Did you (he) have anything to eat or drink during the night?

Was intake unusual in any way? Yes _____ No _____

(If answer is yes) Why? _____

            In what way? _____

What time did you (he) go to bed last night? _____

Do(es) you (he) take vitamin or mineral supplements?

          Yes _____ No _____

(If answer is yes) How many per day? _____

          Per week? _____

What kind? (insert brand name if known)

Multivitamins _____

Ascorbic acid _____

Vitamins A and D _____

Iron _____

Other _____

SUGGESTED FORM FOR RECORDING FOOD INTAKE

Time	Where eaten*	Food	Type and/or preparation	Amount	Food code†	Amount code†

*Code

  H—Home

  R—Restaurant, drugstore, or lunch counter

CL—Carried lunch from home

CC—Child care center

†Do not write in these spaces.

OH—Other home (friend, relative, baby-sitter, etc.)

  S—School, office, plant or work

FD—Food dispenser

SS—Social center, e.g., Senior Citizen, etc.

Fig. 8-3. 24-hour recall. (From Screening children for nutritional status: suggestions for child health programs, Washington, D.C., 1971, U.S. Government Printing Office.)

DIETARY QUESTIONNAIRE FOR CHILDREN

Name _____

Date _____

1. Does the child eat at regular times each day? _____
2. How many days a week does he eat—

   a morning meal? _____

   a lunch or midday meal? _____

   an evening meal? _____

   during the night?† _____
3. How many days a week does he have snacks—

   in midmorning? _____

   in midafternoon? _____

   in the evening? _____

   during the night?* _____
4. Which meals does he usually eat with your family?

   None _____ Breakfast _____ Noon meal _____ Evening meal _____
5. How many times per week does he eat at school, child care center, or day camp?

   Breakfast _____ Lunch _____ Between meals _____
6. Would you describe his appetite as Good? _____ Fair? _____ Poor? _____
7. At what time of day is he most hungry?

   Morning _____ Noon _____ Evening _____

8. What foods does he dislike? _____

   _____

9. Is he on a special diet now? Yes _____ No _____

   If yes, why is he on a diet? (Check)

   _____ for weight reduction (own prescription)

   _____ for weight reduction (doctor's prescription)

   _____ for gaining weight

   _____ for allergy, specify _____

   _____ for other reason, specify _____

   If no, has he been on a special diet within the past year? Yes _____ No _____

   If yes, for what reason _____

10. Does he eat anything which is not usually considered food? Yes _____ No _____

    If yes, what? _____ How often? _____

11. Can he feed himself? Yes _____ No _____

    If yes, with his fingers? _____ with a spoon? _____

12. Can he use a cup or glass by himself? Yes _____ No _____

13. Does he drink from a bottle with a nipple? Yes _____ No _____

    If yes, how often? _____ At what time of day or night? _____

* Include formula feeding for young children.

Fig. 8-4. Dietary questionnaire for children. (From Screening children for nutritional status: suggestions for child health programs, Washington, D.C., 1971, U.S. Government Printing Office.)

DIETARY QUESTIONNAIRE FOR CHILDREN—cont'd

14. How many times per week does he eat the following foods (at any meal or between meals)?
    Circle the appropriate number:

Bacon _____ 0 1 2 3 4 5 6 7 >7, specify _____
Tongue _____ 0 1 2 3 4 5 6 7 >7, specify _____
Sausage _____ 0 1 2 3 4 5 6 7 >7, specify _____
Luncheon meat _____ 0 1 2 3 4 5 6 7 >7, specify _____
Hot dogs _____ 0 1 2 3 4 5 6 7 >7, specify _____
Liver—chicken _____ 0 1 2 3 4 5 6 7 >7, specify _____
Liver—other _____ 0 1 2 3 4 5 6 7 >7, specify _____
Poultry _____ 0 1 2 3 4 5 6 7 >7, specify _____
Salt pork _____ 0 1 2 3 4 5 6 7 >7, specify _____
Pork or ham _____ 0 1 2 3 4 5 6 7 >7, specify _____
Bones (neck or other) _____ 0 1 2 3 4 5 6 7 >7, specify _____
Meat in mixtures (stew, tamales, casseroles, etc.) ___ 0 1 2 3 4 5 6 7 >7, specify _____
Beef or veal _____ 0 1 2 3 4 5 6 7 >7, specify _____
Other meat _____ 0 1 2 3 4 5 6 7 >7, specify _____
Fish _____ 0 1 2 3 4 5 6 7 >7, specify _____

15. How many times per week does he eat the following foods (at any meal or between meals)?
    Circle the appropriate number:

Fruit juice _____ 0 1 2 3 4 5 6 7 >7, specify _____
Fruit _____ 0 1 2 3 4 5 6 7 >7, specify _____
Cereal—dry _____ 0 1 2 3 4 5 6 7 >7, specify _____
Cereal—cooked or instant _____ 0 1 2 3 4 5 6 7 >7, specify _____
Cereal—infant _____ 0 1 2 3 4 5 6 7 >7, specify _____
Eggs _____ 0 1 2 3 4 5 6 7 >7, specify _____
Pancakes or waffles _____ 0 1 2 3 4 5 6 7 >7, specify _____
Cheese _____ 0 1 2 3 4 5 6 7 >7, specify _____
Potato _____ 0 1 2 3 4 5 6 7 >7, specify _____
Other cooked vegetables _____ 0 1 2 3 4 5 6 7 >7, specify _____
Raw vegetables _____ 0 1 2 3 4 5 6 7 >7, specify _____
Dried beans or peas _____ 0 1 2 3 4 5 6 7 >7, specify _____
Macaroni, spaghetti, rice, or noodles ___ 0 1 2 3 4 5 6 7 >7, specify _____
Ice cream, milk pudding, custard or cream soup ___ 0 1 2 3 4 5 6 7 >7, specify _____
Peanut butter or nuts _____ 0 1 2 3 4 5 6 7 >7, specify _____
Sweet rolls or doughnuts _____ 0 1 2 3 4 5 6 7 >7, specify _____
Crackers or pretzels _____ 0 1 2 3 4 5 6 7 >7, specify _____
Cookies _____ 0 1 2 3 4 5 6 7 >7, specify _____
Pie, cake or brownies _____ 0 1 2 3 4 5 6 7 >7, specify _____
Potato chips or corn chips _____ 0 1 2 3 4 5 6 7 >7, specify _____
Candy _____ 0 1 2 3 4 5 6 7 >7, specify _____
Soft drinks, popsicles or Koolaid _____ 0 1 2 3 4 5 6 7 >7, specify _____
Instant Breakfast _____ 0 1 2 3 4 5 6 7 >7, specify _____

16. How many servings per day does he eat of the following foods? Circle the appropriate number:
    Bread (including sandwich), toast, rolls, muffins
    (1 slice or 1 piece is 1 serving) _____ 0 1 2 3 4 5 6 7 >7, specify _____
    Milk (including on cereal or other foods)
    (8 ounces is 1 serving) _____ 0 1 2 3 4 5 6 7 >7, specify _____
    Sugar, jam, jelly, syrup (1 tsp. is 1 serving) ___ 0 1 2 3 4 5 6 7 >7, specify _____

17. What specific kinds of the following foods does he eat most often?

Fruit juices _____

Fruit _____

Vegetables _____

Cheese _____

Cooked or instant cereal _____

Dry cereal _____

Milk _____

Fig. 8-4, cont'd

DIETARY QUESTIONNAIRE FOR ADULTS AND ADOLESCENTS

Name _____ Sex _____ Date of birth _____

Address _____ Marital status _____ Date _____

1. Grade of school   2. Still in
   completed? _____   school? _____ 3. Occupation _____

4. Are you employed? _____ Full time? _____ Part time? _____

5. Income level $ _____ Sources of income _____
   Where appropriate:

6. Are you pregnant? _____ Stage? _____ Lactating? _____
   If pregnant have you changed the way you eat or drink? How? _____
   _____
   On whose advice? _____

7. Where do you usually get your food supplies? _____
   If home produced, what? _____
   Do you home preserve? What? How much? _____
   _____

   If purchased:
   Kind of store? _____ Cash or credit? _____
   Distance to store? _____ Transportation? _____
   How often shop for food? _____ Why? _____
   Are food stamps available? _____ Do you purchase? _____
   How much do you pay? $_____ Value get? $ _____
   Are donated or surplus foods available? _____ Do you use? _____

8. Do you feel you have adequate storage facilities for food in your home? _____

9. Do you feel you have adequate cooking facilities? _____
   Kind? _____ Working oven? _____

10. Do you feel you have adequate refrigeration? _____ Kind? _____

11. Do you eat at regular times each day? _____

12. How many days a week do you eat:
    a morning meal? _____
    a lunch or midday meal? _____
    an evening meal? _____
    during the evening or night? _____

13. How many days a week do you have snacks, and what do you have then?
    in midmorning _____
    in midafternoon _____
    in the evening _____
    during the night _____

14. Where do you usually eat your meal?
    Morning _____ Midday _____ Evening _____

Fig. 8-5. Dietary questionnaire for adults and adolescents. (From Screening children for nutritional status: suggestions for child health programs, Washington, D.C., 1971, U.S. Government Printing Office.)

spoiled. Estimates of such losses vary but usually have been reported to be in the vicinity of 10% of the total energy value of the diet.

In this connection a study was performed in which garbage was examined. Anthropology students at the University of Arizona chose various census tracts in the Tucson area and analyzed the garbage found in each particular census tract.[4]

Figs. 8-1 to 8-5 describe the household record of food used in 1 week—the 24-hour recall of the dietary questionnaire for children, adults, and adolescents.

DIETARY QUESTIONNAIRE FOR ADULTS AND ADOLESCENTS—cont'd

15. With whom do you usually eat?

   Morning _____ Midday _____ Evening _____

16. How many times a week do you usually eat away from home? _____

17. Would you say your appetite is Good? _____ Fair? _____ Poor? _____

18. What foods do you particularly dislike? _____

19. Are you on a special diet? _____ If yes, what kind? _____ Who prescribed? _____

20. Are there foods you don't eat for other reasons? _____

21. Do you eat anything not usually considered food (e.g., clay, dirt, starch, other)? _____

   If yes, what? _____; when? _____; how much? _____

22. Do you add salt to your food at the table? _____

23. Do you have any difficulty chewing? _____

24. How many times per week do you eat the following foods (at any meal or between meals)? Circle the appropriate number:

   Bacon _____ 0 1 2 3 4 5 6 7 >7, specify _____
   Tongue _____ 0 1 2 3 4 5 6 7 >7, specify _____
   Sausage _____ 0 1 2 3 4 5 6 7 >7, specify _____
   Luncheon meat _____ 0 1 2 3 4 5 6 7 >7, specify _____
   Hot dogs _____ 0 1 2 3 4 5 6 7 >7, specify _____
   Liver—chicken _____ 0 1 2 3 4 5 6 7 >7, specify _____
   Liver—other _____ 0 1 2 3 4 5 6 7 >7, specify _____
   Poultry _____ 0 1 2 3 4 5 6 7 >7, specify _____
   Salt pork _____ 0 1 2 3 4 5 6 7 >7, specify _____
   Pork or ham _____ 0 1 2 3 4 5 6 7 >7, specify _____
   Bones (neck or other) _____ 0 1 2 3 4 5 6 7 >7, specify _____
   Meat in mixtures (stew, tamales, casseroles, etc.) ____ 0 1 2 3 4 5 6 7 >7, specify _____
   Beef or veal _____ 0 1 2 3 4 5 6 7 >7, specify _____
   Other meat _____ 0 1 2 3 4 5 6 7 >7, specify _____
   Fish _____ 0 1 2 3 4 5 6 7 >7, specify _____
   Cheese and cheese dishes _____ 0 1 2 3 4 5 6 7 >7, specify _____
   Eggs _____ 0 1 2 3 4 5 6 7 >7, specify _____
   Dried beans or pea dishes _____ 0 1 2 3 4 5 6 7 >7, specify _____
   Peanut butter or nuts _____ 0 1 2 3 4 5 6 7 >7, specify _____

25. How many servings per day do you eat of the following foods? Circle the appropriate number:

   Bread (including sandwich), toast, rolls, muffins
   (1 slice or 1 piece is 1 serving) _____ 0 1 2 3 4 5 6 7 >7, specify _____
   Milk (including on cereal or other foods)
   (8 ounces is 1 serving) _____ 0 1 2 3 4 5 6 7 >7, specify _____
   Sugar, jam, jelly, syrup (1 tsp. is 1 serving) _____ 0 1 2 3 4 5 6 7 >7, specify _____
   Butter or margarine (1 tsp. is 1 serving) _____ 0 1 2 3 4 5 6 7 >7, specify _____

Fig. 8-5, cont'd

Continued.

DIETARY QUESTIONNAIRE FOR ADULTS AND ADOLESCENTS—cont'd

26. How many times per week do you eat the following foods (at any meal or between meals)?
Circle the appropriate number:

Fruit juice _____ 0 1 2 3 4 5 6 7 >7, specify _____
Fruit _____ 0 1 2 3 4 5 6 7 >7, specify _____
Cereal—dry _____ 0 1 2 3 4 5 6 7 >7, specify _____
Cereal—cooked or instant _____ 0 1 2 3 4 5 6 7 >7, specify _____
Pancakes or waffles _____ 0 1 2 3 4 5 6 7 >7, specify _____
Potato _____ 0 1 2 3 4 5 6 7 >7, specify _____
Other cooked vegetables _____ 0 1 2 3 4 5 6 7 >7, specify _____
Raw vegetables _____ 0 1 2 3 4 5 6 7 >7, specify _____
Macaroni, spaghetti, rice, or noodles _____ 0 1 2 3 4 5 6 7 >7, specify _____
Ice cream, milk pudding, custard, or cream soup _____ 0 1 2 3 4 5 6 7 >7, specify _____
Sweet rolls or doughnuts _____ 0 1 2 3 4 5 6 7 >7, specify _____
Crackers or pretzels _____ 0 1 2 3 4 5 6 7 >7, specify _____
Cookies _____ 0 1 2 3 4 5 6 7 >7, specify _____
Pie, cake, or brownies _____ 0 1 2 3 4 5 6 7 >7, specify _____
Potato chips or corn chips _____ 0 1 2 3 4 5 6 7 >7, specify _____
Candy _____ 0 1 2 3 4 5 6 7 >7, specify _____
Soft drinks, popsicles, or Koolaid; sherbets _____ 0 1 2 3 4 5 6 7 >7, specify _____
Instant Breakfast _____ 0 1 2 3 4 5 6 7 >7, specify _____
Artificially sweetened beverage _____ 0 1 2 3 4 5 6 7 >7, specify _____
Coffee or tea _____ 0 1 2 3 4 5 6 7 >7, specify _____
Beer _____ 0 1 2 3 4 5 6 7 >7, specify _____
Wine _____ 0 1 2 3 4 5 6 7 >7, specify _____
Whiskey, vodka, rum, scotch, gin _____ 0 1 2 3 4 5 6 7 >7, specify _____

27. What specific kinds of the following foods do you eat most often?

Fruit juices _____
Fruit _____
Vegetables _____
Cheese _____
Cooked or instant cereal _____
Dry cereal _____
Milk _____
Cream or cream substitute _____
Butter or margarine _____
Salad dressings _____

Fig. 8-5, cont'd

Data collection methods

Whether it is a nutritionist or a nutrition aide who is completing a 24-hour recall, proper training is necessary to obtain maximum information from a client by using this method. Actually, for group comparisons 1-day records on a large number of people will be more revealing of dietary patterns than will studies conducted over long periods on a limited number of people. The 24-hour intake is fairly simple to obtain, either by recall or in a 15- or 20-minute interview conducted by personnel with relatively little technical background.

Certain equipment may be used in conducting the 24-hour recall, such as various-sized glasses, spoons, bowls, or food models that will help the client indicate quantities more accurately. A notation of whether an individual has a typical or atypical daily food pattern should be indicated on the form.

The 24-hour intake recall questionnaire (Fig. 8-3) and the dietary questionnaire (Fig. 8-4) may also be used by trained interviewers under the supervision of a nutritionist experienced in obtaining dietary recalls. The dietary questionnaire is often called a frequency determination, and it can provide both a check on the completeness of the 24-hour recall and additional information on dietary patterns and food practices. Variations appropriate to different cultural groups may be and should be devised. A dietary questionnaire or frequency is often useful in individual counseling, as well as in nutrition education and community programs.

Interpreting the data—analysis of dietary information

One of the simplest analyses of the 24-hour recall is a comparison of the client's food consumption with the recommended dietary allowance according to the standard basic food groups. The 24-hour recall may also be calculated in terms of specific nutrients, using food composition data from sources such as *Composition of Foods,* Agriculture Handbook 8,[5] *Nutritive Value of American Foods in Common Units*[6] and *Food Values of Portions Commonly Used.*[7]

If the limitations of the 24-hour recall are kept in mind, gross calculations of nutrient intake are valid. Comparisons with the basic food groups are at best a convenient tool for indicating possible weak areas in the diet, but they have severe limitations if the diet has small variety, unconventional foods, or special cultural components. The use of food composition tables is somewhat more precise but still only a crude quantitative expression of nutrients consumed.

Failure to meet the Recommended Dietary Allowances (RDA) standard does not indicate malnutrition, since with the exception of calories, the RDAs are calculated to be above average physiologic requirements for each nutrient. Since the RDAs are revised periodically, the survey results will be more meaningful for later reference if they are described in terms of absolute quantities of nutrients consumed. The 1974 Recommended Daily Dietary Allowances appear in Table 8-2. The next edition of the Recommended Dietary Allowances is expected to be published in early 1979.

An example of one nutrition-intervention program developing its own dietary information system was developed in Arizona (Appendix 8-1). This 24-hour dietary evaluation method was devised mainly for use by nutritionists, nutrition aides, nurses, physicians, and other allied health personnel to evaluate a person's dietary intake and also for determining the adequacy of dietary intake in a population before and after participation in the Nutrition Delivery System.

Foods are categorized into eighteen groups, utilizing a system of standard measuring units (SMU), for each food item. Eight particular nutrients are evaluated to determine possible risk based on comparing units with 1974 RDA for various age groups. The nutrients are protein, iron, cholesterol, calcium, vitamin A, vitamin C, empty calories, and fat. Age groups include infants, 1 to 10-year-olds, 11 to 18-year-olds, adults, and pregnant or lactating women. This information should be gathered by trained nutrition aides who monitor the clients and complete the dietary recalls.[8]

Limitations of diet history methodology

A word of caution was indicated previously about assuming malnutrition if there is evidence of not meeting the Recommended Dietary Allowances. In addition to this there are several other points to keep in mind when making dietary studies, including the following:

1. Differences in nutritional requirements among individuals.

2. So-called conditioning factors such as concurrent disease, genetic or enzyme defects, which may interfere with or modify an individual's ingestion, absorption, utilization, requirement, or excretion of nutrients.

3. The skill of the history taker and the degree of cooperation and memory of the client.

4. The inadequacy of short-term studies, which may not reflect total nutrient intake over long periods. Another consideration is that present knowledge of absolute nutri-

Table 8-2. Food and Nutrition Board, National Academy of Sciences National Research Council Recommended Daily Dietary Allowances,[a] revised 1974

	Age (yr)	Weight (kg)	Weight (lb)	Height (cm)	Height (in)	Energy (kcal)[b]	Protein (g)	Vitamin A activity (RE)[c]	(IU)	Vitamin D (IU)	Vitamin E activity[e] (IU)
Infants	0.0-0.5	6	14	60	24	kg × 117	kg × 2.2	420[d]	1,400	400	1
	0.5-1.0	9	20	71	28	kg × 108	kg × 2.0	400	2,000	400	5
Children	1-3	13	28	86	34	1,300	23	400	2,000	400	7
	4-6	20	44	110	44	1,800	30	500	2,500	400	9
	7-10	30	66	135	54	2,400	36	700	3,300	400	10
Males	11-14	44	97	158	63	2,800	44	1,000	5,000	400	12
	15-18	61	134	172	69	3,000	54	1,000	5,000	400	15
	19-22	67	147	172	69	3,000	54	1,000	5,000	400	15
	23-50	70	154	172	69	2,700	56	1,000	5,000		15
	51+	70	154	172	69	2,400	56	1,000	5,000		15
Females	11-14	44	97	155	62	2,400	44	800	4,000	400	12
	15-18	54	119	162	65	2,100	48	800	4,000	400	12
	19-22	58	128	162	65	2,100	46	800	4,000	400	12
	23-50	58	128	162	65	2,000	46	800	4,000		12
	51+	58	128	162	65	1,800	46	800	4,000		12
Pregnant						+300	+30	1,000	5,000	400	15
Lactating						+500	+20	1,200	6,000	400	15

[a]The allowances are intended to provide for individual variations among most normal persons as they live in the United States which human requirements have been less well defined.
[b]Kilojoules (kJ) = 4.2 × kcal.
[c]Retinol equivalents.
[d]Assumed to be all as retinol in milk during the first six months of life. All subsequent intakes are assumed to be half as retinol as β-carotene.
[e]Total vitamin E activity, estimated to be 80% as α-tocopherol and 20% other tocopherols.
[f]The folacin allowances refer to dietary sources as determined by *Lactobacillus casei* assay. Pure forms of folacin may be effective
[g]Although allowances are expressed as niacin, it is recognized that on the average 1 mg of niacin is derived from each 60 mg of
[h]This increased requirement cannot be met by ordinary diets; therefore, the use of supplemental iron is recommended.

tional requirements is rapidly evolving. Food composition tables are often incomplete and not necessarily accurate, and additional laboratory and clinical investigations are in order before nutritional deficiencies can be determined with confidence.

Dilemma of dietary histories

There are two schools of thought in dietary data. In one camp, workers in the field question the validity of collecting dietary data on individuals for epidemiologic purposes in that (1) direct measurement of food intake is feasible only for small groups; (2) food records may cause the client to change his nor-

mal eating habits; (3) dietary histories are subject to problems of memory; and (4) although 24-hour recalls may be more objective than dietary histories, they fall short because only one day is measured. The other school of thought is that repeated 24-hour recalls are indeed valuable aids in the difficult and complex area of classifying dietary intakes and should be used more frequently, particularly for populations with specific nutrients which do not have variability.

A list of selected references reflecting the dilemma of diet histories as a tool in nutritional assessment follows the references at the end of this chapter.

Water-soluble vitamins							Minerals					
Ascorbic acid (mg)	Folacin[f] (μg)	Niacin[g] (mg)	Riboflavin (mg)	Thiamin (mg)	Vitamin B6 (mg)	Vitamin B12 (μg)	Calcium (mg)	Phosphorus (mg)	Iodine (μg)	Iron (mg)	Magnesium (mg)	Zinc (mg)
35	50	5	0.4	0.3	0.3	0.3	360	240	35	10	60	3
35	50	8	0.6	0.5	0.4	0.3	540	400	45	15	70	5
40	100	9	0.8	0.7	0.6	1.0	800	800	60	15	150	10
40	200	12	1.1	0.9	0.9	1.5	800	800	80	10	200	10
40	300	16	1.2	1.2	1.2	2.0	800	800	110	10	250	10
45	400	18	1.5	1.4	1.6	3.0	1,200	1,200	130	18	350	15
45	400	20	1.8	1.5	2.0	3.0	1,200	1,200	150	18	400	15
45	400	20	1.8	1.5	2.0	3.0	800	800	140	10	350	15
45	400	18	1.6	1.4	2.0	3.0	800	800	130	10	350	15
45	400	16	1.5	1.2	2.0	3.0	800	800	110	10	350	15
45	400	16	1.3	1.2	1.6	3.0	1,200	1,200	115	18	300	15
45	400	14	1.4	1.1	2.0	3.0	1,200	1,200	115	18	300	15
45	400	14	1.4	1.1	2.0	3.0	800	800	100	18	300	15
45	400	13	1.2	1.0	2.0	3.0	800	800	100	18	300	15
45	400	12	1.1	1.0	2.0	3.0	800	800	80	10	300	15
60	800	+2	+0.3	+0.3	2.5	4.0	1,200	1,200	125	18+[h]	450	20
80	600	+4	+0.5	+0.3	2.5	4.0	1,200	1,200	150	18	450	25

under usual environmental stresses. Diets should be based on a variety of common foods in order to provide other nutrients for

and half as β-carotene when calculated from international units. As retinol equivalents, three fourths are as retinol and one fourth

in doses less than one fourth of the recommended dietary allowance.
dietary tryptophan.

CLINICAL ASSESSMENT: A TOOL OF NUTRITIONAL ASSESSMENT
Clinical assessment of nutrition status and dental appraisal

Until more sensitive indicators of subclinical malnutrition can be identified, public health practitioners will be unable to identify the more subtle forms of malnutrition. The more overt physical signs and symptoms of malnutrition, however, are clearly defined in dietary malnutrition.

In 1962 the World Health Organization Expert Committee on Medical Assessment of Nutritional Status proposed a classification of physical signs to be used in nutrition surveys.

Updated in 1966, this has proved to be a most valuable guide. Table 8-3 has been adapted from this classification. No chapter on nutrition assessment is complete without this classic chart; however, these physical signs are rarely seen in ambulatory populations throughout the United States.

The WHO Expert Committee[32] classified the physical signs most often associated with malnutrition into three groups:

Group one. Signs that are considered to be of value in nutritional assessment. These are often associated with nutritional deficiency states. Signs of malnutrition may often be mixed and may be

Table 8-3. Physical signs indicative or suggestive of malnutrition*

Body area	Normal appearance	Signs associated with malnutrition
Hair	Shiny; firm; not easily plucked	Lack of natural shine; hair dull and dry; thin and sparse; hair fine, silky and straight; color changes (flag sign); can be easily plucked
Face	Skin color uniform; smooth, pink, healthy appearance; not swollen	Skin color loss (depigmentation); skin dark over cheeks and under eyes (malar and supra-orbital pigmentation); lumpiness or flakiness of skin of nose and mouth; swollen face; enlarged parotid glands; scaling of skin around nostrils (nasolabial seborrhea)
Eyes	Bright, clear, shiny; no sores at corners of eyelids; membranes a healthy pink and are moist; no prominent blood vessels or mound of tissue or sclera	Eye membranes are pale (pale conjunctivae); redness of membranes (conjunctival injection); Bitot's spots; redness and fissuring of eyelid corners (angular palpebritis); dryness of eye membranes (conjunctival xerosis); cornea has dull appearance (corneal xerosis); cornea is soft (keratomalacia); scar on cornea; ring of fine blood vessels around corner (circumcorneal injection)
Lips	Smooth, not chapped or swollen	Redness and swelling of mouth or lips (cheilosis); especially at corners of mouth (angular fissures and scars)
Tongue	Deep red in appearance; not swollen or smooth	Swelling; scarlet and raw tongue; magenta (purplish color) of tongue; smooth tongue; swollen sores; hyperemic and hypertrophic papillae; and atrophic papillae
Teeth	No cavities; no pain; bright	May be missing or erupting abnormally; gray or black spots (fluorosis); cavities (caries)
Gums	Healthy; red; do not bleed; not swollen	"Spongy" and bleed easily; recession of gums
Glands	Face not swollen	Thyroid enlargement (front of neck); parotid enlargement (cheeks become swollen)
Skin	No signs of rashes, swelling, dark or light spots	Dryness of skin (xerosis); sandpaper feel of skin (follicular hyperkeratosis); flakiness of skin; skin swollen and dark; red swollen pigmentation of exposed areas (pellagrous dermatosis); excessive lightness or darkness of skin (dyspigmentation); black and blue marks due to skin bleeding (petechiae); lack of fat under skin
Nails	Firm, pink	Nails are spoon-shaped (koilonychia); brittle, ridged nails
Muscular and skeletal systems	Good muscle tone; some fat under skin; can walk or run without pain	Muscles have "wasted" appearance; baby's skull bones are thin and soft (craniotabes); round swelling of front and side of head (frontal and parietal bossing); swelling of ends of bones (epiphyseal enlargement); small bumps on both sides of chest wall (on ribs)—beading of ribs; baby's soft spot on head does not harden at proper time (persistently open anterior fontanelle); knock-knees or bow-legs; bleeding into muscle (musculoskeletal hemorrhages); person cannot get up or walk properly
Internal systems		
Cardiovascular	Normal heart rate and rhythm; no murmurs or abnormal rhythms; normal blood pressure for age	Rapid heart rate (above 100 tachycardia); enlarged heart; abnormal rhythm; elevated blood pressure
Gastrointestinal	No palpable organs or masses (in children, however, liver edge may be palpable)	Liver enlargement; enlargement of spleen (usually indicates other associated diseases)
Nervous	Psychological stability; normal reflexes	Mental irritability and confusion; burning and tingling of hands and feet (paresthesia); loss of position and vibratory sense; weakness and tenderness of muscles (may result in inability to walk); decrease and loss of ankle and knee reflexes

*Modified from Christakis, G., editor: Nutritional assessment in health programs, Am. J. Public Health **63** (suppl.):1-82, 1973.

due to the deficiency of two or more micronutrients.

Group two. Signs that need further investigation. They may be related to malnutrition, perhaps of a chronic type, but are often found in populations of developing countries where other health and environmental problems such as poverty and illiteracy are coexistent.

Group three. These include physical signs that have no relation to malnutrition, although they may be similar to physical signs found in persons with malnutrition and must be carefully delineated from them.

Physical signs should be recorded as precisely and practically as possible. Such terms as "poor," "fair," or "good" in terms of nutritional status should be avoided unless criteria for these terms are properly identified. An effective teaching tool that can assist the public health practitioner in identifying and standardizing signs of physical deficiencies is a series of color slides, "How to Diagnose Nutritional Deficiences in Daily Practice."[9]

The signs of malnutrition are multiple. A notice of one sign will at least alert the observer to continue with a more careful assessment of the body for other signs. Environmental factors such as excessive heat or sun, wind or cold air, lack of personal hygiene, and various cultural factors can cause or contribute to the physical signs that are associated with malnutrition.

The age of the person being examined also plays a role in the way the signs present themselves and in their interpretation. Any physical finding that suggests a nutritional abnormality should be considered a clue rather than a diagnosis and should be further explored.

The detailed clinical examination for signs of malnutrition must also include a search for signs related to metabolic diseases that may have a nutritional component. In the United States they tend to manifest themselves to a greater degree than undernutrition. For example, summarized below are the physical findings and laboratory evidence of hyperlipidemia that indicate high levels of serum cholesterol and/or triglyceride in a nutritional assessment study.

Small, yellowish lumps around eyes (xanthelasma)

Small or large tumors around joints of hands, legs or skin (xanthomas)
White ring around both eyes (corneal arcus)
Early coronary heart disease
Enlargement of liver and spleen
Turbid or creamy appearance of serum
High serum levels of cholesterol and/or triglycerides
Abnormal blood lipoprotein patterns[1]

Problems in clinical assessment. Two major problems encountered in the clinical assessment of nutrition status are (1) a low rate of prevalence in developed countries, except among high-risk groups, and the non-specificity of clinical signs among most populations in these countries, and (2) the substantial differences in the prevalence of physical signs as recorded by different examiners.

Despite these difficulties, physical examinations must be an integral part of most nutrition surveys for the following reasons:

1. Physical examination may reveal evidence of certain nutritional deficiencies that will not be detected by dietary or laboratory methods.
2. The identification of even a few cases of clear-cut nutritional deficiency may be particularly revealing and provide a clue to other pockets of malnutrition in a community.
3. The nutritional examination may reveal signs of a host of other diseases that merit diagnosis and treatment.

ANTHROPOMETRIC ASSESSMENT: A TOOL OF NUTRITIONAL ASSESSMENT

Anthropometry, the study of human body measurements, comprises a valuable part of forming the nutritional assessment profile. Problems of stunting, undernutrition, and overnutrition can be identified with the use of anthropometric methods.

The American Public Health Association guide, *Nutritional Assessment in Health Programs*, recommends the following for anthropometric measurements[1]:

Neonates and infants
    Weight
    Recumbent length (crown-heel)
    Head circumference
    Chest circumference
    Triceps skinfold

Pre-schoolers
    The same as the preceding category with standing height replacing recumbent length
    Arm circumference
School age through adolescence
    Delete head and chest circumferences
    Standing height
    Otherwise, the same as the preceding categories
Adulthood and aging
    Standing height
    Weight
    Triceps skinfold
    Subscapular skinfold
    Arm circumference

Weight

Body weight should be measured to the nearest 10 grams, or ½ ounce, for infants or 100 grams, or ¼ pound, for children. A beam balance scale should be used. Zero should be checked prior to every session and whenever the scale is moved. The scales should be calibrated at least every few months using reference weights.[10]

Height and length

Measurements of height and length remain the most important measurement for the assessment of skeletal linear growth.[11] Height or length generally correlates better with socioeconomic status than do measures of weight.[12]

Length is usually indicated for children up to 36 months of age and height thereafter. For length and height measurement a special board such as that designed by Fomon is highly desirable as opposed to a table.[13] Fig. 8-6 illustrates the technique of measuring height.

In measuring height, readings are recorded to the nearest 1 cm or ¼ inch. Recording to the nearest ½ to 1 inch is too crude, especially for children at borderline levels of low stature.

Height and weight of individuals over 60 years of age may not be accurate indices of body composition and nutritional status because of osteoporotic changes. Height always should be measured without shoes.

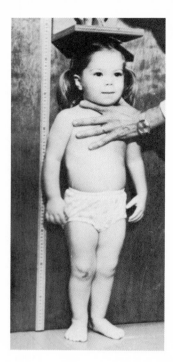

Fig. 8-6. Technique of measuring height. (From Fomon, S. J.: Infant nutrition, Philadelphia, 1974, W. B. Saunders Co.)

Head circumference

The purpose of the head circumference measurement in infants and toddlers is to screen for microcephaly and macrocephaly. It is considered to be a good index of brain growth, but caution is required when interpreting head circumference data because of familial and general body size factors.

An insertion tape provides adequate positioning and fixation of the tape around the head. Any springy hair should be compressed. A hair layer ¼ inch thick around one half of the head will theoretically increase head circumference by almost 1 inch. Increments in head circumference at various age levels are shown in Table 8-4.

Skinfold measurements

Lean body mass can be determined by calculating tricep skinfold thickness and arm circumference (Figs. 8-7 and 8-8). The prevalence of childhood obesity in the United States is at least 10%.[14] The limitations of fat-

Table 8-4. Increment in head circumference in various age intervals*

Age interval (months)	Percentiles	S.D.	Increment in head circumference (cm)		Age interval (months)	Percentiles	S.D.	Increment in head circumference (cm)	
			Males	Females				Males	Females
0-1		−2	1.0	0.8	9-12		−2	0.5	0.4
	10		2.0	1.5		10		0.8	0.8
	25		2.5	2.6		25		1.0	1.0
	50		3.6	3.3		50		1.3	1.2
	75		4.3	4.0		75		1.6	1.6
	90		5.3	4.7		90		1.8	1.7
		+2	6.2	5.6			+2	2.1	2.0
1-3		−2	1.9	1.9	12-18		−2	0.6	0.4
	10		2.4	2.5		10		1.0	0.7
	25		2.8	2.6		25		1.3	1.1
	50		3.3	3.1		50		1.6	1.5
	75		3.7	3.4		75		1.8	1.7
	90		4.2	3.8		90		2.1	1.9
		+2	4.7	4.3			+2	2.6	2.4
3-6		−2	1.7	1.8	18-24		−2	0.0	0.0
	10		2.2	2.3		10		0.2	0.5
	25		2.6	2.5		25		0.6	0.7
	50		3.0	2.9		50		0.9	0.9
	75		3.3	3.2		75		1.3	1.2
	90		4.0	3.4		90		1.7	1.5
		+2	4.5	3.8			+2	2.0	2.0
6-9		−2	1.1	0.9	24-36		−2	0.0	−0.5
	10		1.3	1.4		10		0.5	0.5
	25		1.6	1.6		25		0.7	0.8
	50		1.9	1.9		50		1.0	1.1
	75		2.1	2.2		75		1.3	1.3
	90		2.3	2.5		90		1.5	1.6
		+2	2.7	2.9			+2	2.0	2.7

*Data of Karlberg et al., 1968; from Fomon, S. J.: Infant nutrition, ed. 2, Philadelphia, 1974, W. B. Saunders Co.

fold measurements have been documented by Tanner[15]; nevertheless, it is the most convenient method to assess body fat bulk objectively.

Measurements of weight for age and weight for height are used in assessing obesity, but they do fail to distinguish muscle and soft tissue bulk from fat. On the other hand, serial weight measurements do give a reasonable indication of excessive weight gain and likely obesity.[13] Increments in skinfold thickness at various age levels are shown in Table 8-5.

In general, one limb (left triceps) and one trunkal (left subscapular) measure are advised to account for differing distribution of fat.[16,17] When a single measure is used, tri-

ceps has been favored for adolescents.[18] Either the Lange caliper, which is the only one produced commercially in the United States, or the Harpenden, manufactured in England, can be used to record triceps or subscapular skinfold thickness.

Quality control

Erroneous information regarding specific indices such as height and weight measurements can lead to inappropriate conclusions and poor decisions in patient care management.

Even with the Center for Disease Control surveillance system, certain observations led to questioning the accuracy of the anthropometric data that were collected. There was

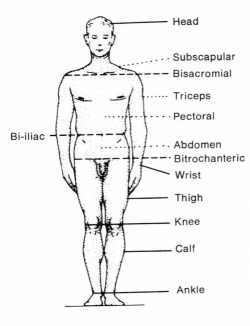

Head

Subscapular

Bisacromial

Triceps

Pectoral

Bi-iliac

Abdomen

Bitrochanteric

Wrist

Thigh

Knee

Calf

Ankle

– – – – – – Diameter

——————— Circumference

· · · · · · · · · · Skinfold thickness

Fig. 8-7. Anthropometric measurements used in various formulas for evaluating nutritional status. (From Guthrie, H. A.: Introductory nutrition, ed. 3, St. Louis, 1975, The C. V. Mosby Co.)

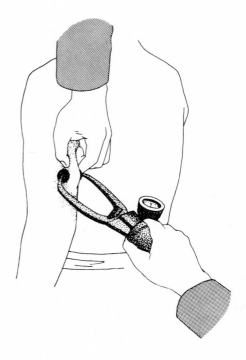

Fig. 8-8. Measuring triceps skinfold with calipers. (From Guthrie, H. A.: Introductory nutrition, ed. 3, St. Louis, 1975, The C. V. Mosby Co.)

Table 8-5. Increments in skinfold thickness in various age intervals*

Age interval (months)	Percentiles	S.D.	Triceps (mm)		Subscapular (mm)	
			Males	Females	Males	Females
1-3		−2	−0.6	−0.9	−1.8	−1.4
	10		0.7	0.1	−0.5	−0.7
	25		1.5	1.4	0.2	0.5
	50		2.5	2.5	1.4	1.6
	75		3.6	3.4	2.2	2.6
	90		4.7	4.4	3.1	3.4
		+2	5.8	5.9	4.6	4.6
3-6		−2	−1.5	−1.7	−3.3	−2.3
	10		−0.1	−0.1	−1.5	−1.2
	25		0.8	0.7	−0.7	−0.6
	50		1.8	2.1	0.2	0.2
	75		2.8	3.3	1.2	1.1
	90		3.6	4.4	2.3	2.0
		+2	5.3	5.9	3.9	2.9
6-9		−2	−3.0	−3.5	−2.9	−3.3
	10		−1.7	−2.2	−1.5	−2.0
	25		−0.7	−1.1	−0.8	−1.1
	50		0.2	−0.2	0.0	−0.2
	75		1.4	0.8	0.8	0.5
	90		2.6	1.6	1.9	1.2
		+2	3.8	3.3	3.1	2.7
9-12		−2	−3.7	−3.6	−3.2	−2.5
	10		−2.4	−2.4	−1.4	−1.6
	25		−1.5	−1.4	−0.6	−1.0
	50		0.0	−0.2	0.0	−0.3
	75		1.2	1.0	0.7	0.4
	90		2.4	2.1	1.8	1.1
		+2	3.5	3.2	3.2	1.9
12-18		−2	−3.2	−3.0	−3.3	−3.1
	10		−2.0	−2.2	−2.1	−2.1
	25		−1.0	−0.9	−1.0	−1.3
	50		−0.1	0.2	−0.4	−0.6
	75		1.4	1.3	0.4	0.2
	90		2.3	2.1	1.3	1.5
		+2	3.6	3.4	2.7	2.1
18-24		−2	−3.4	−3.0	−3.2	−2.7
	10		−2.0	−2.0	−1.7	−1.6
	25		−1.3	−0.8	−1.2	−1.1
	50		0.0	0.1	−0.5	−0.6
	75		1.2	1.2	0.2	0.2
	90		2.4	2.5	0.9	0.9
		+2	3.4	3.4	2.4	1.7
24-36		−2	−3.5	−4.2	−2.9	−3.5
	10		−2.3	−2.7	−1.9	−1.8
	25		−1.2	−1.2	−1.2	−0.9
	50		−0.2	0.3	−0.6	−0.4
	75		1.2	1.3	0.0	0.3
	90		2.3	2.3	0.4	1.2
		+2	3.3	4.2	1.5	3.3

*Data of Karlberg et al., 1968; from Fomon, S. J.: Infant nutrition, ed. 2, Philadelphia, 1974, W. B. Saunders Co.

Table 8-6. Common errors of measurement*

All measurements	Inadequate instrument
	Restless child (procedure should be postponed)
	Reading part of instrument not fixed when value taken
	Reading
	Recording errors
Length	Incorrect age for instrument
	Footwear or headwear not removed
	Head not in correct plane
	Head not firmly against fixed end of board
	Child not straight along board
	Body arched
	Knees bent
	Feet not vertical to movable board
	Board not firmly against heels
Height	Incorrect age for instrument
	Footwear or headwear not removed
	Feet not straight nor flat on vertical platform or wall
	Knees bent
	Body arched or buttocks forward (body not straight)
	Shoulders not straight on board
	Head not in correct plane
	Headboard not firmly on crown of child's head
Weight	Room cold, no privacy
	Scale not calibrated to zero
	Child wearing unreasonable amount of clothing
	Child moving or anxious due to prior misregard
Head circumference	Occipital protuberance/supraorbital landmarks poorly defined
	Hair crushed inadequately, ears under tape
	Tape tension and position poorly maintained by time of reading
	Headwear not removed
Triceps fatfold	Wrong arm (should be left arm)
	Mid-arm point or posterior plane incorrectly measured or marked
	Arm not loose by side during measurement
	Examiner not comfortable nor level with child
	Finger-thumb pinch or caliper placement too deep (muscle) or too superficial (skin)
	Caliper jaws not at marked site
	Reading done too early or too late (should be 2 to 3 seconds)
	At time of reading, pinch not maintained, caliper handle not fully released
Arm circumference	Tape too thick, stretched or creased
	Wrong arm (should be left arm)
	Mid-arm point incorrectly measured or marked
	Arm not loosely hanging by side during measurement
	Examiner not comfortable nor level with child
	Tape around arm, not at midpoint; too tight (causing skin contour indentation), too loose (inadequately opposed)

*Modified from Zerfas, A. J., Shorr, I. J., and Neumann, C. G.: Office assessment of nutritional status, Pediatr. Clin. North Am. **4:** 253, 1977.

considerable concern because some of the reported data contained improbable grouping of heights and weights for age and weight for height when compared with the expected standard. This may have resulted from inaccurate measurements or recording errors or both. Also, health department personnel reported that inadequate weighing and measuring equipment and incorrect techniques are common in clinic settings.

Because of these problems, a study was designed by the Center for Disease Control, Bureau of Training, which was conducted in the state of Washington. Its purpose was to provide information on the frequency and causes of inaccurate measurements.[19]

Significant findings included the following:

1. Reference teams results differed considerably from the heights, weights, and lengths obtained by clinical personnel.
2. Clinic measures tended to measure children less than 2 years old too short.
3. Although accurate weights are generally obtained, clinics tended to report an artificially high percent of children as being stocky and overweight.
4. Clinic measures tended to measure standing children too tall.
5. Equipment problems were considered to be the principal cause of inaccurate measurements.
6. Technique errors were less significant contributors to measurement inaccuracies, although they occurred.
7. The most common technique error noted was that young children were not properly stretched on the board for measuring.
8. Recording errors contributed significantly to inaccuracy.
9. The amount of errors is heavily influenced by motivation.

This study demonstrated the need to do more careful appraisals of anthropometric measurements on a regularly scheduled basis. Staffs must be trained and kept motivated to perform these measurements accurately. Table 8-6 depicts the Common Errors of Measurement.[10]

Table 8-7 shows some anthropometric measurements applied in nutritional assessment. It also indicates some of the advantages and disadvantages of the particular measurements.[20]

Use of growth charts in child health screening procedures
Charting of growth in the United States

The Stuart (Boston) and the Meredith (Iowa) growth charts are the instruments familiar to nutritionists who have worked with children during the past 30 years. The vast majority of infants and children in the United States have been clinically evaluated by comparing their measurements of length or height and weight with such growth charts.

In the 1870s, studies of Boston school-age children were conducted by H. P. Bowditch, who is credited with having developed the first growth chart for the average height and weight of American children.[21] In 1921 Woodbury[22] reported average stature and weight for 172,000 children under 6 years of age from all over the United States and thus provided the first broadly based physical growth reference data for this age group. However, throughout the past 50 years many growth charts have had only short-term usefulness because of the nature of the population sample, lack of expert agreement on broad applicability, or lack of effective dissemination.[23]

Although the Stuart-Meredith growth charts have survived the test of time, their usefulness in contemporary society is limited. Responding to the identified needs of many researchers throughout the country, the National Center for Health Statistics (NCHS) in 1975 compiled data and prepared a series of percentile curves reflecting the growth of contemporary infants, children, and youth in the United States. These recent percentile curves are based on large, nationally representative samples of children. They represent a broad consensus of experts in physical growth, pediatrics, and clinical nutrition. These charts explain the NCHS percentile curves for length or stature, body

Table 8-7. Some anthropometric measurements applied in nutritional assessment*

Measurements	Age groups	Nutritional indication	Reproducibility	Advantages	Disadvantages	Observer error	Interpretation
1. Weight	All groups	Present nutr. status; under and over	Good	Common in use	Difficult in field; can't tell body composition; need accurate age; need proper scales	<100 g in children <250 g in adults	60% severe 60-80% moderate 80-90% mild 90-110% normal 110-120% over 120% & over obese
2. Height	All groups; 7 yr child	Chronic nutr. status (under) Chronic under nutr. in early childhood	Good	Common in use Simple to do in field	Differs by daytime Other factors play a role	<0.5 cm child <3.0 cm in adults	<80% dwarf 80-93% short 93-105% normal >105% giant
3. Head circumference	0-4 yr	Intrauterine & childhood nutr. (chronic undernutrition mental abilities)	Good	Simple	Other factors play a role	<0.5 cm	
4. Mid-arm circumference	All groups	Present under- and overnutrition	Fair	Simple, age independent; child need not be denuded; suitable for rapid survey	No limits for overnutrition no standard for adult	<0.5 cm	<75% severe 75-80% moderate 80-85% mild >85% normal
5. Skin-fold thickness subscapula	All groups	Present under- and overnutrition	Fair	Measure body composition, detect obesity—adults	Needs expensive callipers; difficult with child and in the field	1.0-1.5 mm	Similar to item (1)
6. Weight/height for age ratio	All ages	Present under- and overnutrition	Good	Index of body build; age independent, 1-4 yr and adults	Need proper scales; need trained personnel		<75% severe 75-85% moderate 85-90% mild 90-110% normal 110-120% over >120% obese
7. Mid-arm/head ratio	3 mo-48 mo	Present undernutrition	Good	Simple; age independent; sex independent; any person can do it for field	No standard for adults		<0.25 severe 0.25-0.28 moderate 0.28-0.31 mild 0.31-0.35 normal >0.35 obese
8. Chest/head circs. ratio	1-2 yr	Present undernutrition	Fair or poor	Simple; age independent	For limited age; no classification method		<1 malnourished >1 normal

* Reprinted from Bengoa, J. M.: In Berg, A., Scrimshaw, N. S., and Call, D. L., editors: Nutrition, national development and planning, Massachusetts and London, 1972, The M.I.T. Press, p 110. By permission of The M.I.T. Press, Cambridge, Mass., © 1972.

weight, head circumference, and body weight for length or stature and should stand as a significant milestone in the study of human growth. These charts should be effective in facilitating uniformity in the clinical appraisal of growth and nutritional status and should help to simplify comparative interpretation of growth data. Figs. 8-9 and 8-10 are examples of the growth charts for boys and for girls, prepubescent and 2 to 18 years.

Data sources and measurement techniques

Owen[24] answered the following two questions concerning the new NCHS growth charts, which became available for use in 1976: (1) How do new growth charts differ from the old charts? (2) Do the new charts offer advantages over the old charts? To answer these questions, Owen addressed himself to several areas, including data sources

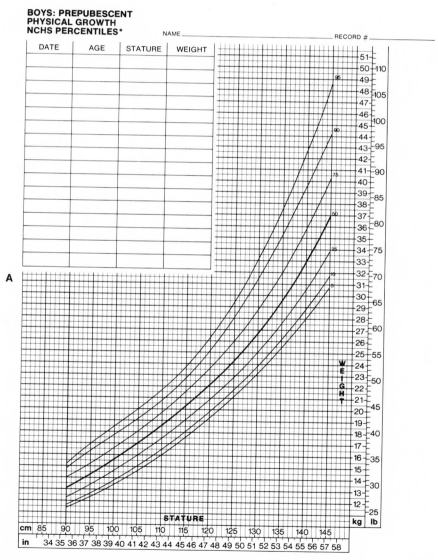

BOYS: PREPUBESCENT PHYSICAL GROWTH NCHS PERCENTILES*

Fig. 8-9. A, Physical growth NCHS percentiles in prepubescent boys. (From Ross Laboratories, Columbus, Ohio.)

Continued.

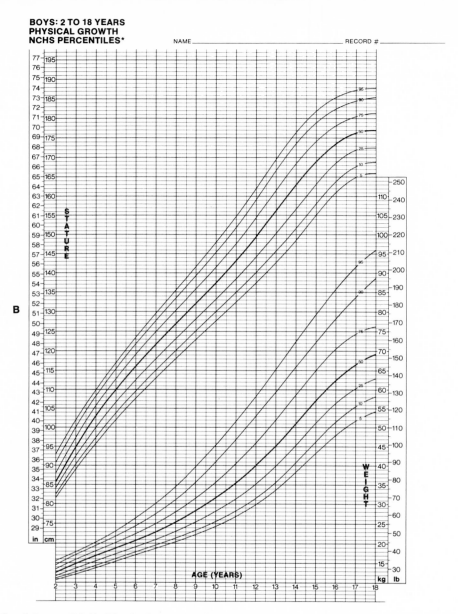

BOYS: 2 TO 18 YEARS
PHYSICAL GROWTH
NCHS PERCENTILES*

Fig. 8-9, cont'd. B, Physical growth NCHS percentiles in boys ages 2 to 18 years. (From Ross Laboratories, Columbus, Ohio.)

and measurement techniques, differences in size and growth chart construction, weight-for-height charts, and anthropometry in the clinical setting.

The old growth charts (Meredith and Stuart) were based on length or height and weight measurements collected in longitu-dinal studies conducted between 1925 and 1945. Measurement techniques were well described, and quality control ensured that there was no question that the cumulative data were accurate and precise. However, relatively small numbers of children were represented in the growth charts derived

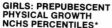

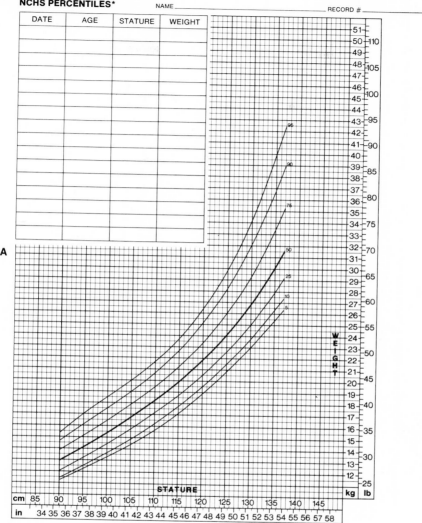

Fig. 8-10. A, Physical growth NCHS percentiles in prepubescent girls. (From Ross Laboratories, Columbus, Ohio.)

Continued.

from the longitudinal studies in Boston, and the studies were characterized by decreasing numbers of children at successive age intervals. In the case of the Iowa charts, the actual number of infants and children represented and the methods of construction of the charts are difficult to discern.[25,26]

The new growth charts are based on data from two major sources. In the charts encompassing the period from birth to 36 months, longitudinal measurements of 866 children at the Fels Research Institute were used. These recumbent lengths and nude weight measurements collected between 1929 and 1975 were made in the same manner as those in the Boston and Iowa longitudinal studies. New charts for children 2 to 18 years of age were constructed using NCHS data collected between 1962 and 1974. These were based on a nationally rep-

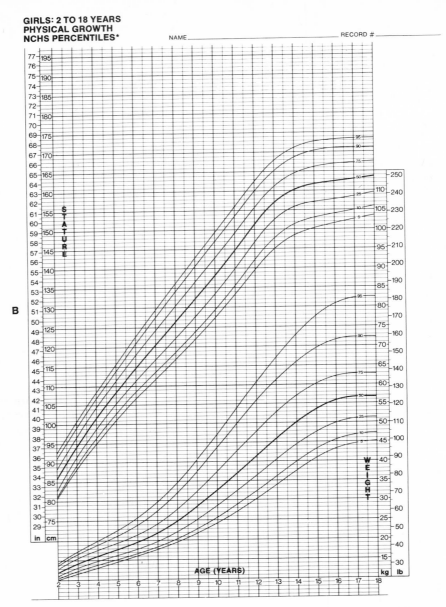

GIRLS: 2 TO 18 YEARS
PHYSICAL GROWTH
NCHS PERCENTILES*

NAME_____   RECORD #_____

Fig. 8-10, cont'd. B, Physical growth NCHS percentiles in girls ages 2 to 18 years. (From Ross Laboratories, Columbus, Ohio.)

resentative sample of some 18,000 individuals. Great care was taken to ensure accurate measuring and recording of height and weight using well-described, standardized techniques.

In the Boston and Iowa studies, recumbent length was measured up to 6 years of age and is so represented in the old charts. This is often forgotten, as is the fact that recumbent length is 1 or 2 cm greater than stature, standing height, by persons plotting standing height of youngsters 3 or 4 years of age on the old charts. Currently, in virtually all clinical settings, children of more than 1 or 2 years of age are measured in the standing position, since the new growth charts (2 to 18 years) are based on stature.

Differences in size and growth chart structure

Secular growth, increasing size, and earlier maturation of a population in middle and upper income children in the United States have occurred at an average rate of 1 cm per decade for the 4-year-olds since the late 1880s. However, it appears to have ceased in the mid-1960s.[27,28] The only real change in stature is reflected in the lower percentiles (5th and 10th) and probably indicates changes among lower socioeconomic groups. In contrast, and not surprisingly, the 95th percentile of weight for age is somewhat greater in the mid-1970s than in the mid-1960s. Thus the user of the new growth charts must be aware that the charts represent the population as it exists and not that which is ideal or optimal, especially with respect to body weight.

Examination of the old and new growth charts with respect to the average (median, mean, or 50th percentile), weight- or height-for-age shows some fairly consistent trends toward greater height and greater weight in the 1960s and 1970s when compared with the 1930s and 1940s. Yet it is inappropriate to compare the extreme percentiles in the old and new charts because of the differences in sample sizes, class intervals according to age, and methods used to derive the percentiles. The use of relatively small samples, as in the Boston and Iowa charts, may attenuate the variance at the extremes, especially when the same children comprising a relatively homogeneous population (socioeconomically) are measured at successive relative precise ages. The loss of either end or both ends of the distribution will result in underestimation of height and of weight variability for clinical work.

Furthermore, the extreme percentiles in the old growth charts corresponded to mathematical approximations or curves that were smoothed by hand. In contrast, weight-for-age and weight-for-height curves of 5th,

10th, 25th, 50th, 75th, 90th, and 95th percentiles were produced and plotted by the computer in the new growth charts. This was possible because of the large number of individuals represented in the new data.

Weight-for-height charts

The availability of the large number of measurements of height and weight represented in the NCHS data has allowed the development of weight-for-height charts. The NCHS charts provide a visual depiction and descriptive quantitation of the relation between weight and height. For reasons alluded to earlier, it appears likely that major attention will be focused on the upper 90th and 95th percentiles of the weight-for-height charts as indicators of fatness or obesity.

From a practical point of view, it appears that the nutritionist and clinician might find a weight-for-height chart, used in a serial manner, helpful in earlier identification of trends in body composition (fatness), which would be less evident if only weight-for-age and height-for-age are plotted as has been the traditional practice. Although contemporary measures and standards for skinfold thickness of infants and young children in the United States are not readily available, it would be useful if the clinician were able to correlate increasing weight for height with such independent measurements of fat.[13,29]

Anthropometry in the clinical setting

Anthropometry is the most frequently performed child health screening procedure. There have been a number of anthropometric studies with large population groups that have indicated associations between socioeconomic status, dietary adequacy, and growth among young children. Larkin and associates recently compared a small group of children (2 to 77 months of age) with growth failure, that is, height or weight measurements below and 3rd percentile, with children (2 to 59 months of age) who demonstrated a higher level of achievement in weight and height for age. Although families of children with inadequate growth purchased more food stamps and had higher monthly credit payments, the major differences between the two groups was in birth weight. There were five times as many low birth weight (below 2,500 grams) children among the study group than among a control group.[30]

Because size at birth may influence size throughout the first several years of life, it is important to obtain the best information possible concerning weight and gestational age at birth. Similarly, among families where income is considered adequate, parents' stature must be taken into account when evaluating growth of children.[31]

The new NCHS growth charts better represent the United States childhood population today than did the old growth charts. The availability of the new NCHS growth chart should stimulate new interest in anthropometry as a screening procedure for growth failure and for obesity.

BIOCHEMICAL ASSESSMENT: A TOOL OF NUTRITIONAL ASSESSMENT

Laboratory methods of nutritional assessment are considered to provide a more objective and precise approach to nutritional status, that is, when compared with community assessment, dietary methodology, or clinical assessment methods. They principally consist of biochemical tests performed in a laboratory as follows:

1. Appropriate biochemical tests should be selected for the particular survey contemplated.

2. Tests for field surveys are usually confined to two obtainable body fluids—blood and urine.

3. Generally, intricate biochemical tests are costly and time consuming to carry out. In all surveys the expected value of results to be obtained by particular methods in the assessment of status must be weighed against the problem of collection, transport, laboratory, and interpretation.

4. Frequently the interpretation of laboratory data is difficult and does not necessarily correlate with either clinical or dietary findings. In contrast, there is a significant degree of correlation between some nutrient intakes and selected biochemical measures as shown in Table 8-8. In addition, although some checks are of considerable assistance, they have as yet uncertain standards for less advanced forms of malnutrition, especially in young children.[1,32] Laboratory indicators of current dietary intake and of the nutritional status of young children are presented in Table 8-9.

Objectives of laboratory assessment

Laboratory tests have two primary purposes, one of which is to detect marginal nutritional deficiencies in individuals. Their use is especially important in early detection, before overt clinical signs of disease appear, thus permitting indications of appropriate remedial steps. Their other purpose is to supplement or enhance other studies such as dietary or community assessment among specific population groups to identify nutritional problems. Table 8-10 indicates biochemical

Table 8-8. Correlation between dietary intakes and some biochemical variables*

Dependent variable (biochemical)	Independent variable (dietary)	Correlation coefficient	Analysis of variance	
			df	F ratio
Urea nitrogen	Protein	.13	1/1270	23†
Ascorbic acid	Vitamin C	.46	1/1351	371†
Riboflavin	Riboflavin	.26	1/1282	97†
Thiamin	Thiamin	.23	1/1305	95†
Vitamin A	Vitamin A	.05	1/1516	4

*From Owen, G. M., and Lippman, G.: Nutritional status of infants and young children: U.S.A., Pediatr. Clin. North Am. **24**:211, 1977.

†Significant ($p < .001$).

Table 8-9. Laboratory indicators of current dietary intake and of nutritional status of the young child*

Dietary component	Current intake	Nutritional status	Comments
Protein	Serum or urine urea nitrogen	Serum albumin	Urea nitrogen in serum or urine correlates reasonably well with current net intake of protein if renal function is normal. Creatinine values in serum <6 mg/dl or in urine <8 mg/gm suggest low recent intake of protein. Serum albumin is a rather insensitive and nonspecific indicator of protein status, but values <3.2 gm/dl suggest a poor protein nutritional status.
Iron	Transferrin saturation	Hemoglobin, hematocrit, cell indices	Levels of transferrin saturation (iron/total iron-building capacity × 100) <16% suggest iron deficiency even when the concentration of hemoglobin is >10.5 gm/dl. Hemoglobin concentration <10.5 gm/dl (hematocrit 32%) is suggested as lower limit of normal for 6-year-old child. A mean corpuscular hemoglobin concentration (MCHC) <30 gm/dl of packed erythrocytes suggests iron deficiency.
Vitamin A	Serum carotene	Serum vitamin A	Approximately one half of total vitamin A intake from foods is supplied by fruits, vegetables, and cereal grains in the form of carotene. A level of serum carotene <40 μg/dl suggests low net intake of carotene. A level of serum vitamin A <20 μg/dl suggests low stores in vitamin A or may indicate failure of transport of retinol out of liver into blood.
Ascorbic acid	Serum ascorbate or whole blood ascorbate	Leukocyte ascorbate	At usual levels of intake of ascorbic acid from foods there is good correlation between intake and serum ascorbate; levels in serum <0.3 mg/dl suggest that recent intake has been low. Whole blood ascorbate levels <0.3 mg/dl indicate low intake and reduction in body pool of ascorbic acid. Leukocyte ascorbic acid levels <20 mg/100 gm suggest poor nutritional status.
Riboflavin	Urinary riboflavin	Erythrocyte glutathione reductase	There is a reasonably good correlation between intake and urinary excretion of riboflavin. Excretion of <250 μg/gm creatinine suggests low recent intake of riboflavin. Glutathione reductase–FAD (flavin-adenine dinucleotide) effect expressed as a ratio >1.2 suggests poor nutritional status.
Thiamin	Urinary thiamin	Erythrocyte transketolase	Excretion of <125 μg/gm creatinine suggests low intake of thiamin. Transketolase–TPP (thiamin pyrophosphate) effect expressed as a ratio >15 suggests poor nutritional status.
Folacin	Serum folacin	Erythrocyte folacin, formiminoglutamic acid (FIGLU)	Level of serum folacin <6 μg/dl suggests low intake. Levels of erythrocyte folacin <20 μg/dl or increased excretion of FIGLU in urine following a histidine load suggests poor nutritional status.
Iodine	Urinary iodine	Protein-bound iodine (PBI)	Urinary excretion of <50 μg/gm creatinine suggests low recent intake of iodine. PBI <3 μg/dl suggests poor nutritional status.

*From Owen, G. M., and Lippman, G.: Nutritional status of infants and young children: U.S.A., Pediatr. Clin. North Am. **24:**211, 1977.

Table 8-10. Biochemical tests applicable to nutrition surveys[*]

Nutritional deficiency	First category[a]	Second category
1. Protein	Amino acid imbalance test Hydroxyproline excretion test (F) Serum albumin Urinary urea (F)[b] Urinary creatinine per unit of time (T)	Serum protein fractions by electrophoresis
2. Vitamin A	Serum vitamin A Serum carotene	
3. Vitamin D	Serum alkaline phosphatase (in young children)	Serum inorganic phosphorus
4. Ascorbic acid	Serum ascorbic acid	White blood cell ascorbic acid Urinary ascorbic acid Load test
5. Thiamin	Urine thiamin (F)[b]	Load test Blood pyruvate Blood lactate Red blood cell hemolysate transketolase
6. Riboflavin	Urinary riboflavin (F)[b]	Red blood cell riboflavin Load test
7. Niacin	Urinary N-methylnicotinamide (F)[b]	Load test Urinary pyridone (n-methyl-2-pyridone-5-carbonamide)
8. Iron	Hemoglobin Hematocrit Thin blood film	Serum iron Percentage saturation of transferrin
9. Folic acid } Vitamin B_{12}	Hemoglobin Thin blood film	Serum folate *(L. casei)* Serum B_{12} *(E. gracilis)*
10. Iodine		Urinary iodine (F) Tests for thyroid function

[*]From Jeliffe, D. B.: The assessment of the nutritional status of the community, Geneva, 1966, World Health Organization· adapted from WHO Expert Committee on Medical Assessment of Nutritional Status, 1963.
[a]Urinary creatinine used as reference for expressing other urine measurements in first category.
[b]Expressed per gram of creatinine.
(F) In a single urine specimen, preferably fasting.
(T) In timed urine specimens.

tests applicable to nutrition surveys as suggested by Jelliffe.[32]

In general, laboratory methods indicate deficiencies in the following areas: (1) serum protein, the albumin level; (2) the blood-forming nutrients such as iron, folacin, vitamin B_6, and vitamin B_{12}; (3) water-soluble vitamins such as thiamin, riboflavin, niacin, and vitamin C; (4) the fat-soluble vitamins A, D, E, and K; (5) minerals such as iron, iodine, and other trace elements; and (6) levels of blood lipids, glucose, and various enzymes that are duplicated in heart disease, diabetes, and other chronic diseases.

Generally, two types of tests are employed in laboratory surveys: measurement of circulating levels of nutrients in blood or urine and/or functional tests. After the presence of nutritional problems are recognized, the functional tests measure the effectiveness of the body's use of its nutrient intake. For example, if deficiencies are detected in the urine, measurement of the enzymes transketolase and red blood cells will provide a more accurate indicator of its severity.

Preparation for biochemical study

Collection of samples. When the appropriate biochemical tests for a particular kind of survey have been chosen, a decision must be made about the number of steps required for processing. This will determine the amount of necessary equipment. The number of specimens will depend on statistical considerations in relation to the total number of persons examined clinically, in the field, and on the limitations imposed by facilities for transport, storage, and actual analysis.

Blood samples. Plasma is required for the examination of albumin, vitamin A, carotene, ascorbic acid, and alkaline phosphatase. Blood tests are often carried out using macromethods, although the large quantities usually can be obtained only from adults or school children. Venous samples are best taken by vacuum tubes such as vacutainer or by using disposable needles to avoid contamination and the need for cleaning and sterilizing syringes. The latter is the easiest and cheapest method of obtaining blood samples, especially if used with a sphygmomanometer rather than a tourniquet. It also permits several samples of blood to be made into different containers during one venipuncture, if required. Equipment for washing out and unplugging syringes and needles must be immediately available when samples are taken. Blood samples are collected into stoppered or screw-capped glass vials, containing an anticoagulant such as heparin lithium. For those biochemical tests carried out by micromethods, blood obtained will be collected in heparinized capillary tubes and sealed by using commercial clay, especially prepared for a cover, or by heating in a flame. All such samples must be refrigerated.

Urinary analysis. For urinary analysis (e.g., urea, thiamin, riboflavin, N-methylnicotinamide), fasting samples passed in different time periods are ideal but not too practical under field conditions, especially with children. Single random specimens must often suffice. However, when urine is used as a measure of body-muscle mass, creatinine estimation must be collected over a timed period, minimally 3 hours and preferably 24 hours.

Urine should be stored in sturdy screw-capped glass or, even better, plastic bottles containing hydrochloric acid, which acts as a preservative and inhibitor of bacterial growth. The quantity of hydrochloric acid should not be enough to dilute the sample greatly; 1 drop of concentrated hydrochloric acid should be enough for about 25 ml of urine. The specimen can then be kept at room temperature or stored in the refrigerator.

Laboratory considerations site. Various laboratory tests differ in requirements regarding staff and facilities and the time in which they must be performed once the sample has been taken. Three kinds of laboratory sites are necessary for the ideal situation: First, there should be a survey site with facilities for taking, labeling, packaging, and refrigerating samples. Second, the field laboratory should be adjacent to, or not far distant from, the survey site with adequate bench or table space, water supply, a refrigerator, cylinders of gas, and if possible, electricity. Third, a base laboratory is often situated in a central institution such as a medical school, state health department laboratory, or an agricultural research station.

The success of a given survey depends on the tests planned, the availability and location of existing laboratories, the distances and communications facilities involved, and the funds available. In some surveys it may be possible to build up a new laboratory to help an existing one develop or expand. However, in many shorter surveys it is easier and more economical to make it a rule that whenever possible, specimens should be collected in the field, preserved and refrigerated suitably, and taken back to a central laboratory at the end of the survey.

Equipment. The equipment initially needed should be calculated as far as possible according to an estimation of the amount of samples and their necessary storage and transport. For field work a 20% excess is desirable to cover breakage, loss, and initial underestimation of attendance. Supplies should be standardized as far as possible.

Techniques. Laboratory techniques must be selected for their accuracy, sensitivity, reproducibility, and practicability within the technical resources available. Methods commonly used and approved vary with individual nutrients being tested.

Interpretation of laboratory data. The significance and accuracy of results of biochemical tests are related to standards of collection, methods of transport and storage, which

Table 8-11. Biochemical methods and remarks regarding interpretation*

Substance	Method	Quantity required	Comment
Hemoglobin (blood)	Cyanmethemoglobin (O'Brien et al., 1968)	20 μl	Concentration of hemoglobin less than 11.0 gm/dl for children below 10 years of age and less than 12.0 gm/dl for older children (less than 13.0 gm/dl for males over 14 years of age) indicates anemia.
Hematocrit (blood)	Capillary tube (O'Brien et al., 1968)	40 μl	Hematocrit less than 34 children below 10 years of age and less than 37 for older children (less than 41 for males over 14 years of age) indicates anemia.
Iron and iron-binding capacity (serum)	Manually by method of Fischer and Price (1964) or automated (Garry and Owen, 1968)	200 μl 100 μl	Concentration of iron, iron-binding capacity and percent saturation of transferrin may require different interpretation in infants than in older individuals.
Free erythrocyte porphyrins (blood)	Method of Piomelli et al. (1976) with filter paper disc	100 μl	Free erythrocyte porphyrin/hemoglobin ratio greater than 5.5 μg/gm indicates iron deficiency.
Total protein (serum)	Microbiuret manually (O'Brien et al., 1968) or automated (Failing et al., 1970)	50 μl	With manual method, a serum blank is desirable.
Albumin (serum)	Electrophoresis on cellulose acetate (Fomon et al., 1970)	10 μl	Concentration of albumin less than 2.9 gm/dl suggests poor protein nutritional status.
Ascorbic acid (plasma)	2.6 Dichloroindophenol reaction manually (O'Brien et al., 1968) or automated (Garry et al., 1974)	20 μl 50 μl	Concentration less than 0.3 mg/dl suggests that recent dietary intake has been low.
Vitamin A (plasma or serum)	Fluorometry (Garry et al., 1970; or Thompson et al., 1971)	200 μl	Concentration less than 10 μg/dl suggests deficiency and concentration less than 20 μg/dl indicates low stores.
Alkaline phosphatase (serum)	Liberation of p-nitrophenol manually (O'Brien et al., 1968) or automated (Morgenstern et al., 1965)	100 μl	Activity greater than 25 Bodansky units/dl is suggestive of rickets.
Inorganic phosphorus (serum or plasma)	Modification of method of Fiske and Subba Row (1925) manually (O'Brien et al., 1968) or automated	50 μl	Concentration less than 4.0 mg/dl is abnormal and suggestive of rickets. However, normal concentration does not rule out the presence of rickets.
Urea nitrogen (serum)	Urease manually (O'Brien et al., 1968) or diacetyl monoxime manually or automated (Marsh et al., 1965)	100 μl 50 μl	Concentration less than 8 mg/dl suggests low recent dietary intake of protein. However, concentrations as low as 3.5 mg/dl are sometimes found in breastfed infants.
Cholesterol (serum)	Manually by method of Carr and Drekter (1956) or automated (Levine and Zak, 1964)	100 μl	Concentration of cholesterol more than 230 mg/dl indicates hypercholesterolemia.
Lipoproteins (serum)	Agarose electrophoresis (Laboratory Methods Committee, 1974)	100 μl	For interpretation, see Fredrickson and Levy (1972).
Creatinine (urine)	Alkaline picrate manually (O'Brien et al., 1968) or automated	100 μl	Serves as reference for other urine determinations.
Riboflavin (urine)	Fluorometry (Horwitz, 1970)	2 ml	Excretion less than 250 μg/gm of creatinine suggests low recent dietary intake.
Thiamin (urine)	Thiochrome fluorometry (Horwitz, 1970)	10 ml	Excretion of less than 125 μg/gm of creatinine suggests that dietary intake has been low for weeks or months.
Iodine (urine)	Automated ceric ionarsenious acid system (Garry et al., 1973)	5 ml	Excretion of less than 50 μg/gm of creatinine suggests low recent dietary intake.

*From Fomon, S. J.: Nutritional disorder of children: prevention, screening and follow-up, Washington, D.C., 1976, publication no. HSA 76-5612, Government Printing Office.

would include possible exposure to ultraviolet light, heat, and shaking, and the actual technique utilized, which would include consideration of laboratory controls, using control sera.

The accurate interpretation of results depends on knowledge of the unique metabolism of each particular nutrient, including its storage in the body and the possibility of synthesis in the mode of excretion. The tests employed usually assess one of two aspects of nutritional inadequacy, although their specificity may be less than is at present appreciated.

Table 8-11 provides a useful summary for the practitioner.[33]

The interpretation of laboratory data will always provide areas for some disagreement, since the prime objective is to detect risk of deficiency before clinical evidence of disease develops. Standards may also vary somewhat according to the methods used, since they vary in specificity and reproducibility. All methods used should be standardized and an appropriate design developed so that the results do not vary beyond acceptable limits during the course of the program. This is best accomplished by repeating evaluation of standards that have been previously checked by a recognized standard laboratory. The best single source for advice on standards and controls is the Nutritional Biochemistry Section of the Center for Disease Control, although there are other laboratories that can be consulted also.

The criteria used in the Ten State Nutrition Survey are included in Appendix 8-2 for current information and reference purposes. These standards may well be modified in the future as better methods and more data about the physiologic significance of different intake of various nutrients and their functions are obtained.

Precaution in laboratory evaluation

Certain considerations must be recognized when evaluating the results of laboratory nutritional assessments. Nutrient levels vary from time to time and may reflect immediate rather than usual intake. Biologic fluid levels and functional operation vary from person to person, even when they are taking similar diets or are apparently suffering equally from nutritional depletion. Furthermore, intercurrent disease may affect nutrient levels.

It also must be kept in mind that the "cutoff points" selected as representing some degrees of risk of deficiency are and perhaps always will be a somewhat arbitrary decision. As Christakis[1] points out, the controversies will remain until there are more simple and reliable tests, an extension of the range and specificity of laboratory evaluation of nutrients, and better data on the physiologic significance of the tests used.

Laboratory assessment for individual nutrients*

Certain methods are employed to assess those nutrients that can be measured by laboratory evaluation. Appendix 8-3 contains references for nutritional laboratory assessment. These should be available prior to the performance of any survey techniques.

Protein deficiency in the United States is uncommon. Pregnant women tend to have reduced levels, but it is uncertain whether "normal" criteria for nonpregnant women also apply to pregnant women. Protein deficiency may be indicated by a decrease in serum protein levels, especially serum albumin, but this finding is not specific for protein deficiency. Also, serum protein levels may be maintained for a considerable period of time, despite limited protein intake. Nevertheless, total serum protein and serum albumin determinations provide some information and are standard clinical chemical procedures.[1]

Water-soluble vitamins

Vitamin C (ascorbic acid). Clinical scurvy, the disease associated with severe vitamin C deficiency, is uncommon in the United

---

*This section has been quoted from two sources: (1) Christakis, G., editor: Nutritional assessment in health programs, Am. J. Public Health **63**(suppl.):1-82, 1973; (2) Jellife, D. B.: Assessment of nutritional status of the community, Geneva, 1966, World Health Organization.

States, although infants, alcoholics, the elderly, and neglected persons may be scorbutic. On the other hand, reduced levels of vitamin C in blood plasma have been reported in a significant portion of people in many nutrition surveys. Serum levels of vitamin C vary substantially and depend, to a considerable degree, on the intake immediately preceding the test. This is important to remember when interpreting the results of plasma vitamin C levels.

Thiamin. Although clinical evidence of thiamin deficiency is very uncommon in most United States populations, it is probably an important cause of morbidity in alcoholics. The usual test is the determination of thiamin excretion in the urine, ordinarily made on "spot samples" collected in the field or in the clinic rather than 24-hour collection. However, thiamin content in spot samples from the same individual varies substantially, and this is a relatively insensitive test of the nutritional status.

A functional enzyme test is preferable. Transketolase is an enzyme that requires thiamin (as thiamin pyrophosphate, TPP) to function. Transketolase in red blood cells and the "TPP effect" (the increase in activity due to the addition of TPP) may be measured, and this is probably the best procedure, since activity does change with a moderate depletion of thiamin. It has not yet been applied to broadly based surveys. Microbiologic assays are also used to estimate thiamin in blood.

Riboflavin. A variety of lesions associated with riboflavin deficiency are not uncommon in many parts of the world. The specificity of such lesions as indicators of riboflavin depletion is, however, in doubt. The usual method of estimating riboflavin adequacy is by examination of urinary excretion. These tests also are not completely satisfactory because of the variability in riboflavin excretion.

Niacin. Pellagra, the disease caused by niacin deficiency, is now rare in the United States, although it may occasionally be seen in alcoholics or other persons with severely restricted diets. Niacin is derived from the amino acid, tryptophan, and thus pellagra is ordinarily associated with the consumption of little tryptophan, such as is found in populations with corn and sorghum-based diets.

Estimation of N-methylnicotinamide in the urine has been the traditional method of determining adequacy of niacin intake. As with thiamin, urinary excretion is not a generally satisfactory method for surveys. Microbiologic methods are available for the estimation of circulating niacin.

Folacin. Folate deficiency results in anemia. Low circulating levels of folacin have been reported to be common in pregnant women and in women taking birth control pills and other estrogenic medications. The circulating level of folate in plasma or red blood cells is utilized in estimating adequacy of intake, although the standards for interpreting data are controversial. Folate deficiency increases excretion of formiminoglutamic acid (FIGLU) in the urine, but this also may occur in vitamin B_{12} deficiency.

Vitamin B_6 (pyridoxine). Thus far, vitamin B_6 has received little attention in relation to its effects on nutritional status. This is unfortunate because dietary surveys have indicated that vitamin B_6 intake may be marginal in some population groups in the United States. Evidence indicates that vitamin B_6 requirements may be increased during pregnancy and in women taking birth control pills. Tests suggested for evaluating vitamin B_6 status include measurement of various B_6 metabolites in the urine, estimation of tryptophan metabolites in the urine after a tryptophan dose, estimation of transaminase in blood cells or plasma, the response to additional pyridoxal phosphate, and estimation of vitamin B_6 in the blood.

Vitamin B_{12}. Vitamin B_{12} deficiency causes anemia, and an inability to utilize the vitamin B_{12} in food is the cause of pernicious anemia. Vitamin B_{12} deficiency due to inadequate intake has been reported in some vegetarians. Reduced blood levels of vitamin B_{12} have been reported in pregnant women and those taking birth control pills. Analytic estimation of vitamin B_{12} is by microbiologic techniques or by radioisotopic methods.

Other water-soluble vitamins. Pantothenic acid, biotin, and choline are the other water-soluble vitamins. These appear to be essential, but they do not seem to present practical nutritional problems in most populations. However, this may be a false assumption, since methods for estimating nutritional status with regard to these nutrients have not been developed and little is known of the probable requirement. Microbiologic or chemical methods for their estimation are available.

Fat-soluble vitamins

The fat-soluble vitamins A, D, E, and K are best absorbed in the presence of some fat in the diet. Thus diseases that interfere with fat absorption may also impair absorption of fat-soluble vitamins. Patients with sprue, gluten enteropathy, and other absorption problems may manifest deficiencies even though the dietary intake appears to be adequate. It should also be noted that vitamins A and D are known to be toxic when consumed in excess, and they could represent a potential problem in the vitamin-conscious society of the United States.

Vitamin A and beta-carotene. Vitamin A does not occur directly in plant foods, but the body converts plant pigment, beta-carotene, into Vitamin A. Both are ordinarily measured in serum to indicate vitamin A adequacy. A low carotene level, of course, only demonstrates limited consumption of green leafy and yellow vegetables, not necessarily vitamin A deficiency.

Surprisingly, substantial numbers of people examined in the Ten State Nutrition Survey had low serum vitamin A levels, indicating some degree of vitamin A deficiency. Autopsies have shown that a significant number of children in Canada and the United States had no vitamin reserves in their livers, the primary site of vitamin A storage. Yet xerophthalmia, caused by severe vitamin A deficiency, is rare in the United States. Thus the significance of the low levels of vitamin A is open to some debate. Night blindness, an early sign of vitamin A deficiency, which may be assessed by dark adaptation

tests, has not yet been adequately investigated.

Vitamin D. Rickets, the childhood deficiency disease resulting from an inadequate vitamin D intake, is relatively rare in the United States but does occur occasionally. Osteomalacia in the elderly, possibly due to a lack of vitamin D, is reported to be relatively common in many countries.

Elevated serum alkaline phosphatase levels were once thought to indicate vitamin D deficiency, but this is not an infallible test. No suitable methods are available to survey populations for this deficiency. Although there is relatively little evidence to indicate that vitamin D deficiency is a general problem, the situation is somewhat uncertain. Since vitamin D may be supplied by synthesis when the body has exposure to sunlight, dietary evaluation is also unsatisfactory.

Vitamin E. Clinical evidence of vitamin E deficiency has only been reported in infants. Deliberate restriction of vitamin E in adults may result in increased red blood cell fragility under certain conditions. Since there is abundant evidence in animals that increased consumption of unsaturated fats increases the need for vitamin E, this vitamin deserves more study than it has received in the past.

Vitamin E may be measured in the serum directly. Methods also exist for estimating the fragility of red cells.

Vitamin K. Since vitamin K is synthesized by the flora in the intestinal tract, deficiency is thought to occur only in very young infants before the flora are established and in diseases in which fat absorption or the utilization of vitamin K is abnormal. There is no evidence that tests for vitamin K function need to be included in general nutrition surveys.

It might be noted that whereas most nutrients—carbohydrate, fat, protein, vitamins, and minerals—are supplied by diet, some portion of human vitamin needs is supplied from synthesis by gastrointestinal microorganisms. Such is the case for vitamins K, B_1, B_{12}, folacin, biotin, and other micronutrients. Thus any pathology of the intestinal tract will reduce availability of these vitamins, as will antibiotic therapy, which modifies intestinal flora.

Minerals

Iron. A deficit of iron eventually results in anemia. The most common method of detecting anemia is by measuring the hemoglobin level in the blood or the hematocrit, but of course, anemia may be caused by a variety of nutritional or nonnutritional factors other than iron deficiency.

Modest degrees of anemia caused by inadequate iron intake are common in the United States, especially in women and children, since iron requirements are increased by growth and menstrual blood loss. The extent of iron deficiency in adult men is a matter of considerable interest and debate. Several different standards have been recommended for the evaluation of hemoglobin and hematocrit, and the extent of anemia observed in any population depends, of course, on the standards used.

Hematocrit. The determination of the hematocrit, or the percentage of packed red cells in whole blood, is a standard clinical procedure available in all community hospitals and other laboratories.

Hemoglobin. Hemoglobin determination is a simple colorimetric procedure that is standard in all clinical laboratories. Ordinarily, both hemoglobin and hematocrit tests are made. They are preferable to blood cell counts, since they involve less laboratory error.

Serum iron and transferrin. Iron is carried in the plasma by a specific protein called transferrin. A reduced saturation of transferrin and a reduced serum iron level provide more specific evidence of iron deficiency and will detect reduced iron stores before anemia develops. If iron levels and transferrin saturation are normal in the face of anemia, the anemia does not represent iron deficiency.

Calcium. Although substantial numbers of people in the United States consume less calcium than ordinarily recommended, there is little or no evidence of calcium deficiency. Blood levels of calcium are essentially constant over a wide range of intakes, and measurement of blood calcium does not provide adequate evaluation of dietary calcium. No suitable laboratory or clinical methods for surveys are available for monitoring the adequacy of calcium intakes.

Iodine. The adequacy of iodine intake is usually estimated by the clinical evaluation of thyroid enlargement or goiters. However, not all goiters are the result of iodine insufficiency. An approximation of iodine intake may be determined by relating urinary iodine to urinary creatinine. Other clinical determinations, for example, of plasma-bound iodine (PBI), reflect the functional utilization of iodine and are standard clinical laboratory tests.

Other minerals. A number of trace minerals are not discussed in detail here, although they are essential. They include magnesium, manganese, zinc, fluoride, chromium, selenium, copper, sodium, potassium, phosphorus, and chloride, among others.

Currently, there is widespread interest and research into the nutritional and metabolic aspects of certain of these trace elements. Clinical evidence of magnesium and zinc deficiencies has been found in hospital populations, and relatively low levels of intake of both these minerals are not uncommon in the United States. However, methodology to evaluate the nutritional status of these and other trace elements has not been standardized, and criteria for adequacy have not been developed.

Lipids and other serum determinations. Circulating levels of cholesterol, triglycerides, glucose, various enzymes, and hormones such as insulin and glucagon, also have significant implications with regard to nutritional status and certain diseases, especially coronary heart disease and diabetes. Measurements of these and other elements have been included in some surveys and should be considered as integral parts of nutrition surveys in the future.

PUBLIC HEALTH SIGNIFICANCE AND THE ROLE OF THE NUTRITIONIST

The methodology and the depth undertaken in completing a nutritional assessment will depend on the amount of manpower

Text continued on p. 241.

Table 8-12. Levels of nutritional assessment for infants and children*

Level of approach†	History		Clinical evaluation	Laboratory evaluation
	Dietary	Medical and socioeconomic		
Birth to 24 months				
Minimal	1. Source of iron 2. Vitamin supplement 3. Milk intake (type and amount)	1. Birth weight 2. Length of gestation 3. Serious or chronic illness 4. Use of medicines	1. Body weight and length 2. Gross defects	1. Hematocrit 2. Hemoglobin

Mid-level	1. Semi-quantitative
	  a. Iron-cereal, meat, egg yolks, supplement
	  b. Energy nutrients
	  c. Micronutrients—calcium, niacin, riboflavin, vitamin C
	  d. Protein
	2. Food intolerances
	3. Baby foods—processed commercially; home cooked
		1. Family history:
		  Diabetes
		  Tuberculosis
		2. Maternal
		  Height
		  Prenatal care
		3. Infant
		  Immunizations
		  Tuberculin test
			1. Head circumference
			2. Skin color, pallor, turgor
			3. Subcutaneous tissue paucity, excess
				1. RBC morphology
				2. Serum iron
				3. Total iron binding capacity
				4. Sickle cell testing

In-depth level	1. Quantitative 24-hour recall 2. Dietary history	1. Prenatal details 2. Complications of delivery 3. Regular health supervision	1. Cranial bossing 2. Epiphyseal enlargement 3. Costochondral beading 4. Ecchymoses	Same as above, plus vitamin and appropriate enzyme assays; protein and amino acids; hydroxyproline, etc., should be available
For ages 2 to 5 years				
	Determine amount of intake	Probe about pica Medications	Add height at all levels Add arm circumference at all levels Add triceps skinfolds at in-depth level	Add serum lead at mid-level Add serum micronutrients (vitamins A, C, folate, etc.) at in-depth level
For ages 6 to 12 years				
	Probe about snack foods Determine whether salt intake is excessive	Ask about medications taken; drug abuse	Add blood pressure at mid-level Add description of changes in tongue, skin, eyes for in-depth level	All of above plus BUN

*From Christakis, G., editor: Nutritional assessment in health programs, Am. J. Public Health 63(suppl.):46, 1973.

†It is understood that what is included at a minimal level would also be included or represented at successively more sophisticated levels of approach. However, it may be entirely appropriate to use a minimal level of approach to clinical evaluations and a maximal approach to laboratory evaluations.

Table 8-13. Levels of nutritional assessment for adolescents*

Levels of approach	History		Clinical evaluation	Laboratory evaluation
	Dietary	Medical and socioeconomic		
Minimal level	1. Frequency of use of food groups 2. Habits-patterns 3. Snacks 4. Socioeconomic status	1. Previous diseases and allergies 2. Abbreviated system review 3. Family history	1. Height 2. Weight	1. Urine, protein and sugar 2. Hemoglobin
Mid-level	1. Above 2. Qualitative estimate 3. 24-hour recall	1. Above in more detail	1. Above 2. Arm circumference 3. Skinfold thickness 4. External appearance	1. Above 2. Blood taken by vein for albumin (serum), serum iron and TIBC; vitamins A and beta carotene; RBC indices; blood urea nitrogen (BUN); cholesterol; zinc
In-depth level	1. Above 2. Quantitative estimate by recall (3-7 days)	1. Above	1. Above 2. Per ICNND Manual 3. X-ray of wrist and bone density	1. Above 2. *Blood tests:* folate and vitamin C; alkaline phosphatase; RBC transketolase; RBC glutathione; lipids 3. *Urine:* creatinine; nitrogen; zinc; thiamine; riboflavin; loading tests (xanthurenic acid/FIGLU) 4. *Hair root:* DNA; protein; zinc; other metals

*From Christakis, G., editor: Nutritional assessment in health programs, Am. J. Public Health **63**(suppl.):55, 1973.

Table 8-14. Levels of maternal nutritional assessment*

| Level of approach | History | | Clinical evaluation | Laboratory evaluation |
	Dietary	Medical and socioeconomic		
Minimal	Present basic diet; meal patterns; fad or abnormal diets; supplements	Obstetrical Age: parity; interval between pregnancies; previous obstetrical history Medical Intercurrent diseases and illnesses; drug use; smoking history Family and social Size of family; "wanted" pregnancy; socioeconomic status	Pre-pregnancy weight; weight gain pattern during pregnancy; signs and symptoms of gross nutritional deficiencies	Hemoglobin; hematocrit
Mid-level	The above, plus semi-quantitative determination of food intake	The above, plus occupational patterns; utilization of maternity care and family planning services	The above, plus screening for intercurrent disease	The above, plus blood smear; RBC indices; serum iron; sickle preparation
In-depth level	The above, plus household survey data; dietary history; quantitative 24-hour recall		The above, plus special anthropometric measurements of skinfold, arm circumference, etc.	The above, plus folate and other vitamin levels

*From Christakis, G., editor: Nutritional assessment in health programs, Am. J. Public Health **63**(suppl.):62, 1973.

Table 8-15. Levels of nutritional assessment for adults*

Level of approach	History — Dietary	History — Medical and socioeconomic	Clinical evaluation	Laboratory evaluation
Minimal	Present food habits Meal patterns "Empty calories" Dietary supplements	Name, age, sex Address Socioeconomic level Number in family Brief medical history (including family)	Height and weight Blood pressure	Hemoglobin A simplified Dipstix evaluation which would identify presence of protein and glucose in blood, urinary pH
Mid-level	Semi-quantitative determination of food intake	Sequential history Present health, past history, review of systems, family history, social history (e.g. Cornell Medical Index) Smoking history	Anthropometric measurements (skinfold thickness, etc.); brief examination by M.D. or physician's assistant; chest x-ray as indicated	Evaluations for serum cholesterol, vitamin A, vitamin C, and folic acid; urine excretion for thiamine
In-depth level	Household survey data Quantitative 24-hour recall Dietary history Diet patterns as they might influence lipogenic characteristics	All of above; personal interview by physician; family history of cardiovascular disease	Comprehensive health status evaluation by an appropriate health team, by or under supervision of a physician	Serum triglyceride level, plus those nutrients in mid-level; urine or serum evaluation of pyridoxine status (vitamin B_6 nutriture); evaluation of protein nutriture by height, weight, and chronological age indices; serum essentials and nonessential amino acid ratios; evaluation of vitamin B_{12} nutriture by serum analysis; serum iron and serum iron binding capacity; adipose tissue aspiration and fatty acid analysis by gas-liquid chromatography

*From Christakis, G., editor: Nutritional assessment in health programs, Am. J. Public Health **63**(suppl.):65, 1973.

and the monies available. To assist the field worker (the nutritionist and other personnel) in completing various levels of nutritional assessment on specific age groups, Christakis has developed a scheme that includes the minimal, mid-level and in-depth level approaches. These levels of approaches have been designed for infants and children, birth to 24 months of age, 2 to 5 years, and 6 to 12 years; for adolescents; for pregnant women; for adults, and for the elderly. Tables 8-12 to 8-16 depict the Christakis scheme for methods of assessment on the three levels as dietary, medical and socioeconomic, clinical evaluation, and laboratory evaluation.

At the mid-level and in-depth approach for adults and the elderly, the cholesterol and triglyceride evaluations are recommended as an important index for determining the risk of coronary heart disease.

The National Heart and Lung Institute is sponsoring Lipid Research Centers and Centers for Multiple Risk Factor Intervention Trials for the prevention of coronary heart disease. This illustrates the present and future public health significance of the use of serum cholesterol and triglyceride determinations in the screening of persons with elevated levels of lipids, who may be at high risk of developing coronary heart disease. Moreover, physicians who are involved in the evaluation of intervention programs are using serum cholesterol and triglyceride levels to assess response to diets designed to lower these lipid factors. The current interest in serum lipids has been generated primarily by three considerations: (1) the identification by the Framingham Study and other studies of serum cholesterol level as a risk factor in coronary heart disease (along with hypertension, smoking, obesity, and other factors)[34]; (2) the indication of prospective studies (such as one by the Anti-Coronary Club of the City of New York Department of Health) that the lowering of serum cholesterol by nutritional means has been attended by reduced coronary heart disease morbidity and mortality[35]; and (3) the emergence of hyperlipidemia (a condition in which

both genetic and environmental factors collaborate to raise serum lipids) as having possible public health significance.[36]

Lane and White[37] indicate that nutritionists are increasing their roles in screening programs such as WIC and EPSDT. However, it must be remembered that screening is not the same as case finding, surveying, or diagnosing. The authors indicate that nutritionists, more than other types of medical and public health professionals, tend to be sympathetic to the concept of multifactored disease causations and thus should be perfectly at home with the concept of degrees of risk rather than presence or absence of disease. It also indicates that nutritionists, whose status in many health departments until now has been low, should be eager to develop programs in which other people do the screening for them, leaving them more time for intervention programs. This is exactly what happens when nutritionists work with screening programs that are funded by federal agencies such as Social Security and Agriculture and staffed by nurses from county health departments. These nutritionists are in a perfect

STATISTICAL GUIDANCE

If statistically sound sampling procedures based on probability are not followed, the significance of survey results will at best be uncertain, and possibly biased and incorrect.

By contrast, with correct sampling, investigations can provide accurate information on an examination on only a portion of the population, with a consequent saving of time, money and staff and with less disruption of the local community.

T. D. Woolsey, W. G. Cochran, D. Mainland, M. P. Martin, F. E. Moore, and *R. E. Patton:* On the use of sampling in the field of public health, Am. J. Public Health **44**:719, 1954.

However, sampling problems are far from simple and usually require the specialized skill of the statistician. Some understanding by the nutritionist of statistical principles is valuable in order to bridge the gap between the two technical fields of knowledge.

D. B. Jelliffe: The assessment of the nutritional status of the community, Geneva, 1966, World Health Organization, p. 142.

Table 8-16. Levels of nutritional assessment for the elderly*

Levels of approach	History		Clinical evaluation	Laboratory evaluation
	Dietary	Medical and socioeconomic		
Minimal	1. Meals eaten per day, week; regularity 2. Frequency of ingestion of protective foods (four food groups) 3. Supplemental vitamins, protein concentrates, mineral mixes 4. General knowledge of nutrition, sources of information	1. Chronic illness and/or disability; occupational hazard exposure; use of tobacco, alcohol, drugs 2. Symptoms such as bleeding, fainting, loss of memory, dyspnea, headache, pain, changed bowel and/or bladder habits, altered sight and/or hearing, condition of teeth, and/or dentures 3. Therapy (prescribed or self-administered) such as drugs, alcohol, vitamins, food fads, prescription items, eyeglasses, hearing aids 4. Names, addresses, and phone numbers of persons providing medical or health care; close family or friends 5. Lives alone, with spouse, or companion 6. Sources of income	1. Height and weight; cachexia; obesity 2. Blood pressure, pulse rate and rhythm 3. Pallor, skin color and texture 4. Condition of teeth and/or dentures and oral hygiene 5. Affect during interview and examination 6. Vision and hearing appraised subjectively and objectively by examiner 7. Any gross evidence of neglect	1. Hemoglobin 2. Blood and/or urine sugar 3. Urinalysis (color, odor, bile and sediment by gross inspection; pH, glucose, albumin blood, and ketones by stick test) 4. Feces (color, texture, gross blood; occult blood by guaiac test)
Mid-level†	In addition to the above: 1. Food preferences and rejections 2. Overt food fads 3. Meal preparation facilities and knowledge 4. Food budget 5. Usual daily diet: *Protective foods* (meats, dairy products, fruits and vegetables, cereals); *nutrients* (protein, fat, carbohydrates, iron, water and fat-soluble vitamins, minerals, trace elements, and	In addition to the above: 1. Family history of spouse, parents and siblings, other relatives, persons living in same household 2. Pain: location, frequency, character, duration 3. Mental hygiene: attitudes, fears, prejudices, symptoms of psychoses, symptoms of psychosomatic symptoms and signs 4. Income: amount and adequacy for nutrition, housing, health, utilities, clothing, transportation, etc.	In addition include: 1. Head and neck examinations (otoscopic, ophthalmoscopic, dental and oral cavity, nose and throat) 2. Chest (inspection, palpation, auscultation and percussion, bi-manual examination of breast tissue) 3. Abdomen (inspection, auscultation, percussion, and palpation) 4. Rectal and pelvic 5. Inspection and palpation of extremities (evaluation for temperature, edema, pulse, discoloration, ulcers) 6. Gross neurological evaluation; motor and sensory	In addition include: 1. Serum lipids (including B-lipoproteins) 2. Serum iron and iron binding capacity 3. Urinalysis 4. Electrocardiogram 5. Peripheral blood smear for differential white blood cell count and red cell morphology 6. Chest film 7. Post-voiding residual urine by catheterization (if indicated)

In-depth†

water); *empty calorie food* (alcohol, candy, sucrose)

In addition include:

1. 24-hour dietary recall, preferably for each of several widely separated days; analysis of nutrient intake; evaluation of adequacy e.g. relate to activity, body weight, laboratory data, affect, etc.
2. History of past and present food preparation and practices
3. History of dining practices and facilities, including companionship

In addition include:

1. System review
2. Social history
3. Economic history including specifics on sources and amounts of income
4. Mental evaluation (attitudes toward aging)

If indicated, include:

1. Complete sensory and motor neurologic examination
2. Sigmoidoscopy
3. Ophthalmologic examination (ophthalmoscopic examination with pupils dilated, refraction, dark adaptation, color perception, visual field examination)
4. Audiometry

If indicated, include:

1. Serum total protein and albumin; serum creatinine and/or blood urea nitrogen (BUN)
2. Roentgenographic evaluation of bones and joints suspected of being fractured, harboring infection and affected by rheumatic and/or metabolic bone disease and/or metastatic or primary neoplastic disease
3. Glucose tolerance tests
4. Blood and/or urine vitamin assays for water-soluble and fat-soluble vitamins
5. Trace element assays of blood, urine, and/or tissue
6. Kidney-ureter-bladder (KUB) film for stones in urinary tract or gall bladder
7. Bacteriologic cultures of any chronic infections
8. Barium enema, upper gastrointestinal series, gall bladder series and intravenous pyelography
9. Fluoroscopy of chest
10. Angiography for coronary arteries, aorta, peripheral vessels
11. Bone marrow for unexplained anemia
12. Renal clearance studies
13. Histologic evaluation of biopsies of tissue suspected of being neoplastic

*From Christakis, G., editor: Nutritional assessment in health programs, Am. J. Public Health **63**(suppl.):74, 1973.
†The aged, quite unlike children and youth, are the end result of lifetimes of physiologic aging, diseases, and disabilities and cannot be evaluated as if they belonged to younger cohorts. In the above table, it is assumed that Mid-level evaluation procedures may be carried out in ambulatory care settings and that In-depth level procedures may be conducted as hospital or research procedures. The placement of these in actual practice will depend on availability of facilities and personnel.

position to identify persons who are at high nutritional risk and to put them under appropriate supervision. Nutritionists can help in developing the screening package and should encourage the use of simple accurate tests, keeping in mind the reliability, reproducibility, sensitivity, and specificity of the screening tests. It goes without saying that screening by income criteria alone is not an efficient way of discovering nutritional risk.

SUMMARY

The surveillance aspect of a nutritional assessment is vital if one wishes to keep track of a population over a period of time. This enables the nutritionist to make projections about the prevalence of nutritional risk, to plan a rational program, and also to see if existing programs are effective. Surveillance is especially useful on the community level among high-risk population groups. Here, a community diagnosis or profile can be put together using information that considers a number of factors—demographic statistics, cultural and economic data, food supply, transportation facilities, local health records, environmental data, food programs, and many others. These data can be combined to give a detailed portrait of a particular locale. However, as with every level on which nutritional assessment can occur, if the gathering of data becomes the main objective and focus of energy, the true purpose of alleviating nutrition problems is lost.

The role of the nutritionist is vital. Perhaps the most important thing for the nutritionist to understand is that much of what is necessary for the development of a nutrition surveillance system already exists in almost every state. Children are being screened. Referrals are being made. Systems of data management are being created. These data are significant. It is data gathering for the purpose of decision making that enables evaluation and the measurement of outcomes in public health programs that are designed to meet the public needs, which is the subject of the next chapter.

REFERENCES

1. Christakis, G., editor: Nutritional assessment in health programs, Am. J. Public Health **63**(suppl.): 1, 1973.
2. Hollingshead, A. B.: Two factor index of social position, New Haven, Conn., 1957, Yale University Press.
3. Orshansky, M.: The shape of poverty in 1966, Soc. Security Bull. March, 1968.
4. Harrison, G. G., Rathye, W. L., and Hughes, W. W.: Food waste behavior in an urban population, J. Nutr. Educ. **47**:13, 1975.
5. Watt, B. K., and Merrill, A. L.: Composition of foods: raw, processed, prepared, Agriculture Handbook no. 8, rev. ed., Washington, D.C., Dec., 1963, Government Printing Office.
6. U.S. Department of Agriculture: Nutritive value of American foods in common units, Agriculture Handbook no. 456, Washington, D.C., Nov., 1975, Government Printing Office.
7. Church, C. F., and Church, H. N.: Food values of portions commonly used, ed. 12, New York, 1975, J. B. Lippincott Co.
8. Arizona Department of Health Services, Bureau of Nutrition Service, Nutrition Delivery System, Phoenix, Arizona, 1976.
9. Sandstead, H. H., Carter, J. P., and Darby, W. J.: How to diagnose nutritional deficiences in daily practice, Nutr. Today **4**:20, Summer, 1969.
10. Zerfas, A. J., Shorr, I. J., Neumann, C. G.: Office assessment of nutritional status, Pediatr. Clin. North Am. **2**:253, 1977.
11. Falkner, F.: Office measurement of physical growth, Pediatr. Clin. North Am. **8**:13, 1961.
12. Beaton, G. H., and Bengoa, J. M.: Practical population indicators of health and nutrition. In Nutrition and preventive medicine, WHO Report, Geneva, 1973, World Health Organization.
13. Fomon, S. J.: Infant nutrition, ed. 2, Philadelphia, 1974, W. B. Saunders Co.
14. Johnson, M. L., Buche, V. V., and Meyer, J.: The prevalence and incidence of obesity in a cross section of elementary and secondary school children, Am. J. Clin. Nutr. **4**:231, 1956.
15. Tanner, J. M.: The measurement of body fat in man, Proc. Nutr. **18**:148, 1959.
16. American Academy of Pediatrics, Committee on

Nutrition: Measurement of skinfold thickness in childhood, Pediatrics **42:**538, 1968.

17. Owen, G. M.: The assessment and recording of measurements of growth of children: report of a small conference, Pediatrics **51:**461, 1973.

18. Seltzer, C. C., and Mayer, J.: Greater reliability of the triceps skinfolds over the subscapular skinfold as an index of obesity, Am. J. Clin. Nutr. **20:**950, 1967.

19. U.S. Department of Health, Education, and Welfare, Center for Disease Control: Nutrition surveillance sources of error in weighing and measuring children, Washington, D.C., Sept., 1975, Government Printing Office.

20. Kanawati, A.: Assessment of nutritional status in the community. In McLaren, D. J., editor: Nutrition in the community, New York, 1976, John Wiley & Sons, Inc.

21. Roberts, L. J.: Nutrition work in children, Chicago, 1935, The University of Chicago Press.

22. Woodbury, R. M.: Statures and weights of children under six years of age, Washington, D.C., 1921, U.S. Department of Labor, Children's Bureau, Community Child Welfare Service no. 3, publication no. 37, Government Printing Office.

23. Hamill, P. V. V., and Moore, W. H.: Contemporary growth charts: needs, construction and application, Public Health Currents, special source, 1976.

24. Owen, G. M.: The new NCHS growth charts, South. Med. J. **71:**296, 1978.

25. Reed, R. B., and Stuart, H. C.: Patterns of growth in height and weight from birth to 18 years of age, Pediatrics **24:**904, 1959.

26. Jackson, R. L., and Kelly, H. C.: Growth charts for use in pediatric practice, J. Pediatrics **27:**215, 1945.

27. Meredith, H. V.: Change in stature and body weight of North American boys during the last 80 years. In Lepeitt, L., and Spiker, C., editors: Advances in child development and behavior, Vol. 1, New York, 1963, Academic Press, Inc.

28. Marech, M. M.: A forty-five year investigation for secular changes in physical maturation, Am. J. Physical Anthropol. **36:**1, 1972.

29. Owen, G. M., Kram, K. M., Garry, P. J., et al.: Nutritional status of Mississippi preschool children: a pilot study, Am. J. Clin. Nutr. **22:**1444, 1969.

30. Larkin, F. A., Perri, K. P., Bursick, J. H., and Roka, J. M. K.: Etiology of growth failure in a clinic population, J. Am. Diet. Assoc. **69:**506, 1976.

31. Winberg, J., Solomon, I. L., and Shoen, E. J.: Parent-specific-height standards for preadolescent children of three racial groups with method for rapid determination, Pediatrics **52:**555, 1973.

32. Jelliffe, D. B.: The assessment of the nutritional status of the community, Geneva, 1966, World Health Organization.

33. Fomon, S. J.: Nutritional disorders of children: prevention, screening and follow up, Washington, D.C., 1976, HEW publication no. (HSA) 76-5612, Government Printing Office.

34. Dawber, T. R.: Some factors associated with the development of coronary heart disease: six year follow up, Am. J. Public Health **49:**1349, 1959.

35. Christakis, G., Rinzler, S. H., Archer, M., and Kraus, A.: Effect of the Anti-Coronary Club Program on coronary heart disease risk-factor status, J.A.M.A. **198:**597, 1966.

36. Lees, R. S., and Wilson, D. E.: The treatment of hyperlipidemia, N. Engl. J. Med. **284:**186, 1971.

37. Lane, J. M., and White, M.: Personal communication, 1977.

Appendix 8-1

NEW 24-HOUR DIETARY EVALUATION METHOD*

Purpose

1. For the use of nutrition aides, nurses, nutritionists, physicians, and other allied health personnel in evaluating a person's dietary intake.
2. For data collection to determine the adequacy of dietary intake in a population before and after participation in the nutrition delivery system.

Basic knowledge necessary

1. Knowledge of standard measuring units per definition.
2. Nutrient content of food groups and exceptional foods.
3. Dietary interview skills.
4. Basic arithmetic.

Procedure

1. Obtain a 24-hour recall.
2. Categorize each food item by the number of standard measuring units (SMU) into the appropriate food group (18 groups total).
3. Circle foods high in vitamin A if the foods fall in a group that is not a good source of vitamin A. For example, liver is a good source of vitamin A, but other organ meats and shellfish are not.
4. Total the number of SMUs from each food group.
5. Determine the number of SMUs of each nutrient group.
6. Compare the total SMUs from each nutrient group to the risk cutoffs set for the individual.
7. Star those nutrients at risk.
8. For counseling purposes, ask how usual this day was. Also ask about favorite foods, never-eaten foods, etc. Record this information in "Comments" section.

New 24-hour recall—how derived

1. Eighteen food groups based on the nutrients contained in each.

*Arizona State Department of Health, Bureau of Nutrition Services, Nutrition Delivery System.

a. Meat, fish and poultry, organ meat and shellfish, and eggs separated into four groups because of differences in fat and cholesterol content.
b. Beans separated from nuts and peanut butter—no iron or calcium in peanut butter or nuts, and no fat in beans.
c. Milk separated from skim milk—to enable an evaluation of fat and cholesterol intake.
d. Cottage cheese separated from natural cheeses because it is lower in calcium.
e. Leafy greens separated from deep yellow—leafy greens contain iron, calcium, and vitamin C in addition to vitamin A.
f. Other fruits and vegetables—catchall category providing roughage; dried fruits—iron, sometimes vitamin A.
g. Animal fat separated from vegetable fat to enable better evaluation of cholesterol intake. Vegetable fat is not labeled "empty calories" because of essential nature of linoleic acid.
h. Snacks and sweets—a general category to enable an evaluation of frequency of consumption.
i. Alcohol—to enable an evaluation of frequency of intake.

2. Risk indicator standards.
   a. Eight following nutrients are evaluated:

Protein	Vitamin A
Iron	Vitamin C
Cholesterol	Empty calories
Calcium	Fat

   b. Risk indicator standards based on measuring units necessary to meet 1973 RDA for various age groups. Age groups included are as follows:
   Infants
   1-10 years
   11-18 years
   Adults
   Pregnant or lactating women
   c. Where age or sex made a significant difference in nutrient needs, different risk indicator standards were set.
3. Nutrients selected for evaluation.

a. Protein. Standard measuring unit defined as a food containing 7 to 8 grams protein per SMU based on diabetic exchange list.

b. Iron. Standard measuring unit defined as any food containing about 2 mg iron per serving.

c. Vitamin A. Standard measuring unit defined as one serving of deep yellow vegetables (3,500 IU) or one serving of leafy greens (7,900 IU). If intake is inadequate, evaluator reviews dietary recall for circled foods (unique food sources of vitamin A, i.e., liver, butter, etc.)

d. Citrus and others. Standard measuring unit defined as any food that supplies 50 mg vitamin C per serving.

e. Cholesterol. Two forms are defined as follows:

   (1) Ch_1. Standard measuring unit is defined as any food that contains an excess of 200 mg cholesterol per SMU.

   (2) Ch_2. Standard measuring unit defined as any food which contains an excess of 25 mg cholesterol per SMU.

f. Calcium. Two forms are defined as follows:

   (1) Ca_1. Standard measuring unit is defined as any food containing about 250 mg calcium per SMU (dairy products).

   (2) Ca_2. Standard measuring unit is defined as any food containing about 100 mg calcium per SMU (beans, leafy greens). Translate Ca_2 foods to Ca_1 foods before evaluating risk ($2\frac{1}{2}$ Ca_2 = 1 Ca_1).

g. Empty calories. Standard serving size is not defined. Evaluator is interested in the frequency of intake.

h. Fat. Two forms are recognized as follows: (1) animal and (2) vegetable. For both, standard measuring unit is defined as containing an average of 7 grams fat per serving.

Appendix 8-2

TABLE OF CURRENT GUIDELINES FOR CRITERIA OF NUTRITIONAL STATUS FOR LABORATORY EVALUATION*

Nutrient and units	Age of subject (years)	Criteria of status		
		Deficient	Marginal	Acceptable
†Hemoglobin	6-23 mo.	Up to 9.0	9.0- 9.9	10.0+
(gm/dl)	2-5	Up to 10.0	10.0-10.9	11.0+
	6-12	Up to 10.0	10.0-11.4	11.5+
	13-16M	Up to 12.0	12.0-12.9	13.0+
	13-16F	Up to 10.0	10.0-11.4	11.5+
	16+M	Up to 12.0	12.0-13.9	14.0+
	16+F	Up to 10.0	10.0-11.9	12.0+
	Pregnant (after 6+ mo.)	Up to 9.5	9.5-10.9	11.0+
†Hematocrit	Up to 2	Up to 28	28-30	31+
(packed cell volume	2-5	Up to 30	30-33	34+
in percent)	6-12	Up to 30	30-35	36+
	13-16M	Up to 37	37-39	40+
	13-16F	Up to 31	31-35	36+
	16+M	Up to 37	37-43	44+
	16+F	Up to 31	31-37	33+
	Pregnant	Up to 30	30-32	33+
†Serum albumin	Up to 1	—	Up to 2.5	2.5+
(gm/dl)	1-5	—	Up to 3.0	3.0+
	6-16	—	Up to 3.5	3.5+
	16+	Up to 2.8	2.8-3.4	3.5+
	Pregnant	Up to 3.0	3.0-3.4	3.5+
†Serum protein	Up to 1	—	Up to 5.0	5.0+
(gm/dl)	1-5	—	Up to 5.5	5.5+
	6-16	—	Up to 6.0	6.0+
	16+	Up to 6.0	6.0-6.4	6.5+
	Pregnant	Up to 5.5	5.5-5.9	6.0+
†Serum ascorbic acid (mg/dl)	All ages	Up to 0.1	0.1-0.19	0.2+
†Plasma vitamin A (mcg/dl)	All ages	Up to 10	10-19	20+
†Plasma carotene	All ages	Up to 20	20-39	40+
(mcg/dl)	Pregnant	—	40-79	80+
†Serum iron	Up to 2	Up to 30	—	30+
(mcg/dl)	2-5	Up to 40	—	40+
	6-12	Up to 50	—	50+
	12+M	Up to 60	—	60+
	12+F	Up to 40	—	40+

*From Christakis, G., editor: Nutritional assessment in health programs, Am. J. Public Health **63**(suppl.):1-82, 1973.
†Adapted from the Ten State Nutrition Survey.
‡Criteria may vary with different methodology.
§Erythrocyte glutamic oxalacetic transaminase.
‖Erythrocyte glutamic pyruvic transaminase.

TABLE OF CURRENT GUIDELINES FOR CRITERIA OF NUTRITIONAL STATUS FOR LABORATORY EVALUATION—cont'd

Nutrient and units	Age of subject (years)	Criteria of status		
		Deficient	Marginal	Acceptable
†Transferrin saturation (%)	Up to 2	Up to 15.0	—	15.0+
	2-12	Up to 20.0	—	20.0+
	12+M	Up to 20.0	—	20.0+
	12+F	Up to 15.0	—	15.0+
‡Serum folacin (ng/ml)	All ages	Up to 2.0	2.1-5.9	6.0+
‡Serum vitamin B$_{12}$ (pg/ml)	All ages	Up to 100	—	100+
†Thiamine in urine (mcg/gm creatinine)	1-3	Up to 120	120-175	175+
	4-5	Up to 85	85-120	120+
	6-9	Up to 70	70-180	180+
	10-15	Up to 55	55-150	150+
	16+	Up to 27	27- 65	65+
	Pregnant	Up to 21	21- 49	50+
†Riboflavin in urine (mcg/gm creatinine)	1-3	Up to 150	150-499	500+
	4-5	Up to 100	100-299	300+
	6-9	Up to 85	85-269	270+
	10-16	Up to 70	70-199	200+
	16+	Up to 27	27- 79	80+
	Pregnant	Up to 30	30- 89	90+
‡RBC transketolase-TPP-effect (ratio)	All ages	25+	15- 25	Up to 15
‡RBC glutathione reductase-FAD-effect (ratio)	All ages	1.2+	—	Up to 1.2
‡Tryptophan load (mg xanthurenic acid excreted)	Adults (Dose: 100 mg/kg body weight)	25+(6 hrs.) 75+(24 hrs.)	— —	Up to 25 Up to 75
‡Urinary pyridoxine (mcg/gm creatinine)	1-3	Up to 90	—	90+
	4-6	Up to 80	—	80+
	7-9	Up to 60	—	60+
	10-12	Up to 40	—	40+
	13-15	Up to 30	—	30+
	16+	Up to 20	—	20+
†Urinary N-methyl nicotinamide (mg/gm creatinine)	All ages	Up to 0.2	0.2-5.59	0.6+
	Pregnant	Up to 0.8	0.8-2.49	2.5+
‡Urinary pantothenic acid (mcg)	All ages	Up to 200	—	200+
‡Plasma vitamin E (mg/dl)	All ages	Up to 0.2	0.2-0.6	0.6+
‡Transaminase index (ratio)				
§EGOT	Adult	2.0 +	—	Up to 2.0
‖EGPT	Adult	1.25+	—	Up to 1.25

Appendix 8-3

SELECTED REFERENCES FOR DIETARY ASSESSMENT

Abramson, J. H., Slome, C., and Kosovsky, C.: Food frequency interview as an epidemiological tool, Am. J. Public Health **53**:1093, 1963.

Balogh, M., Kahn, H. A., and Medalie, J. H.: Random repeat 24-hour dietary recalls, Am. J. Clin. Nutr. **24**:304, 1971.

Beal, V. A.: The nutritional history in longitudinal research, J. Am. Diet. Assoc. **51**:426, 1967.

Burke, B. S.: The dietary history as a tool in research, J. Am. Diet. Assoc. **23**:1041, 1947.

Hankin, J. H., Reynolds, W. E., and Margen, S.: A short dietary method for epidemiologic studies. II, Am. J. Clin. Nutr. **20**:935, 1967.

Marjonnier, L., and Hall, Y.: The national diet heart study—assessment of dietary adherence, J. Am. Diet. Assoc. **52**:288, 1968.

Marr, J. W.: Individual dietary surveys: purposes and methods, World Rev. Nutr. Diet. **13**:105, 1971.

Pekkarinen, M.: Methodology in the collection of food consumption data, World Rev. Nutr. Diet. **12**:145, 1970.

Reshef, A., and Epstein, L. M.: Reliability of a dietary questionnaire, Am. J. Clin. Nutr. **25**:91, 1972.

Stefanik, P. A., and Trulson, M. F.: Determining the frequency intakes of foods in large group studies, Am. J. Clin. Nutr. **11**:335, 1962.

Taylor, E. C.: The impact of computer analyses on the design of dietary surveys, Proc. Nutr. Soc. **29**:135, 1970.

Wiehl, D. G., and Reed, R.: Development of new or improved dietary methods for epidemiological investigations, Am. J. Public Health **50**:824, 1960.

Young, C. M., Hanan, G. C., Tucker, R. E., and Foster, W. D.: A comparison of dietary study methods. II. Dietary history vs. seven-day record vs. 24-hour recall, J. Am. Diet. Assoc. **28**:218, 1952.

Young, C. M., and Musgrave, K.: Dietary study methods. II. Uses of dietary score cards, J. Am. Diet. Assoc. **27**:745, 1951.

Young, C. M., and Trulson, M. F.: Methodology for dietary studies in epidemiological surveys. II. Strengths and weaknesses of existing methods, Am. J. Public Health **50**:803, 1960.

SELECTED REFERENCES FOR NUTRITIONAL LABORATORY ASSESSMENT*

General references for clinical chemistry and nutrients

Abraham, S., Lowenstein, F. W., and Johnson, C. L.: Preliminary findings of the first health and nutrition examination survey, United States, 1971-1972: Dietary intake and biochemical findings, National Center for Health Statistics, Washington, D.C., 1974, HEW publication no. (HRA) 74-1219-1, Government Printing Office.

California Department of Health, Maternal and Child Health Unit: Nutrition during pregnancy and lactation: a supplement to standards and recommendations for public prenatal care, Sacramento, Calif., rev. ed., 1975, California State Department of Public Health.

Carr, J. J., and Drekter, I. J.: Simplified rapid technic for the extraction and determination of serum cholesterol without saponification, Clin. Chem. **2**:353, 1956.

Fredrickson, D. S., and Levy, R. I.: Familial hyperlipoproteinemia. In Stanbury, J. B., Wyngaarden, J. B., and Fredrickson, D. S.: The metabolic basis of inherited disease, New York, 1972, McGraw-Hill Book Co.

György, P., and Pearson, W. M., editors: The vitamins, 7 vols., 1967-1973, Academic Press, Inc.

Horwitz, W., editor: Official methods of analysis of the Association of Official Analytical Chemists, ed. 11, Washington, D.C., 1970, Association of Official Analytical Chemists.

Laboratory Methods Committee, Lipid Research Clinics Program: Manual of laboratory operations, vol. I, Bethesda, Md., 1974, HEW publication no. (NIH) 75-628, National Heart and Lung Institute.

---

*From Christakis, G., editor: Nutritional assessment in health programs, Am. J. Public Health **63**(suppl.):1-82, 1973.

Levine, J. B., and Zak, B.: Automated determination of serum total cholesterol, Clin. Chim. Acta **10**:381, 1964.

Natelson, S.: Techniques of clinical chemistry, ed. 3, Springfield, Ill., 1971, Charles C Thomas, Publisher.

O'Brien, D., Ibbott, F. A., and Rodgerson, D.O.: Laboratory manual of pediatric micro-biochemical techniques, ed. 4, New York, 1968, Harper & Row, Publishers.

Tietz, N. W., editor: Fundamentals of clinical chemistry, ed. 2, Philadelphia, 1976, London, Toronto, W. B. Saunders Co.

References for individual nutrients

Protein

*Electrophoretic separation of serum proteins. In Interdepartmental Committee on Nutrition for National Defense: Manual for nutrition surveys, ed. 2, Washington, D.C., 1963, Government Printing Office, p. 147.

Failing, J. F., Jr., Buckley, M. W., and Zak, B.: A study on an ultramicro and automated procedure for serum proteins, Am. J. Med. Technol. **27**:177, 1961.

Oberman, et al.: Electrophoretic analysis of serum proteins in infants and children, N. Engl. J. Med. **225**:743, 1956.

*Total serum protein, albumin and globulin by a modified biuret technique. In Interdepartmental Committee on Nutrition for National Defense: Manual for nutrition surveys, ed. 2, Washington, D.C., 1963, Government Printing Office, p. 133.

Hematocrit

Macro. In Interdepartmental Committee on Nutrition for National Defense: Manual for nutrition surveys, ed. 2, Washington, D.C., 1963, Government Printing Office, p. 116.

Micro. In Todd, J. C., and Sanford, A. H., editors: Clinical diagnosis by laboratory methods, ed. 14, Philadelphia, 1969, W. B. Saunders Co.

Hemoglobin

*Interdepartmental Committee on Nutrition Defense: Manual for nutrition surveys, ed. 2, Washington, D.C., 1963, Government Printing Office, p. 115.

Iron

Fischer, D. S., and Price, D. C.: A simple serum iron method using the new sensitive chromogen tripyridyl-s-triazine, Clin. Chem. **10**:21, 1964.

Garry, P. J., and Owen, G. M.: Automated micro determination (100 μl) of serum iron and total iron binding capacity. Technicon Symposium, Automation in Analytical Chemistry, Vol. I, New York, 1968, Mediad, Inc.

Piomelli, S., Brickman, A., and Carlos, E.: Rapid diagnosis of iron deficiency by measurement of free erythrocyte protoporphyrin and hemoglobin: the FEP/hemoglobin ratio, Pediatrics **57**:136, 1976.

Ramsey, W. N. M.: The determination of the total iron binding capacity of serum, Clin. Chim. Acta. **2**:221, 1957.

Scarlata, R. W., and Moore, E. W.: A micromethod for the determination of serum iron and serum iron-binding capacity, Clin. Chem. **8**:360, 1962.

Woodruff, C. W.: A micromethod for serum iron determination, J. Lab. Clin. Med. **53**:955, 1959.

Ascorbic acid

Cheraskin, E., et al.: A lingual vitamin C test, Int. Z. Vitaminforsch. **38**:114, 1968.

Garry, P. J., Owen, G. M., Lashley, D. W., and Ford, P. C.: Automated analysis of plasma and whole blood ascorbic acid, Clin. Biochem. **7**:131, 1974.

*Serum vitamin C (ascorbic acid)—dinitrophenylhyrrazine method. In Interdepartmental Committee on Nutrition for National Defense: Manual for nutrition surveys, ed. 2, Washington, D.C., 1963, Government Printing Office, p. 117.

*Serum vitamin C—micro procedure. In Interdepartmental Committee on Nutrition for National Defense: Manual for nutrition surveys, ed. 2, Washington, D.C., 1963, Government Printing Office, p. 119.

Pyridoxine

Baker, H., and Frank, O.: Vitamin B$_6$. In Baker, H., and Frank, O., editors: Clinical vitaminology: methods and interpretation, New York, 1968, Interscience Publications, Inc.

Brin, M.: A simplified Toepfer-Lehmann assay for the three vitamin B$_6$ Vitamers, Methods Enzymol. **18**:519, 1970.

Hamfelt, A.: Age variation of vitamin B$_6$ metabolism in man, Clin. Chim. Acta **10**:48, 1964.

Luhby, A. L., Brin, M., Gordon, M., Davis, P., Murphy, M., and Spiegel, H.: Vitamin B$_6$ metabolism in users of oral contraceptive agents. I. Abnormal urinary xanthurenic acid excretion and its correction by pyridoxine, Am. J. Clin. Nutr. **24**:684, 1971.

Price, S. A., et al.: Effects of dietary vitamin B$_6$ deficiency and oral contraceptives on the spontaneous urinary excretion of 3-hydroxy anthranilic acid, Am. J. Clin. Nutr. **25**:494, 1972.

Sauberlich, H. E., et al.: Biochemical assessment of the nutritional status of vitamin B_6 in the human, Am. J. Clin. Nutr. **25**:629, 1972.

Tryptophan load test—xanthurenic acid in serum, Manual for Nutrition Surveys, ICNND, ed. 1, Washington, D.C., 1963, Government Printing Office, p. 88. (NOTE: The test is now modified to give a load of 2 gm l-tryptophan. Approximately 67% of the xanthurenic acid is excreted in the first 8 hours.)

Folacin

Jukes, T. H.: Assay of compounds with folic acid activity, Methods Biochem. Anal. **2**:121, 1955.

Luhby, A. L., and Cooperman, J. M.: Folic acid deficiency and its inter-relationship with vitamin B_{12} metabolism, Adv. Metab. Disord. **1**:263, 1964.

Vitamin B_{12}

Baker, H., and Frank, O.: Vitamin B_{12}. In Baker, H., and Frank, O., editors: Clinical vitaminology: methods and interpretation, New York, 1968, Interscience Publications, Inc.

Lau, K. S., Gottlieb, C., Wasserman, L. R., and Herbert, V.: Measurement of serum vitamin B_{12} level using radioisotope dilution and coated charcoal, Blood **26**:202, 1965.

Skeggs, H. R.: Microbiological assay for vitamin B_{12}, Methods Biochem. Anal. **14**:53, 1966.

Thiamin

Baker, H., and Frank, O.: Thiamine. In Baker, H., and Frank, O., editors: Clinical vitaminology: methods and interpretation, New York, 1968, Interscience Publications, Inc.

Brin, M.: Transketolase and the TPP-effect in assessing thiamine adequacy. In Vitamins and coenzymes: methods in enzymology, Vol. 18, New York, 1970, Academic Press, Inc.

Brin, M.: Erythrocyte transketolase activity. In Bergmeyer, H. U., editor: Methods of enzymatic analysis, ed. 2, New York, 1974, Academic Press, Inc.

*Creatinine in urine, picrate method. ibid. In Interdepartmental Committee on Nutrition for National Defense: Manual for nutrition surveys, ed. 2, Washington, D.C., 1963, Government Printing Office, p. 135.

Dreyfus, P.: Clinical application of blood transketolase determinations, N. Engl. J. Med. **267**:596, 1962.

*Thiamine in urine. In Interdepartmental Committee on Nutrition for National Defense: Manual for nutrition surveys, ed. 2, Washington, D.C., 1963, Government Printing Office, p. 136.

Riboflavin

Baker, H., and Frank, O.: Riboflavin. In Baker, H., and Frank, O., editors: Clinical vitaminology: methods and interpretation, New York, 1968, Interscience Publications, Inc.

Bamji, M. S.: Glutathione reductase activity in red blood cells and riboflavin nutritional status in humans, Clin. Chim. Acta **26**:263, 1969.

*Creatinine in urine—picrate method. In Interdepartmental Committee on Nutrition for National Defense: Manual for nutrition surveys, ed. 2, Washington, D.C., 1963, Government Printing Office, p. 135.

Glatzle, D., et al.: Method for the detection of a biochemical riboflavin deficiency: investigations of the vitamin B_2 status in healthy people and geriatric patients, Int. Z. Vitaminforsch. **40**:166, 1970.

*Urinary riboflavin. In Interdepartmental Committee on Nutrition for National Defense: Manual for nutrition surveys, ed. 2, Washington, D.C., 1963, Government Printing Office, p. 140.

Niacin

Baker, H., and Frank, O.: Nicotinic acid. In Baker, H., and Frank, O., editors: Clinical vitaminology: methods and interpretation, New York, 1968, Interscience Publications, Inc.

N-Methyl nicotinamide in urine. In Interdepartmental Committee on Nutrition for National Defense: Manual for nutrition surveys, ed. 2, Washington, D.C., 1963, Government Printing Office, p. 142.

Pantothenic acid

Baker, H., and Frank, O.: Pantothenic acid. In Baker, H., and Frank, O., editors: Clinical vitaminology: methods and interpretation, New York, 1968, Interscience Publications, Inc.

Hatano, M.: Microbiological assay of pantothenic acid in blood and urine, J. Vitaminol. **8**:134, 1962.

Vitamin A

Garry, P. J., Pollack, D., and Owen, G. M.: Plasma vitamin A assay by fluorometry and use of a silicic acid column technique, Clin. Chem. **16**:766, 1970.

Garry, P. J., et al.: Vitamin A: fluorometry and

---

uses of silicic acid technique, Clin. Chem. **16:**766, 1970.

Neeld, J. B., and Pearson, W. N.: Macro- and Micro-methods for the determinations of serum vitamin A using trifluoracetic acid, J. Nutr. **79:**454, 1963.

Thompson, J. N., Erdody, P., Brien, R., and Murray, T. K.: Fluorometric determination of vitamin A in human blood and liver, Biochem. Med. **5:**67, 1971.

Vitamin E

Baker, H., and Frank, O.: Vitamin E. In Baker, H., and Frank, O., editors: Clinical vitaminology: methods and interpretation, New York, 1968, Interscience Publications, Inc.

Hashim, S. A., and Schruttinger, G. R.: Rapid determination of tocopherol in macro- and micro-quantities of plasma, Am. J. Clin. Nutr. **19:**137, 1966.

SELECTED REFERENCES FOR ANTHROPOMETRIC ASSESSMENT

Committee on Nutrition Advisory to CDC, Food and Nutrition Board, NAS-NRC: Comparison of body weights and lengths or heights of groups of children, Nutr. Rev. **32:**284, 1974.

Committee on Nutritional Anthropometry of the Food and Nutrition Board of the National Research Council. Keys, A.: Recommendations concerning body measurements for the characterization of nutritional status, Hum. Biol. **28:**11, 1956.

Falkner, F.: Office measurement of physical growth, Pediatr. Clin. North Am. **8:**13, 1961.

Johnston, F. E., Hamill, P. V. V., and Lemeshow, S.: Skinfold thickness of children 6-11 years, United States, National Center for Health Statistics, Vital and Health Statistics, Series 11, no. 120, Washington, D.C., 1972, HEW publication no. (HSM) 73-1602, Government Printing Office.

Johnston, F. E., Hamill, P. V. V., and Lemeshow, S.: Skinfold thickness of youths 12-17 years, United States, National Center for Health Statistics, Vital and Health Statistics, Series 11, no. 132, Washington, D.C., 1974, HEW publication no. (HRA) 74-1614, Government Printing Office.

Karlberg, P., Engström, I., Lichtenstein, H., and Svennberg, I.: The development of children in a Swedish urban community: a prospective longitudinal study. III. Physical growth during the first three years of life, Acta Paediatr. Scand. **187**(suppl.):48, 1968.

Parizková, J., and Roth, Z.: The assessment of depot fat in children from skinfold thickness measurements by Holtain (Tanner/Whitehouse) caliper, Human Biol. **44:**613, 1972.

GENERAL CONCEPT

Evaluation, the process of determining the value or amount of success in obtaining a predetermined objective, is an integral part of the process of planning and solving problems. The health and nutrition administrator who uses evaluation to assist in solving problems has the best chance of changing tradition, of influencing public opinion, and of persuading political leaders to increase resources to meet health needs as well as improving the rate of success in obtaining the objective.

OUTCOMES

The student should be able to do the following:
- Define evaluation, the need for it, and its component parts.
- Differentiate between the role of the practitioner and the role of the researcher in the evaluation process.
- Apply the principles and process of evaluation to practical situations, action setting, and field activities.
- Describe the most effective methods in collection of data.
- Utilize evaluation results and implications in program administration.

Evaluation: how to measure outcome

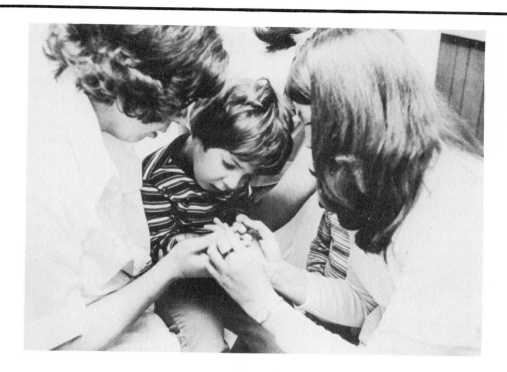

WHAT IS EVALUATION?

The nutrition practitioner's major responsibility is to develop and implement action programs for the community. It has been the practice in the past to consider action without asking the questions: What worked? What did not work? Why? Only when these questions are asked, can change be produced. The cost of health and nutrition programs, which provide services to the public, is generally expensive in terms of manpower and money. Administrators of such programs have the responsibility to account for their accomplishments.

Greenberg[1] in his paper on the "Evalua-

tion of Social Programs" aptly states: "Public accountability requires advance planning such that, for the resources available, the best possible program is implemented at the outset both in design and performance."

In previous chapters we have discussed the analysis required to develop a program plan. Permeating the entire plan should be a realization that evaluation must be built in at all echelons or levels of the program design. (See Fig. 3-3.) Evaluation, though, is a demanding and necessary business, calling for time, money, imagination, tenacity, and skill.[2] The health and nutrition administrator who utilizes evaluation as an integral component of the planning process and the problem-solving process has the best chance of changing provincial thinking, of influencing public opinion, and of persuading political leaders to increase resources to meet the health needs of the public.

Definition of evaluation

A simple and meaningful definition of evaluation has been developed by Knutson,[3] who states, "Evaluation is concerned with determining values or worth." He describes program evaluation as concern specifically with determining the worth or values of efforts expended to achieve a given purpose or objective. He points out that everyone constantly makes evaluations or judgments in terms of right or wrong, good or bad, honest or dishonest, and practical or impractical so frequently and quickly that they are often not consciously aware of it. Individuals draw on the full range of their experiences in making these judgments or evaluations, whether they are objective or intuitive.[3]

Meredith[4] describes program evaluation as the determination of the degree of progress in achieving program objectives. He states that evaluation can and should be used for both planning and control and thus serve as an all-important feedback link between these crucial functions. The American Public Health Association's description of the evaluation process also requires determining the value or amount of success in achieving a predetermined objective. It should include steps such as formulating the objective, identifying the proper criteria to be used in measuring success, determining and explaining the degree of success, and recommendations for continued program activity.[5] In every definition of evaluation, the emphasis on tangible results is evident. Results are the proof of accomplishment and not merely accolades or comments based on subjective data. Simply stated, evaluation is data gathering for decision making.

Evaluation as opposed to evaluative research

To further delineate the term "evaluation" to understand and utilize its component parts effectively, Suchman[6] in *Evaluative Research* makes a distinction between "evaluation" and evaluation research. Evaluation refers to "the social process of making judgments of worth." It is basic to almost every form of social behavior on an individual or organizational level. Generally some logical rational process is used in such judgments, although often there is no systematic procedure for gathering or offering objective evidence to support a judgment. Thus he retains the term "evaluation" in its more common-sense usage as referring to the general process of assessment or appraisal of value.

"Evaluative research" on the other hand, according to Suchman[6] is restricted to the use of scientific research procedures to make an evaluation. Therefore "evaluative" here is an adjective describing a particular kind of research. Evaluative research then emphasizes those procedures needed for collecting and analyzing data that can "prove" rather than "assert" the value of some public program.[6]

Despite the distinction made by Suchman in his comments on evaluation and evaluative research, we are still talking about the same purpose of evaluation, that is judgments of worth or assessments of value, except that the term "research" includes specific, objective procedures for collecting and analyzing data. One additional differentiation should be made that will help practitioners utilize and interpret scientific information for other health professionals and the public.

Weiss[2] in her book on *Evaluation Research* cites the difference between people who are practitioners and those who are evaluative researchers. She states that the researcher is likely to be detached, interested in ideas and abstractions. He thinks in terms of generalization and analytic categories and about the long-term acquisition of knowledge. Instead of being concerned with the practical day-to-day issues of program operation, he seems removed from any program philosophy or position. On the other hand, the practitioner, according to Weiss, is likely to be an outgoing personality, generally intensely concerned about people and specific action. Some observers believe that underlying the personality variables there is a basic difference. Weiss[2] sums it up with her statement, "A practitioner has to believe in what he is doing; a researcher has to question." Of course, this difference in perspective can create tensions between researchers and practitioners.[7] Although these sources of conflict exist because of different role sets, evaluators and practitioners do not have to be at odds. With careful planning, which should include support from the administration and involvement of the practitioner from the initial development of the project, an evaluation can proceed in an atmosphere of cooperation and mutual interest. Good communication and the involvement of personnel at all levels will make the difference between success and failure of an important project.

NEED FOR EVALUATION

To obtain financial support for programs, whether they be social, medical, educational, nutritional, economic, or political, the practitioner is required to provide "proof" of the necessity and effectiveness of the particular program. Health, education, and welfare programs are experiencing great pressures for evaluation at every level of programming. The current trend to determine the benefit of these programs is one way that modern society demonstrates its belief that many social problems can be alleviated through planned action.

Furthermore, expectations by the public have created fundamental changes and trends in public service programs. There is strong demand for evaluation to determine the extent to which currently funded programs are meeting the needs of society.[8] Some of the trends which caused this healthy attitude have been the realization that social problems affect the entire community and not only the victims who have the problems. In general, this represents a recognition that social institutions, rather than individuals alone, bear the major responsibility for the presence of social problems and that institutions, too, must change if individual behavior is to be affected. If society is going to meet this challenge, new programs of preventive

health care will be required. Evaluation of these programs will need to consider new objectives and new criteria for effectiveness. For instance, emphasis on early detection may replace emphasis on rehabilitation as the objectives become prevention of the problem rather than finding cures for the problem.

Another area in which the importance of evaluation is paramount occurs in the changing structure and function of public agencies. The entire trend is toward broader community participation. This is evident in the National Health Planning and Resources Development Act of 1974, where consumer participation is essential to all components of the act. In public service the earlier concerns about the needy and the poor are giving way to concerns about whole segments of the population that are in need, such as the elderly, infants and young children, and pregnant women. This new approach of looking at entire segments of the community has stimulated traditional departments to de-

---

WHY DO WE NEED PROGRAM EVALUATION?

1. To help make decisions—decisions to modify, to expand, to curtail, to continue, or to terminate programs.

2. Any organization using resources should see the most and best service possible is being rendered; in government, to the taxpayer, making sure that public programs meet genuine public needs; that obsolete programs are weeded out and that public revenues are expended wisely.

3. The need for a given program may change with the passage of time. Consequently, there should be a continuing analysis of each program from the standpoint of need, objective, and alternative ways of accomplishing its objectives.

4. Occasional programs are launched which are not really needed and there is a strong tendency for programs once started to be carried along without being seriously questioned.

5. Without program evaluation there is no way of knowing or documenting that public activities are in fact achieving program objectives.

6. Evaluation assists the program manager and the administrator to demonstrate (to the Legislature, to the public, to the client, to the press) that the program is achieving its objectives.

Al Loeb: Evaluating nutrition programs, School of Public Health Social Work, University of California at Berkeley, Jan., 1975.

velop cooperative roles and systems in planning and implementing community programs to meet the needs of the various groups in the population. These changes have produced new kinds of services and problems of organization, and utilization of resources that demand continuous evaluation and reformulation.[9] In turn, new administrative structures, changes in training, and educational requirements produce new objectives that require a broader type of program evaluation. The changes in each of three major considerations in public service—social problems, service agencies, and the public—complement each other in developing a greater demand for evaluation. From the program administrator's point of view, evaluation is necessary in making decisions about whether to develop, continue, expand, terminate, or modify programs, and to determine priorities. Also, evaluation is necessary to demonstrate to the administrator that objectives have been achieved.

In looking specifically at nutrition programs, it has been noted that many of them are not systematically evaluated.[10] Neumann and co-workers[11] have commented that "Most people associated with nutrition programs usually feel what they are doing is worthwhile, that the value is clear to all observers, and that the best has been accomplished with the resources at hand." They have written with the overburdened nutrition program directors in mind, who have, among their many duties, the combined responsibility of organizing, implementing, and evaluating a local or state nutrition program. Gordon and Scrimshaw[12] also comment on the comparatively small effort on scientific evaluation of nutrition intervention programs: "A curious paradox is evident in the care that laboratory and clinical investigators take to establish the validity of newly apparent facts about nutrition and the common absence of evaluation of public health service programs when those findings are turned to practical use."

Gordon and Scrimshaw indicate five broad types of community nutrition programs for which evaluations can be done:

1. A program with the simple objective of food supplementation, that uses a product with a demonstrated capacity to produce a favorable nutritional result. The primary requirements are an identified need, sound administrative conduct, and an appraisal of health benefits limited to nutritional state.

2. A service program that is already underway, for which no provision for evaluation has been made and none has as yet been done. However, partial evaluation is still possible.

3. A comprehensive nutrition program, incorporating related health disciplines, such as infectious disease control, environmental sanitation, public health education, and maternal and child health services. As intervention and preventive care expands, so does the required evaluation.

4. A field trial or action program which is implemented because of favorable conditions in a local area.

5. An action program which presents an opportunity for operational research toward an improved evaluation method. Thus nutrition programs can enhance a general public health return.

The need for evaluation has been described by many investigators, by public health practitioners, by legislators, by the public, yet too little has been done about it. Health practitioners must realize that despite the amount of money, materials, manpower, and frequently limited resources, evaluation, whether simple or complex, can be accomplished.

PRINCIPLES OF EVALUATION

James[13] developed a simple but clear statement on the differences between evaluation and research: "Evaluation differs from research primarily in that it does not seek new knowledge but attempts to mark progress toward a prestated objective." Research often ends with the demonstration of result, whereas evaluation is a circular process, as demonstrated in Fig. 3-3, which analyzes the development of a program plan. In an evaluation process the results are reincorporated into the specific programs from where they were developed. Both evaluation and research utilize the same general statistical, epidemiologic, and technical methods.

Bigman[14] gives six main purposes of evaluation:

1. To discover whether and how well objectives are being fulfilled.
2. To determine the reasons for specific successes or failures.
3. To uncover the principles underlying a successful program.
4. To direct the course of experiments with techniques for increasing effectiveness.
5. To lay the basis for further research on the reasons for the relative success of alternative techniques.
6. To redefine the means to be used for attaining objectives, and even to redefine subgoals, in the light of research findings.

These purposes strongly denote a relationship between evaluation, program planning, and implementation. In addition to determining success or failure with evaluation, these six points indicate that evaluation involves understanding and redefinition. Herzog[15] proposes "a satisfactory evaluation of effort" by posing five questions:

1. What kind of change is desired?
2. By what means is change to be brought about?
3. What is the evidence that the changes observed are due to the means employed?
4. What is the meaning of the changes found?
5. Were there unexpected consequences?

Another way of looking at the evaluation process is proposed by Suchman[6] with this circular scheme:

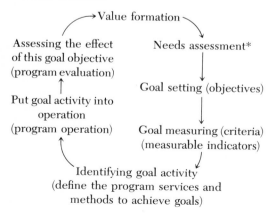

*Added by authors to Suchman's wheel.

Value formation

As each aspect of Suchman's circular scheme is reviewed, the first step considered is value formation. The term "value" has appeared in many definitions of evaluation. One of the preconditions to an evaluation study is the availability of some activities whose objectives may be assumed to have positive value. Most situations, events, or objects may be seen as having some kind of value, whether it be "good," "bad," "desirable," "undesirable," or the like.

Thus the recognition of values helps health practitioners to establish priorities and hierarchies of importance among needs and goals.[16] Such value orientation occurs in all public services. Value determination on the part of the professional and public create the objectives and often the destiny of public service programs. Values may or may not be an actual part of the activity itself, and they may be thought of as being influential whether they are or not.

The relationships between values that are inherent, conceived, and actually operative vary greatly in different circumstances and may be determined only by empirical investigations.[17] For example, any program designed to reduce the incidence of cardiovascular disease by changing the risk factors of individuals must first establish the inherent value of the risk factors as a cause of cardiovascular disease, then it must create those which have these risk factors, a conceived value concerning the undesirability of dying from cardiovascular disease. This then must be translated into the operative value of removing the risk factors of high cholesterol, smoking, obesity, and stress.

Needs assessment

A needs assessment determines the extent and type of problems that certain individuals or groups experience in a community. Health practitioners make the assumption that these people could function at a higher or more efficient level if they receive proper services. According to Mullins,[18] in planning to perform a needs assessment, the following questions should be asked.

1. What do we want or need to know?
2. Why do we want to know it?
3. How will the information be used once it is obtained?
4. How can we obtain the data?
5. What useful data sources already exist at the local, state and federal level?
6. How can we most advantageously compile, analyze, and present the data?
7. What will the program cost?
8. Which needs assessment techniques will be most efficient?

Goal setting (objectives)

A major discussion of goals and objectives has been covered in Chapter 4. Just to recap, goal setting and the later refinement of objectives are always in competition with each other for money, resources, and effort.

Goal measuring (measurable indicators)

The kind of evaluation that is performed will depend largely on the type of measures available for determining the accomplishment of the planner's objectives. If the goal is set to be that the rate of anemia should be reduced in the hypothetical community, then the planner needs some means of determining how many individuals presently have anemia and according to what standards. Is a hemoglobin below 10 gm/dl considered anemic for a child or is it below 11 gm/dl? The more accurate the standard is the more precise will be the evaluation and proof.

Goal-attaining activity

Clearly defining the program plan will assure that an evaluation can be accomplished. The vital steps of planning and defining the program, the services, and methods necessary to achieve the goals and objectives are elaborated in Chapter 4.

Goal activity into operation (program operation)

After identifying what the program plan will be, the plan is set for action and actual operation. Chapter 6 details the method of putting a nutrition program plan into operation. For instance, in dealing with the anemia problem of the hypothetical community, the plan would be implemented by setting up clinic sites to screen and monitor those at risk and so begin to fulfill the goals and objectives.

Assessing the effect of this goal operation

On the basis of an assessment of a goal-oriented operation, a judgment is made as to whether the activity was worth while. This actually brings one back to the value formation. At the end of the evaluation process, one may get a new value, or one may reaffirm, reassess, or redefine an old value. The question of what has been accomplished is the issue here. Values, of course, are consequential factors in deciding on the objectives of public service programs. An evaluation study must consider not only the specific values arising from a nutrition program but also social values, particularly those which might be conflicting.

Categories of evaluation
Paul's categories

To make an evaluation or assessment, it is useful to consider a program according to its various aspects, or categories, and then to measure the success or failure in each. Paul[19] presents three categories for assessment:

1. Assessment of effort, which refers to the energy and activity of the service team, including factors such as number of patients seen, visits made, meetings attended.
2. Assessment of effect, which refers to the results of the effort rather than the effort itself, that is, changes in health information,

---

INTENT TO ACTION IN EVALUATION

Understanding what happens in the political and social complexities or broad-aim intervention programs may well be a priority order of business if we are to learn how to develop programs more realistically to reduce the slippage between intent and action, and to address social problems with greater effect.

Carol H. Weiss: Evaluation research, methods of assessing program effectiveness, Englewood Cliffs, N.J., 1972, Prentice-Hall, Inc. Reprinted by permission of Prentice-Hall, Inc. © 1972.

attitudes, or behavior; reduction in incidence of disease.

3. Assessment of process, which would deal with an analysis of why and how an effect was achieved, including consideration of resistance among community leaders, lack of motivation among potential clients, cultural superstition and fear.

It is important to separate effort, effect, and process in any evaluation. The way in which a service program is established and operates is quite a different consideration from whether or not it does any good or is effective.

As Kandle[20] has said, "A tremendous part of our dollars, staff time and activity in evaluation is still in terms of effort. Many reports, papers, surveys, evaluations, etc. are still written and thought of only in terms of personnel, hospital beds, visits of patients, slides examined, or good intentions proclaimed. We still do not have many practical indices of accomplishments."

Suchman's categories

Suchman[6] proposes five categories of criteria according to which the success or failure of a program may be evaluated. These are (1) effort, (2) performance, (3) adequacy of performance, (4) efficiency, and (5) process. These categories, first presented by James[21] in 1961, are all interrelated, with the evaluation of effort and performance necessarily preceding those of adequacy, efficiency, and process. Briefly, each of these categories presented by James in 1961 may be described as follows.

Effort (or activity). Effort is measured in terms of the quantity and quality of activity that is occurring. It is concerned with the input of energy rather than output or result. The evaluation should answer the following questions: What did you do? How well did you do it?

The measures in this category are based on the capacity for effort itself. The assumption is that this kind of effort will enable the program to reach its objectives. This is usually an easy type of evaluation and can be valuable. To judge the capacity of the effort,

generally the presence of a sufficient number of specific kinds of qualified personnel is considered.

Other examples of evaluation of effort would be the number of nutrition visits made to clients, the number of patients seen in a specific clinic, the number of public health nursing visits, and consideration of the amount of money spent for a given health program.

Performance or accomplishment. Measuring the performance or effect is really measuring the results of the effort more than the amount of effort. The results must be assessed according to one's objective in terms of what kind of change has been effected, if any, and whether certain intermediary goals have been achieved.

Such an evaluation is especially necessary when seeking or justifying supportive funding. In any program that is set up to meet a specific need, the problem ought to be shown to have been solved, or at least alleviated.*

The performance or result evaluation could also be a measure of very specific and concrete outcomes, for example, the number of patients treated or cured after discovery and screening for a certain disorder. The reliability and standards of the outcome, for example, the duration and degree of clientele health, are also necessary considerations in measuring results.

Adequacy of performance or impact. This category measures the total effective performance relative to the total amount of need. A program must be large or adequate enough to meet the needs of a community if it is to be a worthwhile public service

---

*Sometimes a program will involve a great deal of effort but have a negligibly beneficial outcome when looking at behavioral change. This is especially true, as Paul[19] demonstrates when the problem concerns trying to change public attitudes. To give an example of this situation, there was a case where one community was flooded with educative materials, monies, and meetings about the mentally ill. Support to this effort was also given by local physicians and other influential citizens. Another community received no such campaign. When the results were evaluated, neither community had changed their opinions appreciably.[19]

COMPARISON OF IMPACT AND PROCESS EVALUATION

	Process evaluation	Impact evaluation
Answers the question:	How to implement?	Should you implement?
Method:	Documentation and description. Asks what is going on, what are the problems.	Systematic observation. Emphasizes design and analysis to determine causality.
Site selection:	Select sites to *maximize* variation along important dimensions.	Select sites to *minimize* variation along important dimensions.
Example:	Evaluate the Experimental Medical System Policy (EMS): This policy is designed to reduce community mortality rates (unattended deaths in public and private places) and disability rates by creating a system of linkages between emergency room and communication systems, upgrading ambulance equipment, training ambulance and emergency room personnel, and implementing consumer health education programs	
Information obtained from two types of evaluation:	How is political and legal cooperation obtained? How is a system set up? (technical and personnel questions) What new facilities are set up? What do they cost? How are new training programs developed? Who has responsibility for what?	To what extent is there a reduction in mortality and disability due to the operation of the EMS program? What is the impact of the EMS program on costs of emergency care?

Noralou P. Roos: Evaluating health programs: Where do we find the data? J. Community Health **1**:40, Fall, 1975.

rather than an excellent service for only a select few. It is thus necessary to have some idea of unmet needs, an awareness of what is possible in terms of resources, and how progress and expansion toward the objective might be built into the program.

Efficiency (output relative to input). Efficiency refers to the ratio between effort and performance, or output divided by input. Input is the cost in terms of time, money, personnel, and public convenience. To be efficient, the results of a program ought to be in a good proportion with the efforts made. In evaluating this category, the questions to be concerned with are: Does the program work? Is there a better (or more efficient) way to attain results? For instance, it is to be considered that the same end might be achieved in less time, or with less skilled personnel.

Process or specification of conditions of effectiveness. An analysis of the processes involved in a program is particularly necessary if a program has failed to achieve its goals. If a weakness can be located, it is possible that it may be rectified so that the program can succeed. According to James,[21] the analysis should look at the following aspects of the program:

1. The specific causes of success or failure within the program.
2. The recipients of the program, including the amount of the population reached, and the part of the population most beneficially affected.
3. The conditions under which the program

GREATER RATIONALITY TO SOCIAL DECISION MAKING

Evaluation can be a partner in improving social programs if it is given the funds and the conditions to test out small-scale experimental projects. As programs are developed on better knowledge foundations, with better structural arrangements, and greater integration with allied institutions and overall policies, evaluation has a further role to play. It can gauge the effectiveness of the innovations and determine which features are ineffective and which should be retained for further development. With all its failings, evaluation research still has a potential for bringing greater rationality to social decision-making.

Carol H. Weiss: Evaluation research, methods of assessing program effectiveness, Englewood Cliffs, N.J., 1972, Prentice-Hall, Inc. Reprinted by permission of Prentice-Hall, Inc. © 1972.

operates or its context, including its location, public attitudes, time allotment.
4. The effects of the program, including the major or primary effects, unintentional or side effects, the duration of effects, and the kind of effects. The kind may refer to changes in attitude, behavior, or knowledge.

The importance of considerations regarding the social setting is presented by the World Health Organization[22] in its analysis of methods of evaluation. The following questions indicate how evaluation works with this priority in mind:

1. What are the specific social changes being sought?
2. What are the conditions in the project area to which a project must be adjusted if it is to attract the active support of the people?
3. What are the channels of social communication that permit the flow of education from those responsible for the project to the people and likewise, what are the channels for the flow of attitudes and responses from the people back to those responsible for the project?
4. What are the social barriers, so often loosely classified as "superstitions," that must be overcome if the project is to achieve its objectives?
5. Who are the leaders—government, family, religions—whose decisions determine support of or resistance to the project, its methods and its expansion?

METHODOLOGY IN EVALUATION
Developing the question and measuring the answer

There are five procedures that will help answer the question: To what extent is the program reaching its goals?

1. Design a needs assessment through community diagnosis.
2. Set program goals and objectives.
3. Translate goals and objectives into indicators (measurable) of goal and objective achievement (independent or input invariables versus intervening variables).
4. Collect data on the indicators for those who participated in the program.
5. Compare the data on participants with the goal criteria.

Each of these methodologies are described in detail.

Procedure 1: Design a needs assessment through community diagnosis

A program in public health is planned and implemented because presumably there is a need for services in a given area. The first issue that must be addressed is the need of the community. This measurement process in public health is termed "community diagnosis."

The first step in a community diagnosis should be the gathering of data for as complete a profile as possible. A complete outline for a community profile has already been given in Chapter 4, but a few pertinent guidelines may be mentioned again here. Statistical data may be obtained from birth and death records, census and demographic studies, special surveys on attitudes and behavior, and surveys of particular groups.

If the interest is in nutritional status, the population below the poverty level should be especially considered, as well as the incidence of nutrition-related diseases and existing nutrition programs. These data are provided by the hypothetical community in Chapter 4. All data should be compared with a standard norm to establish the need of a community. Even if data describing the norm are lacking, some rules or standards

INERTIA

Professions have norms that may not have a rational basis . . . similarly, with tendencies that are called bureaucratization, institutionalization, and so forth, processes once established tend to be maintained by the authority systems in which they reside. Thus, many things may exist where success or failure of the intended action is not at all clear, yet authority, convention, and other forces may tend to keep them as they are.

Edgar F. Borgatta: Research problems in evaluation of health service demonstration. II, Milbank Mem. Fund Q. vol. 42, no. 3, Oct., 1966.

must be created, despite the fact that this will lead to some subjectivity in the evaluation. However, realistic standards, even if they are not absolutely objective, are required if realistic objectives and goals are to be set.[1]

Procedure 2: Set program goals and objectives

The setting or the awareness of specific goals and objectives gives direction to evaluation and is extremely important from a statistical point of view. The goals and objectives should be based on the information collected for the community diagnosis. The objectives must be clear, specific, and measurable, as we have stated earlier and discussed in detail in Chapter 4.

Vague program goals are a common enough problem to warrant attention. On many occasions consensus on the development of a particular goal or objective is difficult to reach. What can the evaluator do when he is faced with a program that is lacking a statement of specific and meaningful objectives? Weiss[2] offers four possibilities for action:

1. He can present the difficulty and wait for program personnel to reach a consensus.
2. He can read everything about the program available, talk to practitioners, observe the program in operation, and then frame the statement of goals and objectives himself.
3. He can set up a collaborative effort for goal formulation, which is probably the best approach.

With the program practitioners, the evaluator can offer his approximations of goal statements.

4. He can table the issue of goals and proceed not with evaluation in the traditional sense, but a more exploratory open-minded study. Occasionally, evaluations may be based on too specific goals and objectives where indicators of success are premature especially in a field in which there is little agreement on what constitutes success.

Short-term and long-term goals. Decision makers and funding organizations who tend to respond to the demands of the budget cycle rather than the research cycle usually need quick answers. If decisions have to be made for next year's budget, then it is this year's results that count.

On the other hand, evaluation, wherever possible, should make an effort to discover long-term as well as short-term effects, especially when there are basic policies and expensive facilities in question. Consideration of short- and long-term effects can also indicate the rate of progress.

Evaluating progress. When the goals are determined, a decision of how much progress toward the goal has been met will determine success or failure. Certain questions are helpful in this evaluation, such as: How do results compare with last year's results, with the results for those who were not in the special programs, or with the results from similar programs?

Procedure 3: Translate goals and objectives into indicators (measurable) of goal and objective achievement

After the specific objectives have been selected for evaluation, the next step is the development of indicators to measure the extent to which they are achieved. These indicators of program outcomes are the *dependent variables* of the study. For example, in the hypothetical community, cardiovascular disease and anemia were two major health problems. One indicator in cardiovascular disease would be the serum cholesterol level; another indicator or risk factor would be a history of smoking. Indicators of anemia would be hemoglobin and hematocrit levels.

The evaluator also must be concerned with

the description and measurement of other factors, the inputs, which are the *independent variables* of the study. There may also be *intervening variables*—factors that mediate between inputs and outcomes.

Independent or input variables. An analysis of independent or input variables can offer clues as to why a program has been a success or failure and which particular aspects are the causes of these effects. Then useful recommendations for the future can be made. The input variables for a program are considerations such as its purpose, principles, methods, personnel, duration, location, size, and funding source. Sometimes certain characteristics of the participants are also classified as input variables, such as their age, sex, socioeconomic status, race, length of residence in the community, motivation, support from family, expectations, and attitudes toward health.[2]

All kinds of characteristics may be thought of as among the input variables that will be helpful in measuring for whom the program is most effective and valuable. However, as Stouffer[23] suggests, since the evaluators usually have limited resources, it is most productive to concentrate on the most concrete, relevant, and measurable variables.

Intervening variables. There can be a further consideration in the measurement effort—the specification and measurement of conditions between program input and outcomes. The reason for giving systematic attention to these intermediate factors is the expectation that they will affect outcomes. If certain conditions prevail, outcomes will improve. If these conditions are absent, the likelihood of positive outcomes is lessened.

There are two kinds of intervening variables: one is the program operation variable, and the other is the bridging variable.

Program operation variables. Program operation variables are concerned with the implementation of the program—how it actually operates. One kind of program operation variable might be the frequency of exposure. Do participants who attend 85% or more of program sessions do better than those with poorer attendance records? Another might

be the degree of acceptance by peers. Do group members who are well liked perform better than those with marginal group status? Or, an important operational factor might be whether or not patients receive all health services at a single health center.[2] Mann[24] offers a list of variables that can affect outcomes in behavioral change programs, which includes the extent of opportunity for the practice of new behavior patterns, the degree of stress, and the amount of participation by the participant and the practitioner.

Bridging variables. Bridging variables are concerned with the attainment of intermediate milestones. A program usually poses a sequence of events from input to outcome, with certain subgoals in between. Bridging variables might be changes in participants' attitudes or knowledge that are sometimes considered necessary preconditions for behavioral change. Bridging variables are presumed to link the events of the program to the desired effects, and in a way they represent the theory behind the program.[25]

Whereas program operation variables may be thought of or discovered as necessary *conditions* for the theory to operate, the bridging variables give information about the relationship of subobjectives to final goals. Identifying these alerts planners to modification in assumptions or alternative theories. It might turn out, for example, that the program should be striving to reach different intermediate objectives which would be more effective links to final outcomes. The program operation variable, on the other hand, contributes to understanding how the program achieves its effects, or the conditions for effective operation.[2]

Procedure 4: Collect data on the indicators for those who participate in the program

Data for evaluation research can come from a variety of sources and be collected through the whole gamut of research techniques. The only limits are the ingenuity and imagination of the researcher. Weiss[2] suggests that some possible sources are interviews; questionnaires; observation; ratings by peers, staff, and experts; psychometric tests of attitudes, values, personality, preferences, norms, and beliefs; institutional records; government statistics; tests of information, interpretation, skills, and application of knowledge; projective tests, situational tests presenting the respondent with simulated life situations; diary records, physical evidence, and clinical examinations; and financial records and documents, such as minutes of board meetings, newspaper accounts of policy actions, and transcripts of trials.

Interview. Much evaluation research relies on interviews and questionnaires to collect information about program participants —who they are, what they are doing in the program, and what their attitudes and behaviors are before and after program participation. Staff are frequently queried too. Tests are a staple ingredient in the evaluation of educational programs. They provide important data on knowledge and funding. Ratings by experts are common in studies of social work and medical and psychiatric programs. In dietary counseling an interview with the family and a nutritional assessment would give considerable information.

Observation. Some investigators find ways of collecting relevant data by unobtrusive methods that do not involve asking anybody anything. For example, in health programs clinical examination and diagnostic tests have been used. Imaginative examples of these kinds of measures may be found in *Unobtrusive Measures* by Webb and associates.[26]

Observation is an important tool for collecting data on both preprogram and postprogram indicators and on the process itself. For maximum reliability, observations should be recorded immediately. If they lend themselves to easy classification, they can also be coded on the spot.

Program records. Program records in agency files are a natural source of evaluation data. Programs usually collect a fair amount of information about the people who participate, whether it is data on patients

in a hospital or a chart in a well child clinic. Many forms are filled out by staff and participants. Some of this information, however, may be incomplete or vague because of improper handling of agencies. On occasions the agencies sometimes change record-keeping procedures, and if this happens during the period under study, it can vitiate all attempts at before-and-after comparisons.

On the other hand, there are compensations to using institutional records. One is the saving of time and money that original data collection requires. Another is the advantage in continuity. Unlike the one-shot evaluation study that collects precise information for a short period of time and then closes up shop, the agency reporting system can provide continuous information.

Generally, the evaluator will have to revamp procedures, introduce new items suited to evaluation requirements, and institute checks for accuracy and completeness. If this can be done and maintained, indicators of program success are constantly available for ongoing evaluation. Someone also has to be able to analyze the product of the information system with an evaluation prospective. Another point to keep in mind is that the evaluator be in a position to bring the interpreted data to the attention of policy makers, particularly when decisions are pending about that particular program. A further need is the opportunity for periodic revision of the content of the information system.

Government records. Some government agencies maintain records on individuals that could be highly useful in evaluation. A prime example is the Social Security Administration, which collects not only payroll deductions but data on how long a person is employed, the kind of employment, the amount of earnings, and other information. School data are another good source. Depending on school regulations, information on achievement scores, attendance, promotion, and similar items may be retrieved for groups of students. Even more relevant might be the data collected on heights, weights, and growth patterns of children in school settings, but these data are rarely used by schools or health personnel.

Government and statistical series. Government and statistical series provide other sources of data for evaluation that usually have to do specifically with the problem that the program is suppose to cure. Thus, if a program is designed to reduce illiteracy or highway accidents or infant mortality, the evaluator can turn to statistical reports on the prevalence of these problems and periodically check changes in the statistics from the time before the program starts to after it is under way. Obviously, if the program is effective, it will presumably push the figures down.

Procedure 5: Compare the data on participants with the goal criteria

Comparison of the data on participants with the goal criteria is the key point and purpose of an evaluation. It is up to the evaluator to determine statistically what portion of the program's goals have been achieved and how much of the achievement was actually because of the program. Sometimes even before gathering and examining data it is helpful to have a preevaluation overview. From this early appraisal an investigator may be able to predict likely outcomes. For example, one of the important considerations in an early appraisal might be the degree of involvement by the community or perhaps the need to have a physician participate in the planning stage. From previous experience an investigator would know that a program without such involvement usually does not have a successful outcome. The following list contains other possible areas of inquiry for a preevaluation review:

1. An organizational chart indicating areas of responsibility, communication channels, and rules for decision making by staff members
2. The way in which positions are staffed, qualifications of personnel, plans for promotion, incentives, and staff morale
3. The way in which the program is funded initially and at later stages of development

4. Relationship with professional groups and other agencies
5. Designs and methods of supervision, quotas, and quality control measures

An early appraisal of a program that uses these general rules of management may avert a failure of weaknesses, which true evaluation would require several months or even years to detect.[1] Evaluation of accomplishment can be seen on a time scale that measures all output in terms of immediate results to long-range and ultimate goals as shown by Table 9-1. Ultimate goals may be specific, such as lowered mortality, or they may be vague and refer to concepts such as increased levels of well-being or healthful living.

Immediate goals. Immediate goals can be based on increments in knowledge about health and disease. Improving the attitude toward the adoption of recommended health practices leads to adoption of the suggested behavioral pattern. Immediate goals can be scored or measured almost spontaneously, and usually most of them are achieved in a period of not more than 6 to 12 months.

Intermediate goals. Intermediate goals concentrate on the early benefits that are supposed to be derived from the recommended health practice. If the health practice is vaccination, for instance, the intermediate goal would be less disease. If the program consists of family planning services, the intermediate goal would be a significant decline in the birth rate or age-specific fertility rates.

During the intermediate phase, there may also be other more subtle changes taking place that reflect less discomfort and deprivation among members of the community. Less disease, for instance, should be responsible for lower absences from school and industry as well as reduced hospitalization for that diagnostic condition. This means that the evaluation might be based on an indirect correlated response variable when measurement of the direct effect is too costly or imprecise. Intermediate changes, direct or indirect, require longer periods of time to appear than immediate outcomes. A three- to five-year

Table 9-1. A listing of input and output variables that are essential in a program of evaluation*

Input (quasi-evaluation)	Output (true evaluation)		
	Immediate goals Increase in knowledge, improved attitudes and practices	**Intermediate goals** More positive health and improved status	**Long-range goals** Reduction in morbidity and mortality

1. Administrative pattern
  a. Organizational chart
  b. Personnel staffing
  c. Funding plans
  d. Relationships with other agencies (horizontal and vertical)
  e. Built-in quality control measures
2. Service statistics
  a. Operations analysis of services provided including crossclassification by characteristics of services, recipients, and providers of service
			→**Ultimate**

	Reduced disinterest Reduced dissatisfaction	Reduced discomfort and deprivation Reduced disease	Reduced disability Reduced in death Reduction in death
b. Feedback and feed forward operations including comparison with standards and quotas	**Other output** 1. Accompanying favorable effects in community other than among recipients of service 2. Untoward side effects		
Final index	Efficiency $= \dfrac{\text{Output (in terms of goal fulfillment)}}{\text{Input (in terms of dollars, services and/or personnel time)}}$		

*From Greenberg, B. G.: Evaluation of social programs, Rev. Int. Stat. Inst. **36**:275, 1968.

period is not unreasonably long to wait for intermediate effects to become detectable.

Long-range goals. The long-range goals focus on the eventual reduction of liability and death. Such effects may require ten years or more before anything is discernible. The output goals listed in Table 9-1 are all characterized by a reduction in undesirable states.

This is because the diagnosis of needs was based on recognitions of these states, since it is easier to measure deviation from health than to characterize well-being or positive health. The evaluator must reckon with the existence of unanticipated side effects, regardless of the desired outcome. Sometimes these accompanying effects are favorable and

MAJOR RULES OF EVALUATION FOR THE PUBLIC HEALTH WORKER

1. The practical objectives of each program to be evaluated should be clearly stated.

2. The underlying assumptions of validity associated with these objectives should be meticulously identified.

3. Evaluations by effort should always be done. Evaluations by performance, adequacy of performance and efficiency, should be done whenever possible.

4. The entire program should be reexamined in the light of the findings arising from the evaluation exercise.

5. To insure the reliability of any standards developed as aids to evaluation, the status of all significant conditions associated with the use of the standard must be specified.

6. The ultimate value of the evaluation to public health programs will depend to a great extent upon research proofs of the validity of the assumptions involved in the established objectives.

7. As in every new field, there is a period of time set aside for clarification of terms and construction of conceptual frameworks. Further progress will then occur only from the performance of actual evaluation projects, carefully designed and analyzed. Public health practitioners today need the stimulation which can be achieved only through the critical appraisal of a large number of such studies. The time for such work is now!

George James: Evaluation in public health practice, Am. J. Public Health **52**:1145, 1962.

might even overshadow the importance of the main program. On the other side of the coin, genuinely untoward results are also possible.

The two possibilities, good and bad, highlight the need for all agencies engaged in any kind of social and health programs to be on the alert for accompanying side effects. Changes in the status quo of a dynamic interacting system is bound to result in many changes beside the one focused on by the target variable. If it is possible to assign a value judgment to the desirable and undesirable effect, the difference between the two might be considered a kind of net output.

Evaluation design

Once the evaluator knows what he is going to study, the next step is to decide how to study it. A plan must be developed to select the people to be studied, set the timing of the investigation, and establish procedures for the collection of the data. In developing a design, the evaluator can aim at the traditional controlled experiment or at one of the less formalized quasi-experiment designs. The investigation can be of just one project or of a number of projects with the same basic goals. It can deal with the traditional social science variables or with an economic analysis of program cost and benefits.

Experimental model

The classic design for evaluation has been the experimental model, which uses both experimental and control groups. The target population units (individuals, work teams, precincts, students, cities) are randomly chosen to be either the group that gets the program or the control group that does not. Differences are computed, and the program is deemed a success if the experimental group has improved more than the control group. Fig. 9-1 illustrates the model graphically.

Usually the control group will receive some program except when the only fruitful comparison can be made between groups on the experimental program and those receiving the usual treatment. In cases where no real treatment can be offered to controls, a "placebo" program can be devised that gives the aura but not the substance of service. This removes the possibility of a Hawthorne or placebo effect*—a positive response that is merely due to the attention that participants receive.

Campbell and Stanley[27] list eight major threats to the internal validity of an experiment, that is, eight classes of outside or nonprogram variables that can affect the outcomes of an experiment if they are not carefully controlled. These are (1) maturation and history of participants; (2) judging the effects of taking a test on the basis of source scores of the second testing; (3) instrumentation or procedure; (4) changes in the calibration of measuring instruments, or changes in the observers or scores; (5) statistical regression, which operates when groups have been selected on the basis of their extreme scores and then, on a second testing, tend to move back toward the mean score of the group; (6) choosing experimental and control units of different characteristics; (7) experimental mortality, or differential loss of respondents from experimental and control groups; and (8) selection maturation interaction, or the differential maturation of members of experimental and control groups.

Organizing randomized designs is a highly effective way to rule out the possibility that

---

*The term "Hawthorne effect" comes from a series of studies made at the Hawthorne Works of the Western Electric Company between 1927 and 1932. Researchers found that when management paid attention of any kind to workers, output increased.

	Before	After
Experimental	A	B
Control	C	D

If the difference between A and B is greater than the difference between C and D, the program is a success.

Fig. 9-1. Illustration of an experimental model. (From Weiss, C. H.: Evaluation research, Englewood Cliffs, N.J., 1972, Prentice-Hall, Inc.) Reprinted by permission of Prentice-Hall, Inc. © 1972.

something other than the program is causing improvements or setbacks which are observed. Randomizations protect against all these sources of possible confusion in analyzing results.

Problems in action programs. But, of course, the controlled experiment is often impossible in action settings. There may be absolutely no extra people to serve as controls; the program serves everybody eligible and interested. Even if there are unserved people, program practitioners may refuse to assign any of them to a control condition because they believe in their professional obligation not to deny service. Occasionally the only possible controls are widely scattered or unlikely to cooperate with a program that offers nothing in return.

The randomized assignment procedure of the experiment also creates problems. Practitioners generally want to assign all people to treatments based on their professional knowledge and experience. To counteract this, imaginative evaluators have made a number of ingenious adaptations. To evaluate a medical school program, Kendall[28] arranged to have half the class receive the new program during the first semester and the other half during the second semester. She took measures at three points—before the program began, at the end of the first semester, and at the end of the year. For the first semester group the then unexposed second group was the control. In the second semester the first group, even though they were now unequal, were the controls. In effect, the experiment was repeated twice. This type of innovation hopefully would have wide applicability.

However, in the last few years the experimental model has come under attack, not only because it is not feasible but because it is counterproductive.

Use of experimental design. The basic need is to fit the research design to the purpose of the study. Experimental design is a good way to find out how well a particular program achieves its goal. The experiment should be able to offer the optimal design. The essential requirement for a true experi-

ment is the randomized assignment of people to programs. Experimentalists suggest that this is much more possible in the real world than many of us suspect.[29]

When resources are scarce and some people must do without, randomization is possible. When new programs are being introduced over a period of time, the delayed receivers can become the controls for those who get the programs early. Often, special pilot projects can be designed on an experimental basis. But however possible the conditions may be—for having such a program and more power to those who can bring them off—experience shows that they often do not materialize. Programs are rarely run for the convenience of the evaluator, and his requirements are only occasionally a factor in the program in funding arrangements. But there is a trend toward quasi-experimental design, which is a possibility to aim for in public health planning.

Quasi-experimental design

Quasi-experimental designs are those which do not meet all the strict requirements of the experiment but nevertheless can be satisfactory. The influential paper of Campbell and Stanley[27] presents the basic criterion for such designs, which is the extent to which they protect against the effect of extraneous variables on the outcome measures. The best designs are those which control relevant outside effects and lead to valid inferences about the effects of the program.

Unlike the experimental design, which protects against just about all possible outside effects, quasi-experiments have the advantage of being practical when conditions prevent true experimentation. However, these are not sloppy experiments, since they recognize in advance what they do and do not control for. Any misrepresentation is understood and allowed for by the evaluator, who draws conclusions carefully.

Two quasi-experimental designs are worth mentioning here—the time series and the multiple time series.

Time series. The time series design, one of the most attractive quasi-experiments, involves a series of measurements at periodic intervals before the program begins and a continuation after the program ends. It is possible to see whether the measures immediately before and after the program are a continuation of previous patterns or whether they indicate a noteworthy change. For example, in the area of nutrition, patients with any disease entity, such as anemia, are followed up with hemoglobin and hematocrit tests. Over a period of time the changes in the patient's biochemical determinations are observable.

Multiple time series. The second kind of quasi-experimental design is the multiple time series, which also has great validity. The evaluator tries to find a similar group or an institution and take the same periodic measurements during the same time span as he is doing for the group in the program. Thus there is a control group to take care of any effects resulting naturally from the elapse of time. This design appears to be particularly appropriate to evaluations of school programs, since repeated testing goes on normally and long series of prescores and postscores are often available.[2]

Nonequivalent control groups

A similar kind of design occurs when there is a nonequivalent control group, which probably is the most common design in practice. Here there is no random assignment to program and control, as there would be in a true experiment, but available individuals or intact groups, such as patients in the clinic with similar characteristics, are used as controls. Such nonrandomized controls are generally referred to as comparisoning groups, since their before and after measures are compared with the program's groups.

Obviously, the evaluator must be aware of possible misrepresentation arising from the control groups, especially if the groups selected for the study had extreme scores or regression effects. A major problem is how to make the comparisoning groups as similar to the experimental group as possible.

Matching. Matching procedures are sometimes resorted to, in which members of the experimental and control groups are paired according to available measures. Sometimes the whole experimental group is matched with a similar group at the start of the program. Then the benefits of the program to the experimental group should be clear, but experience shows that matching is much less satisfactory than randomized assignments.

Frequently, the characteristics on which people should be matched are difficult to determine because the characteristics that will really effect the change are not known. For example, age, sex, race may be matched up, but the important factor in change is motivation. Thus matching sometimes may be done with even more validity on the basis of pretest scores.

Matching is often an essential prelude to randomization when there are few units under consideration, such as cities, but matching as a substitute for randomization can produce pseudoeffects and misleading results, particularly when experimental and control groups are drawn from basically different populations. Then regression effects that occur when making measurements can get in the way of valid interpretation. All measures contain some component of error, and some, such as certain test scores and attitude measures, contain a sizable amount. On any one testing some individuals will score artificially high and others artificially low. On the next testing, however, their scores are likely to be closer to the mean. Thus, if participants and controls are chosen on the basis of their extreme scores, or without due consideration of them, the subjects are likely to regress toward the mean with or without the program. At a second testing, what looked like effect of the program may be simply the artifacts of statistical regression. This is something of which to be highly aware in nonequivalent control group design.[2]

Self-selection. Another problem in selecting a comparisoning group is the factor of self-selection. People who choose to enter a program are likely to be different from those who do not. The problem of self-selections sometimes can be overcome if both experimentals and controls are selected from volunteers, and if the volunteers are randomly assigned to either group. This could be a condition for a true experiment. But even when randomized assignment is not feasible, it is usually better to have some nonequivalent comparison group than no control at all. Health planners are better off being able to rule out some possible explanation for observed effects than not rule out any.[2]

Nonexperimental designs

Sometimes it is impossible to use even a quasi-experimental design. The evaluator then has to resort to one of three common nonexperimental designs: (1) a "before-and-after" study of a single person, (2) an "after-only" study of a program participant, or (3) an "after-only" study of participants *and* nonrandom controls. The inherent weakness is that they fail to control many of the factors which might explain how observed changes were caused by something other than the program. At their best they can be full of details, provocative, and rich in insight. If the data are collected systematically and with care, they certainly offer more information than would have been possible without any study at all. At worst, the data they produce are misleading. In all cases nonexperimental designs leave considerable room for differing interpretations of how much change has occurred and how much of the observed change was due to the operation of the program. But with all the caveats, there are times when they may be worth considering if there are no other alternatives.

One reason for using a nonexperimental design is that it sometimes provides a preliminary look at the effectiveness of a program. If, for example, a before-and-after study, with all the contamination effects of outside events, maturation, testing, and so on, finds little change in participants, the program is probably having little effect. It may not be worth while to invest in more rigorous evaluation. Thus this kind of preliminary work is particularly apt in an evaluation procedure, since experience has shown that many programs produce little gain in the first place, and generally most of the contaminating factors artificially elevate the level of gain so that a small success must take this kind of gain into account.

Another reason for considering nonexperimental design arises from current federal practices for funding evaluations of major programs. Many government agencies tend to demand a one-time ex post facto investigation. They are responding to political pressures and short-term needs, and they want results. Also, the system of competitive contracting for evaluation, where evaluators submit a request for proposal (RFP), leaves this major decision in the agencies' hands.

Frequently, desirable options may not be available to the evaluator. He may not be called in until the program is in midstream, or he may not have access to comparative groups, since a great deal of evaluation is still being done under restrictive unscientific conditions. It is always useful to consider ways to overcome any basic flaws in an evaluation procedure. This is why the nonexperimental design in public health and in nutrition can be an extremely useful tool.[2]

EVALUATION—IT CAN BE DONE IN A BIG WAY OR IN A SMALL WAY

However good the intentions are of those planning, organizing, and implementing a nutrition program, one cannot be satisfied with the assumption that certain results will follow as a result of program input. It is possible to carry out a proper evaluation without a large, specialized staff. The secret of success is to design the evaluation with the program when it is in the earliest planning stage and to seek advice at that point.

A sound evaluation will help improve a program and can be a great morale booster for staff. In this age of budget cuts and operations research, the touching testimonial as a means of insuring continuation of a program is giving way to carefully documented hard facts. Good evaluation which may spell the difference between the termination or continuation of the program can be done relatively easily and is stimulating to do.

Alfred K. Neumann, Charlotte G. Neumann, and *Aaron E. Ifekwunigwe:* Evaluation of small-scale nutrition programs. Am. J. Clin. Nutr. **26:**446, 1973.

EVALUATION IN AN ACTION SETTING

It must be remembered that evaluation research usually takes place while another, more primary, activity is going on—namely, that of the service program. Since evaluation does most often occur in an action setting, it must be adapted to the program environment and cause as little disruption as possible. Some interference is unavoidable, especially in the collection of data where questions must be asked and answered. If the focus of the evaluation is clear, unnecessary intrusion can be avoided. Weiss[2] indicates three features of an evaluation in an action setting of which the researchers should be aware:

1. The tendency of the program to change while it is being evaluated.
2. The relationship between the evaluator and program personnel.
3. The setting of the program, usually within some institution or organization that in some way affects the outcome.

The changing program

Conscientious practitioners within a program will change their methods as they discover areas and means for improvements. As well, there may be changes in clientele and in community conditions. More money may become available; the staff or the political climate may change. All these can affect viewpoints, principles, and the actual activity of any program, whether it is a model or experiment, and especially if it is a complex, long-range program.

The evaluator periodically must step back to observe these changes and also examine records, talk to personnel, and attend meetings having to do with the program. The evaluator, often in some manner an administrator of the program, should be particularly alert to changes in program management. The staff may make changes that they believe will produce more effective results, but the evaluator should be able to see how these fit in with the ultimate objectives. Parsell[30] recommends a dynamic rather than a static program model, one which will allow for movement and development as the program develops. This may be more difficult to conceive and describe in the planning stage, but it is more in keeping with a useful working

relationship between the model and reality.

To counteract the tendency to change, Feirweather[31] suggests that when innovative programs are being tested, the researcher should be in control of the entire operation. Then, of course, evaluation requirements can be more of a priority and random changes can be avoided.

Even if the researcher is not in control, he still can influence program maintenance. Freeman and Sherwood[32] also agree that the evaluator has the responsibility of preventing the program from straying from its original concept and operation. Although this is not always practical, such comments are well taken.

To handle problems of change, Suchman[33] has proposed a fourth stage in the development of a program. He differentiates between a pilot phase, when program development proceeds on a trial-and-error basis; a model phase, when a defined program strategy is run under controlled conditions; a prototype phase, when the model program is subjected to realistic operating conditions; and an institutional phase, when the program is an ongoing part of the organization.

In the model phase the program must be held stable for experimental evaluation, whereas in other stages less rigidity is acceptable and variable input is not only tolerated but expected. If Suchman's course of development could be implemented, it would effectively resolve the issue of the inevitable program shifts. If the reasons for program drifts are classified and analyzed, it seems possible to counteract them to some extent. Weiss[2] offers these seven suggestions:

1. Take frequent periodic measures of the program's progress. For example, monthly assessments of training and therapy, etc., are better than limiting collection of outcome data to one point in time.
2. Encourage clear transitions if a program changes from one approach to another.
3. Clarify and classify the assumptions and procedures of each phase.
4. Keep careful records on the persons who participated in each phase, rather than lumping all the participants together. Ana-

lyze outcomes in terms of the phases of program.

5. Try to recycle or recapitulate earlier program phases. Sometimes this happens naturally. Re-working a phase is a good way to check on earlier conclusions.

6. Seek to set aside funds to get approval for smaller scale evaluations of at least one program phase or component that will remain stable for a given period.

7. If nothing works, and the program continues to meander, consider giving up the evaluation in favor of meticulous analysis of what, how, and why of events.

Relationship with program personnel

The evaluator's relationship to the other professionals in the program can be a delicate area, and may run the gamut from friendly and cooperative to hostile. The very fact of the evaluation itself can be a source of fric-

---

BENEFITS OF SELF-EVALUATION

In general, the staff secures new concepts and becomes much more knowledgeable in the area of the research. They often learn new approaches and techniques that become useful in their daily work. If it is a well-run project, they develop a kind of critical discernment that comes from setting up hypotheses and avoiding conflicting or confusing methods in approaches. They learn to look for erroneous analogies, inadequate hypotheses, and poor design methodology and evaluation. They may not learn enough to be able to design good projects themselves but they become more aware of the good and bad proposals which are presented to them as part of the operating programs.

On the other hand, the possibility of confusing research objectives with those of daily work cannot be eliminated, particularly, if the work involves education or interviewing, such as public health nurses do. Careful indoctrination as part of good research methodology should leave very little of an experimental design open to the chance and influence of daily work. Where it especially defines approaches or denial of supposedly beneficial services to the control groups of the clients, the service-oriented staff may emotionally be unable to comply. The technician when having conflict of emergency duties with research obligations will usually find the research work put aside while clients' needs are being met. This can result in costly deferment or neglect.

Henrik L. Blum and *Alvin R. Leonard:* Public administration: a public health viewpoint, New York, 1963, The Macmillan Co. © 1963, The Macmillan Publishing Co., Inc.

---

tion, aside from the differences that were touched on earlier—differences in roles and their function, goals, values, frame of reference, and also personality.

Basically, as stated before, the practitioner has to believe in what he is doing, and the researcher has to question it. Thus the evaluator may be seen as a possible threat. In addition, the practitioner may be required to assume new roles or tasks that he had not counted on, such as answering questions and collecting data, perhaps assigning people to experimental groups. It is best if these additional responsibilities can be clearly defined, discussed, and agreed on in advance. To the practitioner, the evaluator's primary interest in effective changes may seem to ignore more subtle outcomes, and the effort, time, and money expended on evaluation may not seem worth while. The practitioner, because he works with the individuals rather than looking at the effects on the group as a whole, believes that he is much more sensitive than the researcher in his observation of smaller changes on the individual human level which might not be apparent on the statistical level.

Naturally, if an agency has some kind of internal conflict relating to management or operation, the friction and even suspicion between practitioner and evaluator is likely to increase. The evaluator's secrecy and confidential records seem especially threatening if one faction believes that another is opposed to their methods or management.

Issues that lead to friction

Particular issues which have been known to be sore spots are requests that practitioners administer questionnaires, tests, and interviews, suggestions that they change record-keeping methods, that they select participants randomly instead of on the basis of their ability to help participants, and that there be control groups. The practitioner often thinks that having a group receive no service is a denial of the ethics of the service professions.

Practitioners often also would like to have feedback from the evaluator's information, if these data can help them improve the program. On the other hand, the researcher does not want to change the methods of the program midstream and thus give his evaluation another variable factor to contend with. Occasionally, practitioners also resent what they consider to be the researcher's higher status, especially since they, the practitioners, work on a day-to-day basis in the program with all its problems. The researcher appears as a critical outsider.

Reducing the friction

The best way to avoid and lessen friction between evaluator and practitioner is to establish communication and rapport. Evaluators should involve the administrators and management of the program in the planning of the evaluation and keep them informed about each step of it. Thus the practitioner and his staff will understand the purpose and value of the evaluation, as well as its procedure. Their cooperation, additional ideas, and information can be of enormous aid to the researcher for the whole duration of the program.

On his side, the evaluator should aim at minimizing disruption of the program, recognize its priorities, and make sure of his own priorities so that his demands will be limited to the most necessary issues. The researcher should try not to get in the way of service and also should try to communicate useful findings and data back to the practitioner, even in a nonformal way. An attitude of mutual respect and appreciation of each other's necessity for the success of the program will ensure that the evaluation can proceed smoothly.

USE OF EVALUATION RESULTS— IMPLICATION FOR PROGRAM ADMINISTRATION

Once the evaluation report, with all its data and findings, is completed, it should be given to the administrator of the program. The next issue is the implementation of change, if it is called for. However, as Weiss[2] points out, frequently there are constraints to change that the evaluator ought to consider as he produces his report.

Evaluator's role

Many researchers see themselves as part of an academic community to whom they look for recognition, rather than part of a practical public service program.[34] After the evaluator has determined the results of his investigation, he often does not draw conclusions or propose recommendations for actual implementation of a change for the better. He then may wonder why his work is neglected by practitioners. However, even if the evaluator has not followed through with recommendations, it is up to the practical administrators and decision makers to use the data themselves and thus not waste the large amount of time and money that has no doubt gone into the evaluation.

Resistance by the institution

Sometimes an evaluation report may clearly point to certain revisions, but they are resisted by the program's organization for various reasons. Change is usually difficult and requires some extra effort; it also generally means that more money is spent and the staff is disrupted. This could involve a revision of roles and relationships with personnel, the community, and funders. As well, change might mean a reconsideration of basic ideology, commitments, and methodology—all areas in which change is particularly difficult and threatening.

Revisions and the gap between evaluation and action

Because of such natural resistance, certain specific techniques should be employed to overcome it. It is the administrator's role to make an effort to use the results of the evaluation to improve his program and to reward or encourage staff members who cooperate with him.[35] Other techniques are suggested by Weiss,[36] such as early recognition of the need for particular revisions and of those persons who will put them into practice, selection of issues of special concern, involvement of the staff in planning and conducting the revisions, and also the usefulness of an evaluation in disseminating information. Another consideration in implementing revisions

Table 9-2. Accountability in public health*

Responsible party	Accountable to whom	In the area of	For the purpose of	Measurable by
Program administrators	Public at large	Communicable disease Prevention	Attaining acceptable standards of quality of life	Mortality, morbidity
	Individual consumer	Services provided	Quality, quantity, adequacy of services provided	Mortality, morbidity
	Providers (participants)	Fees, roles in decision making, planning, working conditions	Acceptable life-style, prestige, self-esteem	Provider feedback, staff turnover
	Governmental bodies	Effectiveness, efficiency, adequacy of program	Satisfaction of constituency; funding, legislation	Fiscal, mortality, morbidity assessment; favorable public image
	Parent organization	Program priorities, efficiency, effectiveness	Organizational and financial support to meet consumer needs	Mortality, morbidity, administrative guidelines, standards
	Sister organizations	Communication, cooperation, program assistance	Coordination of efforts to meet community needs; stimulate community interest; better public image	Formation, frequency of meeting of joint councils; degree of cooperation in joint projects
	Professional organizations	Service priorities, patient eligibility, service components, support of professional organizations	Professional recognition; professional and political support	Professional organizations' endorsements and cooperation
	News media	Communication; cooperation	Maintaining public image; political and financial support	Media's support of agency's efforts
	Special interest	Cooperation with efforts in their special interests	Public image, financial and political support	Degree of cooperation sought by special groups

*Modified from Your accountability for health—How much is lots? Presented at 41st Annual Meeting, Southern Branch American Public Health Association, Louisville, Ky., May 9-11, 1973.

should be the timing of the report, especially if it makes use of comparisons of various methods or procedures.[36]

Evaluation results are also of interest to funding agencies and the government. These policy makers are the ones who decide whether or not to continue a program or to decrease or increase its funding. Information on the evaluation should be given to them and also to boards of education, state departments, hospitals, and other public service agencies for the purposes of gaining visibility and publicity for the program being studied and for demonstrating the need and value of evaluation.

Evaluation does not provide all the answers and often presents no clear path for improvement. However, it can show through concrete evidence what is happening in an existing program and the need for change, especially to those in a decision-making capacity. An evaluation can also indicate with some authority what are likely outcomes or consequences of recommended revisions. This is of particular interest if a radical revision is suggested by the evaluation..

Another result of the evaluation of nutrition services is that of accountability. The evaluation process is not complete unless the results are appropriately communicated. Accountable may be defined as "being answerable." But questions may arise; Answerable to whom? In what area? For what purpose? Answers to these questions appear in Table 9-2, which demonstrates the wide variety of persons, areas, and purposes that are implicated in the process of accountability.

PROGRAM EVALUATION—A LAST FRONTIER?

Program evaluation is frequently thought of as a dry, arid and fruitless endeavor, extolled in theory, but ignored in practice. Under conditions of limited resources and limitless requirements, the application of program evaluation is more than an opportunity—it is a necessity. Rather than a wasteland, it is the last main frontier in public administration.

Al Loeb: Evaluating nutrition programs, School of Public Health Social Work, University of California at Berkeley, 1975.

Negative evaluation results

As indicated earlier, and as Elinson[37] points out, there is a significant tendency for a thorough and objective investigative analysis to show negative results, which is to say that it shows that the program has little or negligible effect. This tendency has the unfortunate consequence of making program administrators less open to evaluation and more suspicious of its value. Furthermore, large established programs are the ones that are rarely evaluated; rather, it is the smaller, innovative program that is trying to do something new that usually must undergo an evaluation. Frequently, these are just the programs that ought to be encouraged.

An evaluation with negative results may really be indicating that the more straightforward aspects of medical educational and general social reform have been accomplished but that the more complex problems of efficient use of time and talent need more attention. It is obvious that there are many competing and overlapping programs and that there is a need for interrelated and integrated programs instead of huge, single-minded programs or a number of small, fragmentary programs. Evaluation can be the most useful tool in pointing out the specific needs in the complex area of administration.

SUMMARY

It is clear that, as much as any program needs appropriate planning and administration to succeed, so does the useful evaluation require similar careful attention. An evaluation is the means by which the success and effects of a program can be measured, and it can point out the direction for beneficial changes in a program. It also helps ensure that the program is responsible to both its clientele and its funders. Although the roles and even the personalities of the evaluative researcher and the program practitioners may seem different, every effort at cooperation and planning together should be made so that the work of both proceeds to produce the most beneficial effects.

In doing evaluative research, the investigator must be aware of the needs of the community and the type of problems that the program is supposed to take care of, the goals of the program, and how to assess the effectiveness and efficiency of the operation in achieving desired effects. To do this, it is helpful to break down the assessment into three categories—evaluations of the effort, the effect or results, and the process. Further considerations are the adequacy of the program in terms of total need and its efficiency in terms of cost in time, money, and personnel (Chapter 10).

There are various procedures outlining the indicators and variables that should be considered in any method of collecting data for such assessments. Ideally, an assessment should also take into account the time scale within which the program operates so that a realistic evaluation of immediate, intermediate, and long-range goal achievement is also possible. This kind of evaluation usually occurs in an action setting, which brings with it additional variables and considerations, such as change during the evaluation, the relationship between evaluators and program personnel, and the larger system of which the program is usually a part.

The evaluation research should proceed according to an evaluation design, which is really a plan or model for the investigation. This design can be a classic experimental design in which both control and experimental groups are randomly chosen, a less strict quasi-experimental design, a design that is forced to use nonequivalent control or comparisoning groups, or even a nonexperimental design. This last is usually necessary when an evaluation is required after the completion of a program.

At the conclusion of an evaluation, the next step is the effective utilization of its findings, even if they show negligible results for the program, as is often the case. If there has been a good working relationship between the researcher and the practitioner, the findings of an evaluation will always be of value, particularly in the area of improving the administration of the new program. In addition, this kind of data is of vital importance in publicizing a program. It also demonstrates to funding agencies and decision makers the values of a program and where it can be improved.

Each act performed for the promotion of public health involves the expenditure of money. Evaluation provides data that influence funding agencies. In fact, the very nature and extensiveness of the public health program is determined in the final analysis by the amount of funds available for its conduct. Thus Chapter 10, will present a discussion of budget and fiscal management.

REFERENCES

1. Greenberg, B. G.: Evaluation of social programs, Rev. Int. Stat. Inst. **36**:260, 1968.
2. Weiss, C. H.: Evaluation research, methods of assessing program effectiveness, Englewood Cliffs, N.J., 1972, Prentice-Hall, Inc.
3. Knutson, A. L.: Evaluating program progress, Public Health Rep. **70**:305, 1955.
4. Meredith, J.: Program evaluation techniques in the health service, Am. J. Public Health **66**:1069, 1976.
5. Glossary of administrative terms in public health, Am. J. Public Health **50**:225, 1960.
6. Suchman, E. A.: Evaluative research, New York, 1967, Russell Sage Foundation.
7. Rodman, H., and Kolodny, R. L.: Organizational strains in the researcher-practitioner relationship. In Gouldner, A. W., and Miller, S. M., editors: Applied sociology: opportunities and problems, New York, 1965, The Free Press.
8. Sanders, I. T.: Public health in the community: handbook of medical sociology, Englewood Cliffs, N.J., 1963, Prentice-Hall, Inc.
9. Dixon, J. P.: Developing problems of official services in keeping in tune with the times, Am. J. Public Health **47**:15, 1957.
10. Planning and evaluation of applied nutrition programs, Nutr. Rev. **25**:132, 1967.
11. Neumann, A. K., Neumann, C. G., and Ifekwunigwe, A. E.: Evaluation of small-scale nutrition programs, Am. J. Clin. Nutr. **26**:446, 1973.
12. Gordon, J. E., and Scrimshaw, N. S.: Evaluating nutrition intervention programs, Nutr. Rev. **30**:263, 1972.
13. James, G.: Evaluation in public health practice, Am. J. Public Health **52**:1145, 1962.
14. Bigman, S. K.: Evaluating the effectiveness of religious programs, Rev. Relig. Res. **2**:97, Winter, 1961.
15. Herzog, E.: Some guidelines for evaluative research, Social Security Administration, Children's Bureau, U.S. Department of Health, Education, and Welfare, Washington, D.C., 1959.
16. King, S. H.: Perceptions of illness in medical practice, New York, 1962, Russell Sage Foundation.
17. Morris, C.: Varieties of human value, Chicago, 1956, University of Chicago Press.
18. Mullins, T.: Evaluations—the proof is in the program, Presented at the Behavioral Health Program

Evaluation Conference, Scottsdale, Ariz., Dec., 1976.
19. Paul, B. D.: Social science in public health, Am. J. Public Health **46**:1390, 1956.
20. Kandle, R. P.: The need and place of evaluation in public health, First National Conference on Evaluation in Public Health, University of Michigan, Ann Arbor, Mich., 1955.
21. James, G.: Evaluation and planning of health programs, Administration of Community Health Services, International City Managers' Association, Chicago, 1961.
22. Organizational study on programme analysis and evaluation, Geneva, Jan., 1954, World Health Organization.
23. Stouffer, S. A.: Some observations on study design, Am. J. Sociol. **55**:355, 1950.
24. Mann, J. H.: The outcome of evaluative research. In Mann, J. H.: Changing human behavior, New York, 1965, Charles Scribner's Sons.
25. Deniston, O. L., Rosenstock, I. M., and Getting, V. A.: Evaluation of program effectiveness, Public Health Rep. **83**:328, 1968.
26. Webb, E. J., Campbell, P. T., et al.: Unobtrusive measures: nonreactive research in the social sciences, Chicago, 1966, Rand McNally & Co.
27. Campbell, D. T., and Stanley, J. C.: Experimental and quasi-experimental designs for research in teaching, In Travers, R. M. W.: Second handbook of research on teaching, Chicago, 1973, Rand McNally & Co.
28. Kendall, P.: Evaluating an experimental program in medical education. In Miles, M. P., editor: Innovations in education, New York, 1964, Teachers College, Bureau of Publications.
29. Campbell, D. T.: Reforms as experiments, Am. Psychol. **24**:409, 1969.
30. Parsell, A. P.: Dynamic evaluation: the systems approach to action research, Santa Monica, Calif., 1966, Systems Development Corp.
31. Feirweather, G. W.: Methods for experimental social innovation, New York, 1967, John Wiley & Sons, Inc.
32. Freeman, H. E., and Sherwood, C. C.: Research in large-scale intervention programs, J. Soc. Issues **21**: 11, 1965.
33. Suchman, E. A.: Action for what? A critique of eval-

uative research. In O'Toole, R., editor: The organizational management and tactics of social research, Cambridge, Mass., 1970, Schenkman Publishing Co., Inc.

34. Davis, J. A.: Great books and small groups: an informal history of a national survey. In Hammond, P. E., editor: Sociologists at work: essay in the craft of social research, New York, 1964, Basic Books, Inc., Publishers.

35. Lippitt, R., et al.: The dynamics of planner change, New York, 1958, Harcourt Brace Jovanovich, Inc.

36. Weiss, C. H.: The utilization of evaluation toward comparative study. In The use of social research in federal domestic program, Vol. III, Research and Technical Programs Subcommittee, 90th Congress, 1st Session, Washington, D.C., 1967, Government Printing Office.

37. Elinson, J.: Effectiveness of social action programs in health and welfare. In Assessing the effectiveness of child health services, Report of the 56th Ross Conference, Columbus, Ohio, 1967, Ross Laboratories.

SUGGESTED READINGS

Agency for International Development: Evaluation handbook, Washington, D.C., 1971, Government Printing Office.

American Institutes for Research: Evaluative research strategies in methods, Pittsburgh, 1970, American Institutes for Research.

American Public Health Association: A broadened spectrum of health and morbidity, Am. J. Public Health **51:**20287, 1951.

Andersen, S.: Operations research in public health, Indian J. Public Health **7:**141, 1963.

Andrew, G.: Some observations on management problems in applied social research, Am. Sociol. **2:**84, 1967.

Archibald, K. A.: Three views of experts' role in policymaking: systems and analysis incrementalism in the clinical approach, Policy Sci. **1:**73, 1970.

Badgley, R. F.: Planning implementation, and evaluation of community health services: a commentary, Canad. J. Public Health **55:**527, 1964.

Davies, J. O. F., Brotherston, J., Baily, N., Forsyth, G., and Logan, R.: Toward a measure of medical care—operational research in the health services, London, 1962, Oxford University Press.

Densen, P. M.: Research and the community functions of a health department, N. Engl. J. Med. **269:**781, 1963.

Drohny, A.: Evaluation of health programs, Bol. Of. Sanit. Panam. **57:**112, 1964.

Evaluation instruments in health education, Washington, D.C., 1965, American Association of Health, Physical Education and Recreation.

Feldstein, M. S.: Operational research and efficiency in the health service, Lancet **1:**491, 1963.

Fleck, A. C., Jr.: Evaluation as a logical process, Canad. J. Public Health **52:**185, 1961.

Hilleboe, H. E., James, G., and Doyle, J. T. Cardiovascular health center. I. Project design for public health research, Am. J. Public Health **44:**351, 1954.

Hochbaum, G.: Evaluation—a diagnostic procedure, Int. J. Health Educ. **5:**636, 1962.

James, G.: Program planning and evaluation in a modern city health department, Am. J. Public Health **51:**1828, 1961.

Kraus, A. S.: Efficient utilization of statistical activities in public health, Am. J. Public Health **53:**1075, 1963.

Krauss, I.: An approach to evaluating the effectiveness of a public health program, J. Health Hum. Behav. **3:** 141, 1962.

Levine, A. S.: Evaluating program effectiveness and efficiency: rationale and description of research in progress, Welfare Rev. **2:**11, 1967.

Likert, R., and Lippitt, R.: The utilization of social sciences. In Research methods in the behavioral sciences, New York, 1953, Holt, Reinehart, & Winston, Inc.

Linnenberg, C. L., Jr.: How shall we measure economics benefits for public health services? Washington, D.C., 1974, Public Health Service publication no. 1178, Government Printing Office.

Longood, R., and Simmel, A.: Organizational resistance to innovation suggested by research. In Evaluating action programs: readings in social action and education, Boston, 1972, Allyn & Bacon, Inc.

Macchiavello, A.: Evaluation of the economic impact of public health activities, Bol. Of. Sanit. Panam. **52:**25, 1962.

Miller, S. M.: The study of man evaluating action programs, Trans-Action **2**:38, 1965.

Rivlin, A. M.: Systematic thinking for social action, Washington, D.C., 1971, The Brookings Institution.

Roberts, D. E.: How effective is public health nursing? Am. J. Public Health **52**:1077, 1962.

Robinson, J. P., Athanasion, R., and Head, K. B.: Measures of occupational attitudes and occupational characteristics, Ann Arbor, Mich., 1967, Institute for Social Research, University of Michigan.

Rosenblatt, A.: The practitioner's use in evaluation of research, Soc. Work, vols. 10-13, 1968.

Rossi, P. H.: Booby traps and pitfalls in the evaluation of sociology programs. Proceedings of the Social Statistics Section, Washington, D.C., 1966, American Statistical Association.

Ruderman, A. P.: Lessons from Latin American experience: economic benefits from public health services, Washington, D.C., 1964, Public Health Service publication no. 1178, Government Printing Office.

Sax, S.: The organization and evaluation of health services for the aged, Med. J. Aust. **2**:315, 1966.

Schaefer, M., Hilleboe, H. E., and Longwood, R.: The "sine wave" process—a key to better public health planning, Bol. Of. Sanit. Panam. **55**:377, 1963.

Stewart, W. H.: Partnership for planning. Presented at the Surgeon-General's Joint Conference with State and Territorial Health Authorities, Washington, D.C., 1966.

Weiss, C. H.: The politization of evaluation research, J. Soc. Issues **26**:57, 1970.

Weiss, C. H.: Organizational constraints on evaluation research, New York, 1971, Bureau of Applied Social Research.

Wholey, J. S.: The absence of program evaluation as an obstacle to effective public expenditure policy: a case study of child health programs. In the Analysis and evaluation of public expenditure, 91st Congress, 1st Session, Washington, D.C., 1970, Government Printing Office.

World Health Organization: Measurement of levels of health, Technical Report Series no. 137, Geneva, 1957, World Health Organization.

World Health Organization: Planning of Public Health Services, Technical Report Series no. 215, Geneva, World Health Organization.

GENERAL CONCEPT

The understanding of sound fiscal management and the budget process forms one of the most important responsibilities in public health administration. Good financial management and the concept of cost-benefit analysis are tools to answer questions such as: What is being obtained for the expenditure and effort? What does it cost to perform a certain act or to provide a certain service? What are the alternatives and are they efficient and effective?

OUTCOMES

The student should be able to do the following:
- Define and describe cost-benefit analysis and cost effectiveness.
- Define and describe a performance budget.
- Identify the elements and basic priorities of budget preparation.
- Define the necessary elements and phases in presenting a budget to legislators, City Council, or whomever is responsible for funding the programs discussed in the budget.

Budgeting: how to manage finances

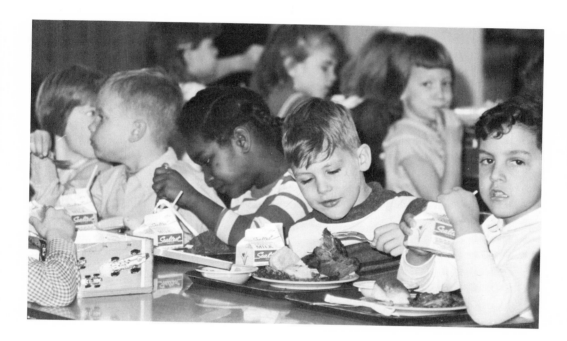

Two areas of fiscal management will be discussed in this chapter. First, cost-benefit analysis will be reviewed as a significant part of the evaluation process, a tool to enhance decision making. Second, the making of fiscal policy and the principles of budgeting will be covered.

In the planning of a program in the public health field, it is up to the administrator to decide which program best meets the local community's needs at the least cost. Here, cost-benefit analysis can be of considerable assistance. This, too, continues to be an essential step in the analysis required in developing a program plan. (See Fig. 3-3.)

COST-BENEFIT ANALYSIS

Cost-benefit analysis is a process whose origin and primary application can be credited to the U.S. Department of Defense. It was an outgrowth of the federal government's desire to determine when to intervene in what had been traditionally considered to be private sector issues.

The development of cost-benefit analysis was based on two economic factors. The first was the recognition that "economists found it increasingly uncomfortable to assume that the basic structure of the economy was that of free competition in which government activities represented only a minor aberration from universal, private decision making."[1] Nevertheless, the federal government accounts for about 20% of the gross national product, which is certainly a considerable expenditure.

The second factor was the government's interest in finding criteria to make best use of its resources. In addition, there was the growing concern of decision makers to improve policy analysis, particularly within the federal government.

Definition of cost-benefit analysis

Cost-benefit analysis has been characterized in the following ways:

1. As an effort to provide more explicit and logically organized information about the effects or outcomes of specific programs or projects.[2]

2. As an attempt "to secure an efficient allocation of resources produced by the governmental system in its interaction with private economy."[3]

3. As a process whereby a public agency in pursuit of economic efficiency allocates its resources in such a way that the most "profitable" projects are executed and developed to the point where marginal benefits equal marginal costs.[4]

4. A process that is based on the assumptions that a specific problem can be identified; that the cost of its consequences can be measured within a permissible range of accuracy; that it can be eradicated or controlled at some predetermined level by a new program; and that the cost of the new program also can be measured.[5]

These descriptions all indicate the purpose and the process of cost-benefit analysis—to best employ the resources at hand by linking the resources to particular goals through coordination of information concerning effectiveness and cost and, finally, being able to recognize at what point the resources are used most efficiently and then implement this information.

The need for cost-benefit analysis occurs because there are always only limited resources available, and choices must be made concerning how to use these most effective-

BASIC HUMAN DESIRES

Good health is one of man's most precious assets. The desire to live, to feel well, to maintain command over one's faculties and to see one's loved ones free from disease, disability, or premature death is one of the most basic of all human desires. In spite of this, no nation can afford or is willing to spend unlimited sums for health preservation. In a climate of limited resources, decision makers must develop priority levels for spending those resources that are available. Although health programs can be amply justified on humanitarian grounds, their competitive position relative to other expenditures may be enhanced by the use of economic justification techniques.

John Amadio, Joyce Mueller, and *Ralph Casey:* Benefit/cost ratios in public health, Is an ounce of prevention really worth a pound of cure? Sponsored by Illinois Department of Health, Southern Illinois University, Carbondale, and Jackson County Health Department, Murphysboro, Ill., Aug., 1976.

ly. Cost-benefit analyses are able to translate alternative choices into a common denominator of dollars and cents. Thus it is a useful tool for comparing the merits of various objectives.[6]

Definition of cost effectiveness

The cost-effectiveness model is a variation of the original cost-benefit analysis model, both of which are pragmatic approaches to very real problems and have little abstract theory underlying their development and application. Decisions based on the data resulting from these analyses are, of course, more objective than the intuitive decisions that otherwise would be made. The purpose of cost-benefit and cost-effectiveness analyses is to improve the decision-making process in real situations.

The following characteristics of cost-effectiveness analysis give an idea of its usefulness:

1. If an issue is a single objective and the aim is to find the best way or alternative (at the least cost) for obtaining this objective, both monetary and nonmonetary data may be reviewed in this process.

2. Because of its fluid conceptual framework, cost-effectiveness analysis includes any study designed to assist a decision maker

USE OF EVALUATION DATA: COST-EFFECTIVENESS

The results of follow-up are used to give an overall evaluation of the effectiveness of the program . . . From such data initial attempts at estimating cost-effectiveness can be made, remembering that we are involved with the reduction of risk rather than the diagnosis and treatment of specific diseases. Thus we get data on the cost-per-child who successfully moves in the direction of lower risk, rather than cost-per-case of disease prevented. If our pediatric and epidemiologic researchers are able to provide us with data on the excess morbidity and mortality associated with such risk factors, then we can go ahead and develop actual cost-effectiveness or even cost-benefit data for the reduction of morbidity and mortality . . . For example, reducing the rate of low birth weight infants, as Arizona has done, prevents a certain amount of infant mortality. The value of each life saved might be expressed in dollar terms as the potential Gross National Product generated by a person over a 70-year lifespan. Using a cost/benefit formula, this value is $105,717.* The maximum cost of WIC services (food, screening, and evaluation, nutrition education and operations at $28/month for 9 months) would be $252. This represents a benefit-to-cost ratio of 419:1, an impressive return on anyone's dollar.

*Amadio, J., Mueller, J., and Casey, R.: Benefit/cost ratios in public health. Is an ounce of prevention really worth a pound of cure? Sponsored by Illinois Department of Health, Southern Illinois University, Carbondale, and Jackson County Health Department, Murphysboro, Ill., Aug., 1976.

J. Michael Lane and *Morissa White:* Personal communication, 1978.

---

identify a preferred choice from among possible alternatives.[7]

3. It is a methodical approach of identifying alternative solutions to a problem (or courses of action) in terms of their costs and effectiveness in attaining some specific objectives. Whereas the costs of the alternatives are always measured in terms of dollars, the effectiveness may be measured in any of a number of terms as long as the term selected is applicable to the alternative under study.[7]

Why use cost-benefit analysis?

Weiss[8] has stated that cost-benefit analysis is most useful in three cases:

1. When existing data (or easily collectible or credibly reconstructible data) indicate the scope and degree of program impact.

2. When the main benefits can be reduced to dollar terms without excessive guesswork or neglect of crucial effects.

3. When general benefit level rather than distributional changes of benefits is the main criterion.

Hyman[6] has stated that cost-benefit analysis is used for three major reasons:

1. It forces the analyst to prepare alternatives, choices, and background analysis concerning the use of scarce resources for the decision maker. Cost-benefit analysis is a tool to aid the decision-maker, not to replace him.

2. It is an excellent tool for conflict management. With many competing interests, proponents of different objectives and programs would be faced with a method that enables the decision-makers to assess their demands, gain perspective and support the decision. Though political and value factors are not eliminated, the decision-maker acquires additional technical knowledge on which to base a decision.

3. It helps integrate the planning-budgeting process by proposing alternatives based on analysis and so greatly improves the analytical capacity required in the planning-budgeting process.

Process of cost-benefit analysis

There are four basic steps in cost-benefit analysis. They include the basic tenets of sound planning:

1. Program objectives must be stated clearly and quantifiably. (Does one want to improve the nutrition services in an ambulatory care setting, or the referral system in the nutrition delivery system to reach a specifically larger number of clients?)

2. After objectives are specified, the outputs expected must be stated. The output implies results. The question should be how many clients maintain their health well enough to perform normally at work, home, and school after their preventive health clinic visits, not how many people attended the preventive health clinic.

3. After objectives and outputs of the program are defined, the total costs of the program for both the first year and as many years as possible should be calculated. This

is necessary because often the first year's expenses will include items such as construction and supply of the facility, whereas subsequently the primary expense will be operating costs. Thus the average yearly cost should be calculated when possible.

4. Finally, the alternatives must be analyzed to determine which has the greatest success in achieving the objectives but at the same time also accomplishes this at the least cost.

In addition to the effects measured in cost-benefit analysis, other side effects must be taken into consideration. Economists refer to these as externalities, which may be either positive or negative.

For example, a new health facility may provide additional jobs for the local community, which would be a positive side effect. However, if the facility is able to offer a higher wage scale than local businesses, this could be seen as a negative side effect by local business. Other side effects could relate to the community's involvement in the facility's operating policies.

Another consideration is the effect of time on the program, which can be measured by a procedure called discounting. If the cost of a service in a year's time will be $105, the present discounted value is about $100, assuming that if the amount were deposited in a bank at an interest rate of 5%, it would be increased to $105 in a year's time. With this procedure, present cost benefits can be compared with future costs, if the latter are discounted to their present value.[9]

Limitations of cost-benefit analysis

Cost-benefit analysis can be extremely helpful to the decision maker, especially if its drawbacks and limitations are kept in mind, as follows:

1. It is difficult to apply a quantifiable measure or a common measure to various kinds of benefits or values. Additionally, it is often difficult to agree on objectives because they, too, involve varying values.

2. Cost analyses are based on the statistically predicted behavior of certain variables, but these variables may behave differently in actuality.[10]

3. Once the analysis has arrived at the point of implementation, there may be a delay in getting the action underway. There may be a number of practical constraints, such as finding a suitable location for a facility, training personnel, or introducing the program to the local community.

4. Cost-benefit analyses are not to be confused with cause-effect analyses. Cost benefit analyses simply give information as to the most economical means of achieving various benefits or objectives, whereas a cause-and-effect analysis would show how a procedure produced a particular effect.

Along with cost-benefit analysis, the decision maker uses his experience and knowledge to make his choices. The cost-benefit procedure will be most useful when the alternatives are specific objectives that are easily quantifiable.

Examples of cost-benefit models
Nutrition model

Dahl[11] points out the cost-effective potential of a nutritional component in health care delivery in a study examining the efficiency of comprehensive health care delivery. The study showed that the presence of a nutritional functional area in a comprehensive health care project for children and youth had the net effect of reducing average registrant cost. He stated that an increase in the allocation of funds to the nutritional functional area by 1 percentage point would be likely to reduce total cost per registrant per year about $1/11$ of a percentage point. In this comprehensive health care delivery system it was found that the average annual registrant cost of $271.52 was $29.30 lower than it otherwise would have been had there been no nutritional functional area in the comprehensive health program.[11]

Another study by Dahl[12] indicated that a major source of nutritional care in the absence of a nutritional functional area was the medical functional area. This study showed that an increase of 1 percentage point of nutritional functional area cost (per registrant per year) would decrease medical functional area cost by $16/100$ or about $1/6$ of a percentage point.

Analysis of the regression components of medical functional area costs showed that the presence of a nutritional functional area was likely to reduce the medical functional area cost by as much as $14.62 per registrant per year, or 13.7%, compared with a situation without a nutritional functional area. In this study the actual nutritional cost per registrant per year for the total program over the project period ranged from $1.81 to $2.66. These figures indicate that the inclusion of a public health nutrition program is a cost-effective strategy in formulating a program of comprehensive health care for children and youths.

Dahl's model used cost-benefit and effectiveness analysis to demonstrate the effectiveness of nutrition services in a comprehensive health care setting. Such rather sophisticated statistical analyses can be used to answer two ever-important questions of "How much money are we saving?" and "How much will it cost the taxpayer?"

Children's health model—study by U.S. Department of Health, Education, and Welfare

At the urging of the President of the United States, in 1966 the Department of Health, Education, and Welfare undertook a study to determine the state of children's health in the country and to see what were the best programs to improve it. The primary concerns were to detect children with correct-able health problems and to determine in what population groups most of them occurred. One of the specific goals was to make maternal and child care services available to health-depressed areas.

Comparative data on the health of expectant mothers and children were not readily available so the study used two criteria to define "health depressed"—maternal and infant mortality and the prevalence of chronic conditions such as mental retardation and hearing and visual problems.

There were at least twelve possible programs aimed at reducing these occurrences. The comparative effectiveness of three such programs is shown in Table 10-1. Two offered comprehensive care to mothers and children, the first with children up to 18 years of age and the second with children up to 5 years. The third program was one of "early case finding," which examined children with specific problems first at 3 years of age and subsequently every other year until 9 years. Each program had an annual budget of $10 million. It is clear that the money was utilized in various ways and produced different results in each program. It would be possible to create, for example, a more effective infant mortality program if all the money were concentrated on reducing this one factor, but then, of course, other benefits would be lost and the amount spent per patient probably would be higher.

Another program analysis by the Depart-

Table 10-1. Yearly effects per $10 million expended in health-depressed areas

	Comprehensive programs to		Case-finding treatment 0,1,3,5,7,9
	18 years of age	5 years of age	
Maternal deaths prevented	1.6	3	
Premature births prevented	100-250	200-485	
Infant deaths prevented	40- 60	85-120	
Mental retardation prevented	5- 7	7- 14	
Handicaps prevented or corrected by 18 years of age:			
Vision problems			
All	350	195	3,470
Amblyopia	60	119	1,140
Hearing loss			
All	90	70	7,290
Binaural	6	5	60
Other physical handicaps	200	63	1,470

Table 10-2. Reduction in number of 18-year-olds with decayed and unfilled teeth per $10 million expended in health-depressed areas

Fluoridation	294,000
Comprehensive dental care without fluoridation	18,000
Comprehensive dental care with fluoridation	44,000

ment of Health, Education, and Welfare, one that aimed at reducing tooth decay and unfilled teeth in 18-year-olds who lived in depressed areas, is illustrated in Table 10-2. It appears that a fluoridation program and comprehensive care with fluoridation greatly reduce the number of patients with dental problems. Thus fluoridation seems the best way to serve the greatest number of people for a given amount of money, although this situation is somewhat simplified, since there were other factors present.

The Department of Health, Education, and Welfare also made analyses of studies that showed the benefits of a family planning program in reducing infant mortality and how the early discovery of handicapping conditions would prevent an acute medical shortage at a future time. Through the useful tool of cost-benefit analysis, the department was instrumental in passing new congressional legislation including the Social Security Amendment of 1967, which provided for early detection of chronic diseases in children and for their treatment and also for research into the training of physician's assistants. Although cost is not the only consideration in deciding about a program, which is also influenced by value judgments and political considerations, such analyses do try to create a more objective viewpoint and clearer issues.[13]

Jackson County public health model

Benefit/Cost Ratios in Public Health[14] by John Amadio and colleagues is an original research report that was sponsored by the Illinois Department of Public Health, Southern Illinois University, Carbondale, and Jackson County Health Department. It is a comprehensive study of public health ser-

vices in a specific area. Amadio states that the objectives of the study were as follows:
1. To develop a formula for determining benefits of basic health programs
2. To apply the formula to known health situations in Jackson County, Illinois, to determine a cash benefit value
3. To derive program benefit-cost ratios for a representative sample of basic public health programs

The study researched about one half of the basic public health services that are provided by the local health department. The programs selected for the study included immunization programs, tuberculosis control program, kidney disease screening, water supply and sewage control, food service inspection, air pollution control, and skilled home nursing care. Preliminary findings indicated that the remaining services would also show positive cost-benefit ratios. Most of the calculations used conservative national or Illinois disease incidence figures. The Amadio study determines a minimum formula needed to calculate the benefits of the public health program and discusses in great detail how the formula is derived.[14]

PERFORMANCE BUDGETING

Performance budgeting is using the cost-benefit analysis in terms of a specific performance.

Performance budgeting and its application to public health has been described by Klepak.[15] It enables the researcher to see how much each unit or individual cost, taking the entire program into account. Thus performance budgeting can save the cost for each immunization in a specific program or the cost of supervising the nutrition aides in a nutrition delivery system.

Advantages

If a cost analysis is possible for all the elements of a program, an effective performance budget can be made. Hanlon[16] points out the following advantages of performance budgeting:
1. Provide effective tools in planning a well-balanced program.

2. Assist in developing short and long-range program objectives.
3. Provide elements for the control of programs and their costs.
4. Provide detailed information concerning work volume and unit cost.
5. Provide a sound basis for comparing past, present, and future activities of programs and performance.
6. Aid greatly in supporting requests for funds on a demonstrable and realistic basis.
7. Discourage padding of the budget by the program directors.
8. Aid in the sound expansion and contraction of program activities.
9. Permit personnel to see relationships among activities and programs.
10. Provide qualitative and quantitative measures of personnel and departmental efficiency.

It must be stressed that such goals for performance budgeting are based on the ideal situation, where measures of performance standards can be clearly and objectively developed, and so the budgeting can imply how specific expenditures can result in certain accomplishments. In the nutrition field such standards are just beginning to be developed. The American Dietetic Association has recently published two documents that represent steps in this area, *Professional Standards Review Procedure Manual* and *Guidelines for Evaluating Dietetic Practice.*

Steps required in developing a performance budget

Generally, however, in any field a performance budget ought to be developed with a good deal of planning that, Michael[17] states, involves consideration of the following steps:

1. Identification and comparison of health problems
2. Determining measurable even if ambitious goals for each of these problems
3. Recognition and analysis of the kind of community the program will be in
4. Analysis of the causes of health problems
5. Development of various plans or programs to combat problems
6. Cost-benefit and cost-effectiveness analyses

for each of the alternative programs, and all of their elements
7. Establishment of both long and short range objectives for these programs
8. Procedure for on-going evaluation

Performance budgeting is most difficult when the programs deal with preventive actions, such as avoidance of an epidemic or reduction of accidents. Here, some evaluation of the net benefits when compared with costs should be made and, difficult as it may seem, some practical measurements usually can be discovered. When thinking about costs in making a performance budget, Hanlon suggests the following guidelines:

1. There should be a record of accumulated costs, reflecting the activity of the program.
2. Fixed costs should be separated from variable costs. In other words, certain expenditures may increase or decrease as the program progresses, whereas others remain fixed.
3. Variable costs should be related to work load and goal achievement, so that the efficiency of the program may be determined and appraised.
4. Often a health program's central activity is offering inter-personal services, rather than using many materials, so that the importance and cost of such services far outweighs that for materials.
5. While specific programs are usually measured, sometimes additional knowledge can be gained if a performance budget is developed for a larger category of programs, such as public health nutrition or laboratory work.

Often measuring services in terms of cost is a simple but effective tool in measuring the efficiency of a program. If, for example, one wished to determine the cost per patient in a maternal health clinic, one would divide the total operating costs per year, which would be mainly manpower, by the total number of patients seen in a year. Or, in the case of laboratory work, the total cost of manpower and materials used in a year divided by the total number of laboratory examinations in a year would give the cost per examination.[16]

DEVELOPMENT OF FISCAL POLICY

To develop any kind of accurate cost-benefit analysis or performance budget, there must be a sound fiscal policy that serves as the backbone of a program. This includes having a clear and informative budget.

Whereas any kind of expenditure issuing from a private source is determined by an accounting of profits and costs, public funds are often allocated with no such guidelines and generally depend on the need for services even more than the desire for such services. In the public sector, fiscal policy making is the legislature's job, which includes the collection of revenues, the establishment of programs, and the efficient operation of these programs. The actual implementation of these programs involves collection of revenues and disbursement of public money, budgeting, accounting, and purchasing. The health administrator is primarily concerned with the last three of these.[16]

Budgeting

As head of a program, the health administrator is responsible for the money it will use, and for this a budget is necessary. All monies received should be in the budget, whether they are from the government, private sector, or grants, and they should be in the custody of the state or local treasurer. Generally, funds belong to one of several categories.[18]

Expendable funds

General fund. Most of the available money is usually here, and its use is unrestricted, as

long as it is within the functioning of the program.

Special funds. This money is usually set aside for special purposes, and so its use is restricted. Therefore it is seldom transferable and should not be considered as part of the general budget.

Sinking funds. These are usually special funds set aside to redeem bonds or repay other kinds of loans.

Under the heading of "working capital funds" are those funds used for the program's activities; they are generally replenished by transfers from other funds.

Endowment funds. The principal usually cannot be expended, but interest accrued from the investment of endowment funds generally can be used for specified purposes.

Suspense funds. These are earmarked for special purposes, and are usable when transferred to another fund.[16]

Purposes of budgeting

The purposes of a budget in a public health nutrition program are to indicate how and at what rate money is to be expended and thus to regulate expenditures over a period of time. A budget can help prevent waste by showing where the responsibility is for each aspect of an organization and the coordination and relationship between the aspects. It also can indicate where expansion is possible and if outcomes are not coinciding with projected estimates. Mainly, it can give an early indication of future financial requirements and possibly where such revenue may come from. It goes without saying that an informative budget is an essential to administrative directors and other persons who are in control of funds.

Prerequisites to budget preparation

Before preparing the budget, there are certain prerequisites to keep in mind. First is a belief in its value as a necessary tool and the desire to follow it. This involves not only the cooperation of the preparers but of their subordinates as well. To ensure a well-coordinated program, the director should request that his divisions or unit heads submit budget

---

HEALTH ECONOMICS

The concepts of demand, supply, the market, and industry are extremely useful tools for organizing analysis of resource allocation problems which underlie many health policy issues. Since health services are much different from those of other commodities, their production and distribution involves an expenditure of limited resources as in the case of any other commodity. Thus economic principles and concepts are relevant and are essential to a fuller understanding of the consequences of most health policy issues.

James R. Jeffers: Health economics: wants, needs, and demands. Reprinted from Kane, R. L., editor: Challenges of community medicine, New York, 1974, Springer Publishing Co., Inc. Copyright © 1974 by Springer Publishing Co., Inc. Used by permission.

proposals for their divisions well in advance of the date on which the final comprehensive budget is due. Each of these should be in accordance with the fiscal policy of the whole program, and there also should be ample time for the staff to go over the proposals for any alterations and refinements that might be necessary. Nevertheless, the responsibility and authority for the supervision of following the budget is usually handled best by a single, highly capable individual.

Second, estimates of future expenditures should be based on past experiences, and estimates of assets should be inclusive but realistic. All expected funds should have their sources indicated. Where relevant, the budget should consider administrative, functional, and depreciation costs, possibilities for expansion of the program, and most emphatically, coordination of various activities.[16]

Third, to prepare the best kind of budget, the health official or budget maker should be aware of the fiscal policies and goals of the many groups that might in some way influence the program, such as various other governmental agencies, the legislative and executive branches of government, political parties, labor organizations, citizens' groups, and business groups.[16]

Budget preparation

A budget may be highly detailed, as in a "line itemed" budget, or more simple, as in a "lump sum" budget. The latter allows more leeway, but it does not have the control and planning offered by a detailed budget. Whatever the choice, or if it is a compromise of the two possibilities, the budget should be organized into separate units, bureaus, or divisions if it is a comprehensive budget for an entire public health service; then it may be broken down further within each unit. For example, the nutrition department would have its own divisions into operating expenses, including supplies, salaries, etc., capital costs, fixed charges, and perhaps the subvention or disbursing of funds to other more local programs. An example of a state budget for the Division of Community

Health Services and the Bureau of Nutrition Services, along with the program's goals, appears on pp. 296 to 298.

Sometimes it is also necessary to have a budget justification, which is a brief but adequate description of the need and reasons for money for a particular area. This is especially necessary if a budget analyst must make decisions about giving certain areas priority over others. An example of a state's budget justification for its Bureau of Nutrition Services appears on p. 299.

Although every budget is different and the health administrator or budget preparer should know of previous budgets for his division and the larger budget of which his division is a part, there are certain basic principles and considerations that every budget should include. These have been delineated by Geiger[19] and in brief they are as follows:

1. Budget or expenditures of the preceding period, which should be equal to the time period of the present budget.
2. Budget of the present period, which of course will include estimates of future expenditures and actual expenditures thus far.
3. Changes in the present budget, which will keep the budget up to date by recording anticipated increases or decreases.
4. Objects of expenditure, including salaries, fees, materials, fixed costs, etc.
5. Estimates for the future budget, based on the present budget, and a comparison between the two.
6. The final adopted and approved budget, including recommendations.

Thus the making of each budget is actually a preparation for the next one as well. After the budget is prepared and reviewed on the administrative level, it often is reviewed and authorized on the legislative level. The next step is implementing it or putting it into operation, and finally there is an evaluation to see that it has been implemented correctly and according to the law.[16]

Frequently, the final budget must be presented and justified at hearings in both the House and Senate in competition with other budgets so that the importance of its clarity and concision cannot be overestimated. Most recently, President Carter has pledged to try and implement zero-based budgeting, which would require justifications of all the money spent at all levels of government programs. This would be done by preparing new budgets annually and accounting for all moneys used in old as well as new programs. Traditionally, only new programs had new budgets, and these were simply superimposed on top of the old programs and budgets. However, zero-based budgeting would force all program directors to start from zero in preparing their budgets.

Presenting the budget

As indicated earlier, a thorough knowledge of the budget's elements, familiarity with past and current health programs, and an awareness of influential groups and pressures are essential in preparing an acceptable budget. It is even more vital to have such information when presenting the budget to a committee. In addition, a knowledge of the biases and preferences of the committee, even their voting records and biographies, is equally vital. Those who are known to be interested in a program's objectives should be kept informed and invited to observe the program's activities in the periods between budget hearings. Committee members may also be asked their advice because of their experience in financial matters. Likewise, the presenter of the budget should have attended other hearings of this committee to be aware of their interests and tone.

It is wise to review pertinent information on committee members, such as their voting records and biographies to speak their language. Draffin[20] suggests that anyone with budget approval authority who shows interest in health and health programs or in the health agencies should be cultivated by providing them with interesting and meaningful information and data, not merely in relation to the budget process but especially between budget periods. They should be invited to attend and, if possible, to participate in various meetings of the agencies, and their ideas and opinions should be solicited.

Generally, after a preliminary hearing, the budget, perhaps after some alterations, will go to the government head or a board of auditors, where it is again reviewed before being sent to the legislature or finance committee. Here the program head and his staff may again have to present and justify it. It is then considered, along with other programs and its adherence to government fiscal policy, and approved. Often there is an advance preliminary hearing much earlier, where the program staff can discuss the budget with government officials.

It should be apparent to the committee that the program is well managed and adheres to its budget with a minimal amount of transfer of funds and deviation from the plan. It should also be shown that the budget is a useful tool in informing the public as to the program's activities, in making requests for grants and other forms of aid, and in demonstrating the value and efficiency of the program and its procedures.[20]

MANAGING FINANCES

It is evident that the health officer, to plan his health programs efficiently, to utilize the health dollar to the best advantage, and to remain within his budget limitations, must assure himself that he has prepared his budget properly, that its terms are applied correctly, and that shifts in programs are adjusted as the funds permit. To do this he must familiarize himself with the principles of the local fiscal requirements and must obtain the best fiscal advice and aid available.

John J. Hanlon: Public health administration and practice, ed. 6, St. Louis, 1974, The C. V. Mosby Co., p. 270.

ACCOUNTING

To know the financial situation of a program, accounting records should be accurate and up to date. This is done by keeping a general ledger, in which all transactions are posted, and detailed accounts of expenditures and receipts. This should include where they come from, where they are going, and the type.

One procedure that is being used more by accounting departments in public health agencies is encumbered control, which is designed to ensure adequate funds for future payment of obligations made in the present. The Emergency Maternity and Infant Care Program, which operated during World War II, provides a convenient example. Lump sum allotments were paid to the state each month on the basis of estimated number of births that would occur during the following month. It was somewhat as if payments were being made before the services were actually rendered rather than on their completion some months in the future. In this way the state could ascertain at any time the total amount of nonobligated funds available with which to provide care for additional individuals. In addition, it provided a basis on which to apply in advance for deficiency allotments.

The program involved various types of services, for example, obstetric, medical, surgical, hospital, and nursing. With cases of uncomplicated pregnancy and childbirth, the procedure was relatively simple. A standard fee was agreed on by the medical profession and each state health department. When a private physician notified the health department that he was assuming the care of a woman who was expected to give birth normally 6 months hence, for example, it was a simple matter immediately to set aside or encumber a sum of money sufficient to cover the physician's standard fee and the anticipated hospital bill. The latter could be rather accurately estimated as the product of the hospital's per diem bed cost and the average number of days that patients in the locality or state stayed in the hospital after giving birth.

In cases such as pregnancy, or situations where the time factor and expense can be fairly well known beforehand, this procedure is effective and uncomplicated in ensuring certain funds for the future. However, in cases where the details are not as predictable, the costs must be estimated, based on standardized fees and expenses. Care must be taken to ensure that too much is not set aside, or else there will be unused funds. On the other hand, too little set aside will mean not enough for future expenses. The accounting records should at all times reflect an up-to-date amount of encumbered and unobligated funds.[16]

PURCHASING

The main point about purchasing that needs to be made here is the recognition that lately there has been a movement away from individual units' expenditures spread out among a variety of business suppliers. Instead, there has been a development of the public purchasing agency that acts as service to centralize purchases. The advantages of this agency are that it can be more efficient by obtaining the best bids and exercising quality control and testing procedures. Financially, delivery and unit costs are reduced, accounting is more efficient, and ordering and disbursement of payments are more efficient.

However, there may be certain disadvantages or problems that have to be considered with such central agencies—increased bureaucracy and red tape, less control over choice of specific materials especially if one brand is substituted for another, and unclear regulations about handling such difficulties.

As in all aspects of efficient program maintenance, an understanding relationship and direct communication among the divisions of the program (including the purchasing agency) are absolutely essential. The requirements for a program should be clearly available and meticulously presented to all those involved so that the purchasers can operate quickly and efficiently. All groups in a program should recognize that the necessity is cooperation in the creation and implementation of fiscal policy, as elsewhere.

SUMMARY

In planning a program in the public health field, it is up to the administrator to decide which particular program best meets the local community's needs at the least cost. To do this, the administrator should have a sound knowledge of the principles of budgeting and the use of various procedures that are helpful in making such decisions.

Among these tools are cost-benefit analysis, which allows the decision maker to see which allocation of resources is most efficient by measuring input of material, personnel, etc., and their effectiveness in terms of cost.

Another tool is cost-effectiveness analysis, which also measures alternative programs in terms of cost. Here, however, the effectiveness does not have to be reduced to dollars and cents but may be presented in other terms that are applicable and comparable to other programs.

One tool that is used in analysis is the development of a performance budget that measures a specific performance. As long as the factors are identifiable and measurable, it can create a ratio that clearly indicates the cost per unit and so shows the efficiency and effectiveness of a particular operation.

These operations and analyses all rely on a sound and informative budget, which acts as a guide and financial plan for a program. A clear, itemized, and thorough budget is essential in obtaining financial support and in setting up and maintaining a program. A budget should include all assets and expenditures and possibly explanations or justifications for these. It should provide indicators for future development as well as showing how it is based on past budgets and experience. A knowledge of the organizational and political complex surrounding the program is vital in the preparation and presentation of a budget, as are other elements in maintaining and managing a program's fiscal needs, such as accounting, purchasing, and implementing the budget.

REFERENCES

1. Haveman, R. H., and Margolis, J.: Public expenditures and policy analysis, Chicago, 1970, Markham Publishing Co.
2. Gross, B. M.: The new systems budgeting, Public Admin. Rev., March-April, 1969.
3. Wildavsky, A.: The political economy of efficiency: cost-benefit analysis, system analysis, and program budgeting, Public Admin. Rev. 26:297, 1966.
4. Hill, M.: A goal-achievement matrix for evaluating alternative plans. In Robinson, editor: Decision-making in urban planning, Beverly Hills, Calif., 1972, Sage Publications, Inc.
5. Steiner, K. C., and Smith, H. A.: Application of cost-benefit analysis to a PKU screening program, Inquiry 10:34, Dec., 1973.
6. Hyman, H. H.: Health planning: a systematic approach, Germantown, Md., 1975, Aspen Systems Corp.
7. Quade, E. S.: Cost-effectiveness: an introduction and overview. Presented at a Symposium on Cost-Effectiveness Analysis, June 14-16, 1965.
8. Weiss, C. H.: Evaluation research, Englewood Cliffs, N.J., 1972, Prentice-Hall, Inc.
9. Galloway, G. M.: The uses of cost-benefit analysis in analyzing recreational facility expenditure, Symposium of Administrative Thinking and Practice in Athletics—Physical Education, University of Michigan, Ann Arbor, Mich., Oct. 31, 1972.
10. Akman, A., and Gordon, J. B.: Systems analysis and operational health, Public Admin. Rev. 60: 1970.
11. Dahl, T.: Economics, management and public health nutrition, J. Am. Diet Assoc. 70:144, 1977.
12. Dahl, T.: The medical functional area in comprehensive health care delivery for children: an economic analysis, Study Service no. 3-2 (20), Minneapolis, Minnesota, 1973, Minnesota Systems Research Inc.
13. U.S. Department of Health, Education, and Welfare, Office of the Assistant Secretary (Planning and Evaluation): Delivery of health services for the poor, Dec., 1967; Nursing manpower program, March, 1968; Public Health Service, Bureau of Health Services, Recommendations and summary: program analysis of health care facilities, Government Printing Office.
14. Amadio, J., Mueller, J., and Casey, R.: Benefit/cost ratios in public health, Illinois Department of Health, Southern Illinois University, Carbondale, and Jackson County Health Department, Murphysboro, Illinois, August, 1976.
15. Klepak, D.: Performance budgeting for the health department, Public Health Rep. 71:868, 1956.
16. Hanlon, J. J.: Public health administration and practice, ed. 6, St. Louis, 1974, The C. V. Mosby Co.
17. Michael, J. M.: Planning—programming—budgeting and health program planning. In The executive process in public health administration, Ann Arbor, Mich., 1968, University of Michigan School of Public Health.
18. Mitchell, W. E., and Walter, S.: State and local finances, New York, 1970, The Ronald Press Co.
19. Geiger, J.: Health officers manual, Philadelphia, 1939, W. B. Saunders Co.
20. Draffin, E. C.: Budget presentation. In Lee, E.,

editor: Proceedings of the Institute on Administration in Crippled Children's Services, Berkeley, Calif., June 24-29, 1962, University of California School of Public Health.

SUGGESTED READINGS

Avnet, H.: Physician service patterns and illness rates, New York, 1967, Group Health Insurance, Inc.

Bogart, E. L.: Economic history of the United States, New York, 1924, Longmans, Green & Co.

Campbell, R. R.: Economics of health and public policy, Washington, D.C., 1971, American Enterprise Institute.

Cohn, E.: Public expenditure analysis, Lexington, Mass., 1972, D. C. Heath & Co.

Cooper, B. S., Worthington, N. L., and McGee, M. F.: Compendium of national health expenditures data, Washington, D.C.; 1972, Government Printing Office.

Cooper, M. H., and Culyer, A. J.: Health economics: selected readings, Baltimore, 1973, Penguin Books, Inc.

Dublin, L. I., and Lotka, A. J.: The money value of a man, New York, 1946, The Ronald Press Co.

Erhardt, C. L., and Berlin, J., editors: Mortality and morbidity in the United States, Cambridge, Mass., 1974, Harvard University Press.

Guttentag, M., and Striening, E. L., editors: Handbook of evaluation research, Beverly Hills, Calif., 1975, Sage Publications, Inc.

Kelly, W. J.: A cost effectiveness study of clinical methods of birth control: with special reference to Puerto Rico, New York, 1971, Praeger Publishers, Inc.

Klarman, H. E.: The economics of health, New York, 1965, Columbia University Press.

Klarman, H. E.: Empirical studies in health economics, Baltimore, 1970, John Hopkins University Press.

Papenfuss, J. K., and Fjelsted, B. L.: Cost-benefit study of selected interventions in control and prevention of tuberculosis in the state of Utah, Salt Lake City, 1969, Utah State Division of Health.

Prindle, R. A.: Economic benefits from public health, objectives, methods and examples of measurements, Washington, D.C., 1973, HEW publication no. 1178, Government Printing Office.

Rice, D. P.: Estimating the cost of illness, Washington, D.C., May, 1966, Public Health Service publication no. 947-6, Government Printing Office.

Ruchlin, H. S., and Rogers, D. C.: Economics and health care, Springfield, Ill., 1973, Charles C Thomas, Publisher.

Weisbrod, B. A.: Economics of public health, Philadelphia, 1961, University of Pennsylvania Press.

Appendix 10-1

THE HYPOTHETICAL STATE PROGRAM INFORMATION

Agency: *Department of Health Services*   Program: *Division of Community Health Services*
(Summary)

Program description

The Division of Community Health Services is responsible for the planning, organization, coordination, implementation, and evaluation of programs concerned with the delivery of health care to the community. The following services are provided: Preventive health care including health education, nutrition, and dental health. Detection, diagnosis, and treatment of disease including venereal disease, tuberculosis, immunization, acute disease control, cervical cancer screening, and the State Laboratory.

Program goal

To provide and promote quality health care to include prevention, detection, diagnosis, and curative services to the hypothetical state in coordination with health care providers.

Program plans

1. To provide leadership and direction for all programs in Community Health Services with emphasis on evaluation of programs in terms of effectiveness, efficiency, need for expansion, and cost containment or discontinuance. These activities will be monitored on a quarterly basis.
2. To complete a review of the Tuberculosis Hospitalization and Subvention Program in the state and program staff utilizing programmatic review and cost containment measures by January, 1977. Recommendations will be made to the Director for further direction of this program.
3. To maintain necessary surveillance systems for monitoring disease occurrence and control activities.
4. To evaluate all licensed laboratory facilities to ensure compliance with licensure statute.
5. To deliver nutrition and supplemental food services to 36,200 individuals and their families, including 1,000 older adults, to reduce the prevalence of malnutrition (undernutrition and overnutrition) by 20% in one year.
6. To develop educational plans for each Department of Health Services division based on needs, goals, and priorities.
7. To provide dental preventive-education services for 1,350 elementary schoolchildren; provide treatment services for 950 indigent elementary schoolchildren; develop and implement multiple topical fluoride mouth rinse programs involving a minimum of 5,000 schoolchildren, resulting in a 30% reduction in dental disease.

Program results

1. Implemented a program of staff development in program planning, evaluation, and management by objectives to assist the manager to develop and achieve the objectives established for the division and for their specific program areas.

THE HYPOTHETICAL STATE PROGRAM INFORMATION—cont'd

2. Completed the 314(d) Plan for the Department of Health Services to fulfill federal requirements to obtain these funds.
3. Surveillance activities in Bureau of Disease Control and Laboratory Services resulted in the reporting and processing of 8,400 cases and suspected cases of reportable diseases other than veneral disease and tuberculosis.
4. The State Laboratory discontinued selected routine services and diverted resources to more critical areas. Each licensed hospital and independent clinical laboratory in the state was inspected during the year.
5. The Nutrition Program screened 30,230 people in 14 counties and 9 Indian tribes. Screening revealed that 58% of the population had a high serum cholesterol, 13% were anemic, 5.2% were underwieght, and 14.6% were overweight. Supplemental food and nutrition instruction was provided to 46,400 WIC recipients—12,280 infants, 11,800 pregnant and lactating women, and 22,320 children.
6. Health education personnel continued coordination of statewide venereal disease education programs, completing the first statewide venereal disease workshop. Health education personnel identified and began assessment of existing health education programs throughout the state.
7. Eight percent (8%) more children received dental preventive and treatment services; 10% more children received free toothbrushes at no cost; 92% more contacts were made at parent and civic group meetings; and 44% more patients received dental services.

THE HYPOTHETICAL STATE PROGRAM INFORMATION

Agency: *Department of Health Services*   Program: *Bureau of Nutrition Services*

Program description

Plans, develops, and implements nutrition services. Priority for services is placed on the following high-risk groups: women in childbearing years, 0- to 5-year-olds, schoolchildren, adults (parents of children), and the elderly. Services are delivered through five systems—screening, referral, monitoring, aide development, and food delivery—to decrease undernutrition and overnutrition. The bureau administers the special Supplemental Food Program for Women, Infants, and Children (WIC), which reaches 60% of the high-risk population; provides training in nutrition to community health workers, allied health personnel, group care facilities, educational institutions, and the public; formalizes training through community colleges and universities to develop indigenous nutrition manpower.

Program goal

To develop and provide quality nutrition services as an integral component of health care, thereby improving nutrition and health in the population with a reduction in the number of people requiring sick care services and a decrease in health care costs.

Continued.

THE HYPOTHETICAL STATE PROGRAM INFORMATION—cont'd

Program plans

1. To deliver nutrition and supplemental food services to 36,200 individuals and their families, including 1,000 older adults, to reduce the prevalence of malnutrition (undernutrition and overnutrition) by 30% in one year.
2. To implement the statewide nutrition surveillance system by January, 1977 for use by local health-related agencies as a tool for monitoring, program planning, and evaluation.
3. Training in nutrition: (a) 90% of community nutrition workers will be able to develop, implement, and evaluate the client nutrition education plan within 7 months of employment; (b) 60% of nutritionists and dietitians and 3% of other health personnel will participate in at least one training session with evaluation mechanism; (c) 90% of the management personnel in aged, day care, and other group care facilities referred for nutritional care and/or food service assistance will be followed to bring at least one previously deficient factor to standard; (d) 75% of those in educational facilities will implement one or more follow-up sessions in which nutrition is related to one or more existing disciplines in the curriculum; (e) 7% of the public will receive nutrition information to improve their diets and/or learn of other sources of help through consultation, group sessions, and mass media.
4. To develop a career ladder for community nutrition workers by June, 1977.

Program results

1. *Screening.* Screened 30,230 people in 14 counties and 9 Indian tribes. Screening revealed that 58% of the population had a high serum cholesterol, 13% were anemic, 16.9% were short for their age, 5.2% were underweight, and 14.6% were overweight.
2. *Monitoring.* Follow-up of those at risk resulted in 41.4% of the population decreasing their high serum cholesterol level, 65% of the population overcoming anemia, 44% making improvements in their height measurements, 51% overcoming underweight, and 22% reducing overweight. A survey on outcome of pregnancy in three projects showed 92% to 100% of WIC mothers delivered full-term mature infants. A computer system to facilitate program evaluation was designed and piloted and will be implemented statewide August, 1976.
3. *Referral.* Approximately 4,500 referrals were made to and from the nutrition program, utilizing over 100 different agencies.
4. *Supplemental Food and Nutrition Instruction* was provided to 46,400 WIC recipients—12,280 infants, 11,800 pregnant and lactating women, and 22,320 children.
5. *Training.* Trained 132 (100%) community nutrition workers; 7 (100% EPSDT) health assistants; 198 (62%) nutritionists and dietitians; 271 (1.5%) other health personnel; 161 (11.5%) of the personnel in aged and group care facilities; 1,061 (0.1%) of those in educational facilities; 455,733 (20%) of the public through 49 workshops, 84 on-the-job inservice programs, 72,099 individual consultation sessions, 3 seminars and 31 mass media presentations. A curriculum was designed for the education of community nutrition workers to improve job skills and mobility; 27 (25%) community nutrition workers are enrolled at a community college in a pilot for evaluation.

THE HYPOTHETICAL STATE SUMMARY OF EXPENDITURES
AND BUDGET REQUESTS

Agency: *Department of Health Services*   Program: *Community Health Services*

Expenditure classification	Actual expenditures 1975-1976	Estimated expenditures 1976-1977	Increase (decrease) requested			Request 1977-1978	Recommended 1977-1978
			A	B	C		
FTE No.	58.00	57.75			8.00	65.75	
Personal services	592.7	717.5	7.2	7.2	111.3	843.2	
Employee related	96.5	115.5	1.1	1.1	11.8	129.5	
Professional services	39.8	31.1	1.4	2.4	5.4	40.3	
Travel—in	41.8	53.3	6.1	3.0	17.1	79.5	
Travel—out	3.0	3.7	0.9	2.4	2.4	9.4	
Food							
Other operating expenditures	359.6	517.2	10.9	25.5	82.0	635.6	
Equipment	19.7	11.0	1.4	1.9	30.7	45.0	
Operations subtotal	1,153.1	1,449.3	29.0	43.5	260.7	1,782.5	
Other	1,173.5	1,112.3			331.0	1,443.3	
Total appropriated	2,326.6	2,561.6	29.0	43.5	591.7	3,225.8	
Add federal funds							
Add other funds	117.3	415.0			(211.5)	203.5	

Total program

THE HYPOTHETICAL STATE SUMMARY OF EXPENDITURES
AND BUDGET REQUESTS

Agency: *Department of Health Services*   Program: *Bureau of Nutrition Services*

Expenditure classification	Actual expenditures 1975-1976	Estimated expenditures 1976-1977	Increase (decrease) requested			Request 1977-1978	Recommended 1977-1978
			A	B	C		
FTE No.	4.75	4.75				4.75	
Personal services	49.5	65.1	0.7	0.6	0.5	66.9	
Employee related	8.0	10.5	0.1	0.1	(0.4)	10.3	
Professional services	1.7	15.1	0.3	0.5		15.9	
Travel—in	5.7	6.0				6.0	
Travel—out	0.3	0.5	0.1	0.2		0.8	
Food							
Other operating expenditures	12.4	24.1	2.1	4.4		91.7	
Equipment		1.3	(0.4)			0.9	
Operations subtotal	77.6	122.6	2.9	5.8	61.2	192.5	
Other	128.8	152.3				263.3	
Total appropriated	206.4	274.9	2.9	5.8	172.2	455.8	
Add federal funds							
Add other funds							

Total program

THE HYPOTHETICAL STATE PROGRAM INFORMATION

Agency: *Department of Health Services*   Program: *Bureau of Nutrition Services*

At A and B level funding: Funds would be insufficient to cover merit increases. Continued lack of opportunity for advancement may result in high staff turnover, especially in the field of nutrition, where nationwide salaries are more competitive.

At C level funding: Five nutrition personnel (4.75 FTEs) will be funded to complete the following duties related to program planning, implementation, and evaluation of nutrition services for 34,795 individuals.

Public Health Nutrition Director

1. Responsible for program planning, direction, and evaluation for delivery of nutrition services to 34,795 clients, which is a 27% increase in the aging and non–WIC eligible segment of the population over the period between 1976 and 1977.
2. Responsible for directing and implementing the hypothetical state's role in national nutrition surveillance and state-based data collection and analysis for use by local health-related agencies. Responsible for collection and evaluation of data on nutritional care services for older adults. Overall direction of $10 million federally funded Supplemental Food Program for high-risk pregnant women and children, serving 27,500 clients.

Public Health Nutrition Specialist II (Training Coordinator)

1. Responsible for coordination of statewide training activities through the identification of need, cataloging of resources, planning of programs, and establishment of evaluation tools to provide training in nutrition for the following:
   a. 90% of community nutrition workers will be trained so that they will be able to develop, implement and evaluate nutrition education plan within 7 months of employment.
   b. 60% of nutritionists and dietitians and 3% of other health personnel should participate in at least one training session with an evaluation mechanism.
   c. 90% of the management personnel in aged, day care, and other group care facilities referred for nutritional care and other group care facilities referred for nutritional care and/or food service assistance will be followed so that at least one previously deficient factor is brought to standard.
   d. 75% of those in educational facilities will implement one or more follow-up sessions in which nutrition is related to one or more existing disciplines in the curriculum.
   e. 7% of the public will receive nutrition information through consultation, group sessions, and mass media.
2. Serves as liaison between Bureau of Nutrition Services and other Department of Health service bureaus, local health departments, and other health agencies in the areas of training statewide.
3. Responsible for the development and implementation of a career ladder for community nutrition workers in conjunction with the local community college.

Public Health Nutrition Specialist II (75% FTE)

1. Provides technical assistance in public health nutrition for persons 55 years of age and older with services to 1,000 aging individuals statewide. Promotes, conducts, and assists in conducting training programs in nutritional care and food services with an evaluation mechanism for 10% of the personnel in aged and group care facilities in fourteen counties.
2. Provides information or counseling in nutrition to the public and other agencies statewide.
3. Participates in coordinating field experience throughout the state for master's students, dietetic trainees, and others from twelve university settings in the United States.

THE HYPOTHETICAL STATE PROGRAM INFORMATION—cont'd

Public Health Nutrition Specialist II (funded by Maternal and Child Health, assigned to nutrition)

1. Integrates and coordinates Special Supplemental Food Program (WIC) with existing health department programs of MCH and nutrition in seven counties.
2. Analyzes nutrition surveillance data for seven counties for program planning, evaluation, and monitoring services for cost effectiveness and contractual compliance.

Secretary III

1. Provides administrative support and prepares a variety of involved statistical and fiscal reports for Public Health Nutrition Director.
2. Maintains correspondence with subvention contractors, other bureaus, and outside agencies and people; maintains filing system for the bureau.
3. Arranges travel schedules, conferences, presentations for Director.

Clerk Typist II

1. Types reports and correspondence for one nutrition specialist.
2. Other responsibilities include answering telephone, greeting visitors, explaining rules and regulations to public, and making appointments.

THE HYPOTHETICAL STATE PROGRAM INFORMATION

Agency: *Department of Health Services*   Program: *Bureau of Nutrition Services*

At B level funding: An additional 2,061 cholesterol determinations at 78.4 cents per test* would be completed for $1,616. This is the estimated number of tests necessary to screen and follow-up the clients to be served at this funding level (34,700 clients). An additional $663 is needed for educational materials.

At C level funding: A total of 34,795 clients would be screened. The additional cholesterol tests would cost $119.* No increase is requested in any category other than institutional supplies.

———

*Cost per test includes standards and controls.

GENERAL CONCEPT

Legislation and related public policies will determine the future of the health system as well as the practice of the health professional. Therefore a knowledge of the legal process and political system is essential.

OUTCOMES

The student should be able to do the following:
- Recognize the need for advocacy skills on the part of health care professionals.
- Know the requirements and procedures for successful lobbying.
- Have an understanding of the legislative process and the branches of government that control it.
- Gain knowledge of previous federal legislation regarding nutrition.

Legislation

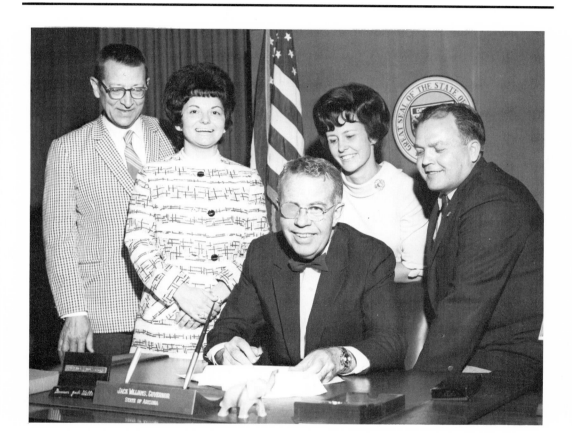

A knowledge and understanding of the legal process and the political system is essential for the public health worker, particularly the nutritionist or the dietitian who may be in charge of planning, initiating, and maintaining a comprehensive program. The importance of nutrition in maintaining health and preventing disease and also the vital role of nutritional care during illness have been established. Now it is necessary that this be communicated to those empowered to enact health legislation so that provision can be made for including nutrition education, nutrition services, and nutrition research as a most significant component in health and consumer legislation.

Legislation and related public policies will determine the future of health programs, the conditions under which health professionals will practice and, indeed, whether they will practice. The government is becoming more and more involved in the delivery of health services.

Public policy is the culmination of activities initiated by individuals or groups that have an effect on the lives of other individuals or groups in society. Public policies are adopted and implemented through public laws, programs, or institutions. Before any desired activity can become a public law or program, however, it must go through a political process.

In a real sense public policy is determined by legislators who make legislative decisions within a framework of personal priorities, limited dollars, constituent concerns, and political compromise. As voters and as representatives of an organized group, health professionals can influence and, in fact, help shape public policy on behalf of the public interest by communicating their concerns, directly and emphatically, to their legislators. It is the operation of the political system that determines the role of government in relation to health. Public health programs are financed and the broad organizational patterns for implementation of these programs are outlined according to basic policy decisions. At a conference held in 1961, sponsored by the American Public Health Association and the U.S. Public Health Service, it was concluded that public health workers were inadequately informed and

---

THE DIETITIAN IN THE LEGISLATIVE ARENA

Every dietitian has responsibility for action in two major areas relating to legislation and public policy: (a) to know what legislation is being considered and to show when and how nutrition services may enhance its effectiveness and (b) to practice so that nutrition services are, and therefore, can be presented to the public as an effective part of other available health services. Action in these two areas is closely related and both are essential for an effective legislative program. One area of action will not be effective without the other. Meeting the responsibility in these two areas is the challenge for every professional dietitian.

Francis E. Fischer: The dietitian in the legislative arena, J. Am. Diet. Assoc. **64**:623, 1974. Reprinted by permission. Copyright The American Dietetic Association.

---

trained in the legal aspects of public health, public policy, and the legal framework within which public health programs are designed and activated.[1]

Awareness of current and proposed health legislation and policies at every level, national, state, and local, in addition to an understanding of the mechanisms of the political process, will enable the nutritionist to become involved in the legislative arena. With this added knowledge the nutritionist and dietitian can advise the legislators how nutrition services, nutrition education, and nutrition research improve the quality and reduce the cost of health services. Such accountability looms uppermost in the minds of many legislators.

Various publications can help keep the public health professional up to date on proposed and current legislation. The *Federal Register* lists changes in USDA food program regulations on Tuesdays and Fridays. Another is the USDA *Program Instructions* for the Food Stamp Program as well as other food programs. USDA has issued a total of 128 instructions related to food stamps alone, and one of these, FNS(FS) Instruction 732-1, is 145 pages long. Copies of these instructions may be requested from USDA–FNS regional offices. Another publication is the Community Nutrition Institute (CNI) *Weekly Report*, which provides reports of major developments in all the federal food programs. A new reference directory is the *National Health Directory, 1977*. This book includes the name, title, address, and telephone number of key information sources on health programs and legislation. Key personnel of the twenty-three federal agencies concerned with health are identified by title, name, address, and telephone number. Finally, the federal regional officials and the governors and top health officials of each state are listed.

ROLE OF THE ADVOCATE

The American Dietetic Association has recommended that the government through legislation take an active role in helping to meet the association's objectives. These are primarily to improve the nutrition of human beings, to advance the science of dietetics and nutrition; and to improve education in these and allied areas. Among other recommendations, The American Dietetic Association[2] has called on the government to assist states and local communities in the following areas:

a. Developing and promulgating national nutrition policies.
b. Recognizing the importance of nutrition to health by establishing an organizational unit with the responsibility for a comprehensive nutrition program coordinated with federal agencies administering health services.
c. Establishing authority at policy-making levels that can be applied to all departments concerned with developing and implementing a coordinated nutrition program.
d. Providing financial assistance for nutrition surveillance and surveys, applied nutrition research and demonstrations, grants-in-aid to support public health nutrition programs, and consumer protection activities.
e. Establishing a uniform system for nationwide reporting of morbidity and mortality from malnutrition which will provide statistics on the magnitude and location of primary, secondary and tertiary malnutrition.

Implementing these recommendations of The American Dietetic Association will require the active participation of the public health profession.

The American Dietetic Association's involvement in legislative activity is a recent movement that started in 1968 with the creation of an Advisory Committee on Legislation and Public Policy.[3] By 1970, chairpersons for each of the fifty-two affiliated dietetic associations were appointed to deal specifically with legislative information and public policy. Position papers began to appear on various subjects, such as food and nutrition services in day care centers[4] and nutrition and aging.[5] The involvement of the membership in the association's legislative programs also began to expand as some of the association's leaders testified before various congressional committees.[6] More members began to talk and write to their legislators. Nevertheless, even though interest has increased, this role of advocacy in the legislative arena still needs strengthening.

Intellectually, most professionals accept the responsibility for advocating on behalf of their clients. Many of them believe that whatever they do for a client is a form of advocacy. The term, "advocacy," however, has come to take on a more specialized meaning than simply meeting the needs of clients. "To advocate" denotes an aggressive form of action. Webster defines an advocate as "one who pleads the cause of another."

Legislative activities provide only one mode of advocacy. There is also the need to ascertain the dietitian's readiness to assume

THE NEW CONSUMERISM

As a pro-consumer nutritionist, I am concerned that the consumer movement has been losing support from the nutrition profession because of lack of firm factual foundations for some of its efforts. Nutrition expertise is useful in order to represent the consumer's viewpoint fairly, without loss of scientific accuracy. And many public interest groups would genuinely appreciate expert assistance—for example in defining issues of nutritional importance, gathering scientific evidence, preparing arguments to back up a case, and writing or reviewing material intended for publication. . .

Advocacy efforts supported by informed, professional nutrition input are much more likely to be taken seriously than those that rely on hearsay or overinterpretation of nutrition research. For example, the case for informing consumers of the sugar content of food products is stronger if it is based on the established links between sucrose and dental caries or risk of excess calorie intake than if it were based on more speculative associations between sucrose and diabetes or heart disease.

The new consumerists should exercise the same kind of nutritional responsibility that is demanded of industry and government. Advocacy efforts should stand up to the tests of accuracy and soundness, fair and unbiased presentation of the facts, and ultimate benefit to the nutritional well-being of the consumer.

Margaret C. Phillips: The new conservatism, J. Nutr. Educ. 9:100, July-Sept., 1977. Reprinted with permission from the Journal of Nutrition Education. © Society for Nutrition Education.

NEEDED: A DEFINITION, LEGISLATION, ACTION

The time is *now* to capitalize on the interest in nutrition and develop nutrition education legislation . . . There are many legislators and others who need to know what nutrition education is before legislation can be passed . . . It is not possible to legislate the motivation of the individual nor to ensure that the educational process takes place. It is possible to develop lines of communication to provide information that is adequate and motivational. It is also possible to identify those areas such as the school community, health care delivery systems, mass media, and food supply sources which have regulatory and informational resources through which nutrition education is either established as an entity or incorporated into the social programs developed for target areas such as cited above.

Helen D. Ullrich: Editorial, J. Nutr. Educ. **5:**224, 1973.

Table 11-1. Preferential focus for association's advocacy role*

Preference	Percent of respondents			
	Yes	May-be	No	No answer
For individuals or groups				
Low-income groups	86	9	2	3
Consumers against improper food label	67	26	2	5
Consumers against improper dietary claims	86	11	2	1
School children	70	22	3	5
In group homes	72	17	6	5
For programs				
Traineeship	56	26	9	8
Research	58	33	3	6
Payment for nutrition services	52	26	19	3

*From Springer, N. S., and Segal, R. M.: Dietitians' attitudes toward advocacy, J. Am. Diet. Assoc. **67:**447, 1975. Reprinted by permission. Copyright The American Dietetic Association.

other roles of advocacy, which was observed by Springer and Segal,[7] who raised some pertinent questions:

What is the stance of the dietetic profession regarding advocacy? Have dietitians moved beyond the role of primarily providing counseling, evaluation and prescriptive service relating to dietary concerns? Have they been willing to challenge the service delivery system that impinges on the legal and human rights of the client? Have they attempted to confront that system directly—at the risk of alienation and reprisals—to guarantee the client's right to quality services? While this may often be regarded as within the scope of professional functioning, by and large, this mode of behavior is neither required nor expected by the organization employing the dietitian.

In a survey to determine the readiness of dietitians to implement such advocacy, Springer and Segal[7] discovered that the majority held positive attitudes. Table 11-1 delineates the respondents' preference regarding the program areas for which The American Dietetic Association should advocate. A majority believed that there was a greater need for the association to advocate for individuals than for programs. This may be related to the fact that the majority of respondents provided direct services to clients, and only a small percentage were involved in training or research.

The respondents had minimal experience in advocacy activities such as assisting in legal suits, demonstrations or sit-ins, presenting testimony at public hearings, and working for welfare rights organizations, as shown in Table 11-2. Many indicated a lack of knowledge about how to effect change as the basis of their inactivity. Thus it is clear that advocacy role models to assist the professional in assuming such roles should be developed.

LOBBYING: WHAT IT TAKES TO PASS LEGISLATION

There are some cardinal rules for working effectively with legislators and other public officials, either when testifying at a public hearing or at a less formal meeting. The first is to be informed. It would be unwise to meet with public officials to advocate a position without first studying the facts and the arguments for and against. Second, there is a need to be realistic. The advocacy of controversial legislation and regulations usually results in compromise. This has always been so and will continue in a democracy. A third principle is to be candid and open. Views should be stated with the reasons behind that

Table 11-2. Members' participation in advocacy roles*

	Percent of respondents							
	Past				Future			
Procedure	Often	Some-times	Never	No answer	Often	Some-times	Never	No answer
Legal court suits	0	3	72	25	17	21	42	20
Participating in demonstrations and sit-ins	0	3	72	25	5	19	59	17
Presenting testimony	0	9	67	24	25	37	22	16
Advising on legal rights	6	19	52	23	34	33	14	19
Changing policy in agency	30	28	30	12	61	22	5	12
Writing or contacting public officials	12	36	33	19	61	25	5	9
Educating the community	25	50	13	12	70	20	2	8
Working with welfare rights organization	3	6	74	17	20	48	16	16
Working with health, education, and welfare agencies	16	38	34	12	53	33	5	9

*From Springer, N. S., Segal, R. M.: Dietitians' attitudes toward advocacy. J. Am. Diet. Assoc. **67**:447, 1975. Reprinted by permission. Copyright The American Dietetic Association.

position, and there should be a willingness to listen to the problems that a particular position may create for the public official. A fourth point is to evaluate and weigh issues, establishing priorities in one's own mind and for the public official.

Communication is always a good way to start. Involve and inform your state legislators between their legislative sessions and give them a chance to meet your group. One nutritionist who was successful in getting state support invited the legislators to have lunch and dinner with her staff and community groups. Kits were prepared for their perusal. It was an opportunity to present problems and needs and to point out how new legislation could help to meet these needs. The nutritionist's request for progress reports from the legislators at regular intervals impressed the officials as to the sincerity of the health professional.

Try to understand the public official's position. Try to see the problems, the outlook, the aims. Recognize that each legislature has commitments and that a certain amount of vote trading goes on in a legislation. There is need for organization, planning, cooperation, and liaison.

A point to be considered is how does one present the case or cause to a public official? Schlossberg,[8] former Staff Director, U.S.

Select Committee on Nutrition and Human Needs, recommends numbers, that is, many people should present the case:

First, you need a good cause; second, you need a good case to promote that cause, and third and finally, you need a good campaign to put your case across the congressional goal line. The first step in any campaign is to reach out and build a coalition with as many groups around the country as you can reach . . . There's no question that the Congress responds to organizations, not individuals. So it is important to engage as many national organizations concerned about children, education and health in the effort, and to have them engage their local chapters around the country.

In New York City the Director of Nutrition Services of Maternity and Infant Care Projects initiated a campaign that resulted in new, beneficial legislation. From a survey of dietary histories she and her staff discovered that the majority of low-income families depend on unenriched white rice as the staple carbohydrate in their diet. Enriched rice was difficult to obtain, especially in larger quantities. To obtain legislation that mandated the enrichment of rice, she prepared a fact sheet and then proceeded to contact and enlist the support of the community, medical and public health leaders, national and local legislators, state and city commissioners of con-

DIETARY HISTORIES INSPIRE LEGISLATIVE ACTION

Since 1966, 30,715 dietary histories of our patients —predominately Negroes and Puerto Ricans, all low income—have been carefully and accurately taken by our staff of professional nutritionists . . . As nutritionists and dietitians, we are sensitive to the concept that we must be the builders of bridges of communication to our patients. This is facilitated when cultural practices are known and respected and when nutritional knowledge is interwoven within the framework of cultural patterns of eating.

From our dietary histories we have learned that white rice, not potatoes, is the staple carbohydrate of both Negro and Puerto Rican families. In food demonstrations for our patients in the waiting rooms of our clinics, our nutritionists, therefore, teach the use of enriched rice. However, market surveys by nutritionists in the communities where our clinics are based revealed that enriched rice was difficult to obtain, especially in the larger size packages, and labeling was often not clear . . . Clearly, a law was needed to mandate the enrichment of rice in our state. Our staff, therefore, decided to initiate a campaign to obtain such a law. To enlist community support, we developed a fact sheet offering information to convince the people of the urgent need. We contacted and enlisted the support of state legislators; medical, nutrition, and public health leaders; national and local legislators; the New York State and City Commissioners of Consumer Protection; and Governor Nelson Rockefeller.

To all, we called attention to the data from our dietary histories on the rice consumption patterns of these families. Responses were all favorable, receptive, and cooperative. Governor Rockefeller, on receiving this information from the President of the New York City Health and Hospitals Corporation, directed the New York State Department of Agriculture and Markets to draft the law.

An impressive fringe benefit was the decision to provide for the cultural practices of other groups by including in the law macaroni and noodle products; wheat flour and related products; and bread, rolls, and related products.

The law was passed last spring and became effective on November 1, 1972.

Implementation of this law, we believe, will make possible a substantial improvement in the nutritional status of the citizens of our state. The law will be of particular benefit to the poor and also to those age and sex groups who are biologically highly vulnerable to malnutrition, i.e., pregnant and postpartum women, the newborn, infants, children, adolescents, and the elderly.

A copy of this law has been placed in the A.D.A. reference library for members who may wish to borrow it.

Stella Hope Page: Dietary histories inspire legislative action, J. Am. Diet. Assoc. **62**:15, 1973. Reprinted by permission. Copyright The American Dietetic Association.

---

sumer protection, and the governors. The law passed required the enrichment not only of rice but of noodle and wheat flour products as well. Thus an individual and organization outside the political-legislative body could influence and determine new policy.

THE POLITICAL SYSTEM

If there is to be a continuing improvement in the governmental process in the United States, it must come from the increased interest and participation of the governed. In no other modern nation are the citizens so instrumental in their own collective political destiny as in the United States. Representative government achieves its greatest expression through the participation of an informed citizenry. The following statement by Senator George McGovern[9] testifies to the strength of informed and active citizens:

The growth of those nutrition programs designed to protect the health of our children and low income citizens has been very encouraging to anyone committed to improving the quality of life in America today. As Chairman of the Senate Select Committee on Nutrition and Human Needs, I have been privileged to both observe and participate in this phenomenon since 1968.

Probably the single most encouraging aspect of this growth has been the critical and absolutely fundamental contribution of concerned citizens at the local, State and Federal levels. Progress without this kind of community energy would not have been possible, at least at the scale we have achieved. And, I am optimistic about the future of these programs for the same reasons. There are now throughout the country thousands of committed and informed nutrition activists who critically analyze and support these programs, and the future growth and improvement in this area will be directly related to their continued commitment.

GOVERNMENT AND PUBLIC HEALTH

The particular political system that exists determines the role of government in relation to health. Public health programs are financed and the broad organizational patterns for implementation of these programs are outlined according to basic policy decisions. In general a governmental system in a democratic society performs two distinct functions. The first function is political . . . The second general function is the provision of service and regulatory activities . . . Individuals involved in public health work are knowledgeable about the service function of government because this is their field of expertise. Often they have had little opportunity in their formal education or experience to obtain a firsthand understanding of the political function of government. Because the political and service functions of government cannot be separated, it is imperative that those who work in public health administration possess an understanding of the political function of government and its relationship to the service function.

John J. Hanlon: Public health administration and practice, ed. 6, St. Louis, 1974, The C. V. Mosby, Co., p. 130.

The purpose of the United States government is expressed in the preamble to the Constitution: "We the People of the United States, in Order to form a more perfect Union, establish Justice, insure domestic Tranquility, provide for the common defense, promote the general Welfare, and secure the Blessings of Liberty to ourselves and our Posterity, do ordain and establish this Constitution for the United States of America."

The Constitution contains provisions in separate articles for three departments of government—legislative, executive, and judicial. There is a significant difference in the grants of power to these departments: The first article, treating of legislative power, vests in Congress "all legislative Powers herein granted"; the second article vests "the executive Power" in the President; and the third article states that "The judicial Power of the United States shall be vested in one Supreme Court and in such inferior courts as the Congress may from time to time ordain and establish."

The legislative process, in the simplest analysis, consists of the interaction among these three basic branches of the government, the legislature, the executive, and the judiciary, which are interlocked by a system of checks and balances. Thus the Executive may veto legislation or sign it into law; the Legislature may introduce and enact a law and can override a veto by the Executive; and the Judiciary may discard a law if it considers it in violation of man's basic freedoms and rights. To these three branches may be added the operating or enforcement agencies that are responsible for carrying out the intent of the legislation and may be a significant source of proposed legislative additions or changes. These major federal regulators are as follows:

Civil Aeronautics Board (CAB). Founded in 1938. Five commissioners determine interstate airline routes, passenger fares, and freight rates.
Consumer Product Safety Commission (CPSC). Founded in 1972. Five Commissioners set product-safety standards and initiate recall notices for defective products.
Equal Employment Opportunity Commission (EEOC). Founded in 1964. Five commissioners investigate and rule on charges of racial and other discrimination by employers and labor unions.
Environmental Protection Agency (EPA). Founded in 1970. An administrator develops and enforces environmental-quality standards for air, water, and noise pollution and for toxic substances and pesticides.
Federal Aviation Administration (FAA). Founded in 1948. An administrator in the Department of Transportation certifies airworthiness of aircraft, licenses pilots, and sets safety standards for airports.
Federal Communications Commission (FCC). Founded in 1934. Seven commissioners license radio and television stations and oversee interstate and international telephone and telegraph operations.
Federal Energy Administration (FEA). Founded in 1974. An administrator regulates price and allocation controls of petroleum products.
Federal Power Commission (FPC). Founded in 1920. Five commissioners set wholesale rates for the interstate transportation and sale of natural gas and for interstate transmission of electricity.
Federal Reserve Board (FRB). Founded in 1913.

A seven-member Board of Governors sets monetary and credit policy and regulates commercial banks belonging to the Federal Reserve System.

Federal Trade Commission (FTC). Founded in 1914. Five commissioners enforce some antitrust laws, protect businesses from unfair competition, and enforce truth-in-lending and truth-in-labeling laws.

Food and Drug Administration (FDA). Founded in 1931. A commissioner in the Department of Health, Education, and Welfare sets standards for certain foods and drugs and issues licenses for the manufacturing and distribution of drugs.

Interstate Commerce Commission (ICC). Founded in 1887. Eleven commissioners set rates, routes, and practices for interstate railroads, truckers, bus companies, and pipelines.

Nuclear Regulatory Commission (NRC). Founded in 1975. Five commissioners issue licenses for the design, construction, and operation of nuclear power plants.

The participation of public health practitioners in the legislative process was encouraged at a World Health Organization Conference of Directors of Schools of Public Health in 1966. The *WHO Technical Report*[10] states that "Legislation is an essential element of public health administration, not only for the control of various activities but increasingly as a means of facilitating or permitting the carrying out of certain activities that promote health."

Executive branch: the President

A President's domination of Washington actually stretches to the other coequal branches of government—the legislative and the judicial. He initiates much of the legislation to be considered by Congress and has the constitutional power to veto bills passed by Congress, and a two-thirds vote by both the Senate and House of Representatives is required to override the veto. In addition, the President sets the important federal money process in motion by proposing to Congress a budget to operate the government.

The President is authorized to appoint federal judges, from the district-court level to the U.S. Supreme Court. Therefore policies and beliefs may be imprinted on the country through judicial decisions handed down years after a President leaves office.

Legislative branch: how Congress passes a bill

The U.S. Congress remains both "the first branch" and "the people's branch" of national government. It consists of the Senate and the House of Representatives and has the primary legislative powers. Its makeup is unique in the federal system in that all its members are elected by the people. In the executive branch, by contrast, only the President and Vice President carry a mandate from the voters, and in the judicial branch all federal judges are appointed, not elected. Congress alone has the authority to levy taxes. These revenues can be spent only under authorization and appropriations bills passed by Congress.

The American Dietetic Association's Advisory Committee on Legislation and Public Policy has published a *Legislative Handbook*, which explains in words and diagrams the tedious steps of the legislative process in Congress. House action is pictorially shown in Fig. 11-1, Senate action is shown in Fig. 11-2, and Conference action is shown in Fig. 11-3.

Actually, the legislative work of Congress is done in committees of the House and Senate. Each committee has a set jurisdiction over an area of public policy. All bills are sent to committees, which normally pass them on to appropriate subcommittees for action. Most bills die at the end of a congressional session for lack of action. Only about 700 become law out of 23,000 introduced in a two-year period.[11] A graphic presentation that summarizes how the United States get their laws is shown in Fig. 11-4.

When a committee decides to consider action on a bill, it usually schedules a public hearing. Here, testimony is taken from the bill's sponsors, administration officials, outside experts, and any special interest groups that want to be heard. It is at this point that the nutrition profession is beginning to take action. However, it is early in the planning

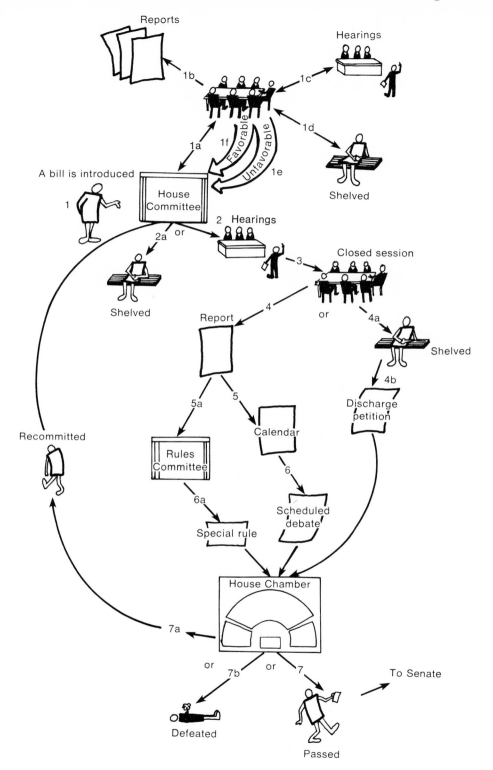

Reports

Hearings

1b

1c

1a

1f

Favorable

Unfavorable

1e

1d

A bill is introduced

1

House
Committee

Shelved

2 Hearings

2a or

Shelved

Closed session

3

Report

4 or 4a

Shelved

5a

5

4b

Rules
Committee

Calendar

Discharge
petition

Recommitted

6a

6

Special rule

Scheduled
debate

House Chamber

7a

or 7b or 7

To Senate

Defeated

Passed

Fig. 11-1. House action.

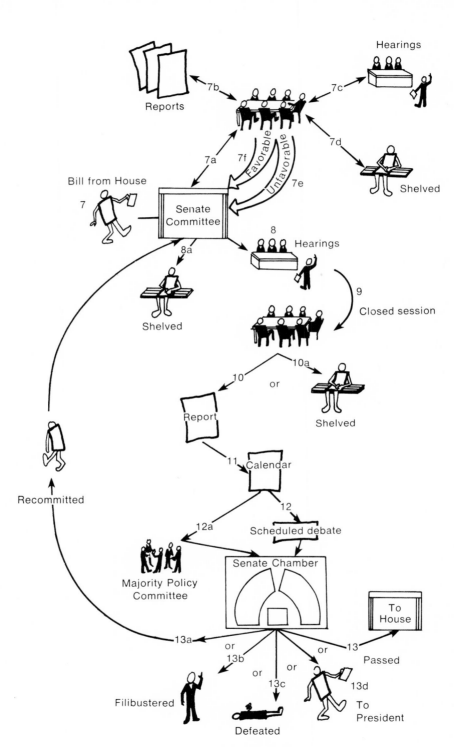

Fig. 11-2. Senate action.

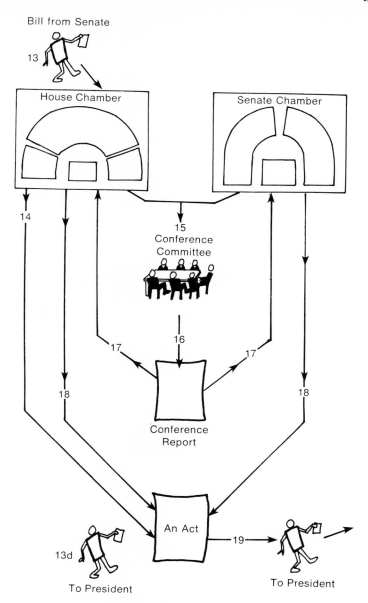

Fig. 11-3. Conference action.

stage, before a bill gets to legislation, that groups such as the American Dietetic Association, American Home Economics Association, American Public Health Association, State and Territorial Public Health Nutrition Directors and Faculties, and Society for Nutrition Education should meet and make their combined views known to senators and representatives. Then these legislators can actually help in the formulation of bills and even present them to other legislators in advance. Meanwhile, it ought to be kept in mind that all legislators are subject to pressures from lobbyists and the administration.

If a bill is approved by both the House and Senate, it is transmitted to the President for approval. If it is vetoed at this level, it can still become law if approved by a two-thirds vote in both the House and Senate. If this

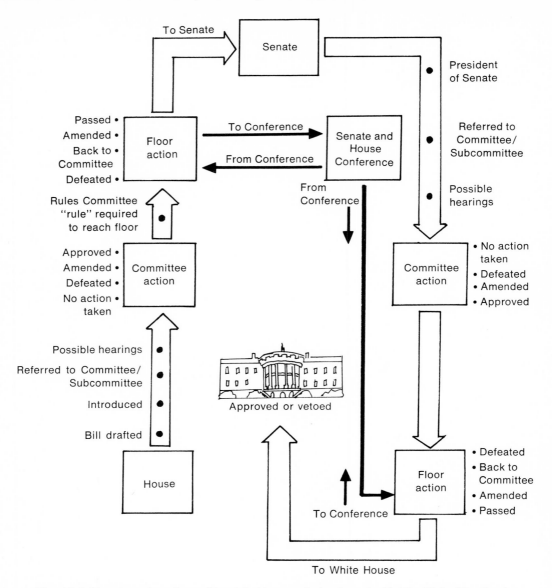

Fig. 11-4. How we get our laws. (Reprinted by permission from the Public Affairs Handbook, copyright 1971, Sperry & Hutchinson Co.)

is not achieved, or if the bill is not sent back to committee for further consideration and amendment, the bill is dropped.

Congressional standing committees

Standing committees were established as early as 1803 for the purpose of ensuring a preliminary check on the flood of bills introduced. These are specialized permanent units that help speed up the legislative process. Committee procedure with witnesses and cross-examinations allows the real merits of a measure to become apparent. The committee presents it in a more workable form for consideration by the entire Congress.

The following is a reference list of the standing committees in the House and Senate.

The Senate. The seventeen standing committees are as follows (the numbers in parentheses indicate the number of committee members allotted for the 92nd Congress):

Aeronautical and Space Sciences (11)
Agriculture and Forestry (14)
Appropriations (24)
Armed Services (16)
Banking, Housing and Urban Affairs (15)
Commerce (18)
District of Columbia (7)
Finance (16)
Foreign Relations (16)
Government Operations (18)
Interior and Insular Affairs (16)
Judiciary (16)
Labor and Public Welfare (17)
Post Office and Civil Service (9)
Public Works (16)
Rules and Administration (9)
Veterans' Affairs (9)

The House. The twenty-one standing committees are as follows (the numbers in parentheses indicate the number of committee members allotted for the 92nd Congress):

Agriculture (36)
Appropriations (55)
Armed Services (41)
Banking and Currency (37)
District of Columbia (25)
Education and Labor (38)
Foreign Affairs (38)
Government Operations (39)
House Administration (25)
Interior and Insular Affairs (38)
Internal Security (9)
Interstate and Foreign Commerce (43)
Judiciary (38)
Merchant Marine and Fisheries (37)
Post Office and Civil Service (26)
Public Works (37)
Rules (15)
Science and Astronautics (30)
Standards of Official Conduct (12)
Veterans' Affairs (26)
Ways and Means (25)

Other committees and their functions. A *select committee* is one established by the House or Senate usually for a limited period and generally for a strictly temporary purpose. Theoretically, when that function has been carried out, the select committee automatically expires.

The *joint committee* comprises members of both the Senate and the House. They can be established by statute or by joint or concurrent resolutions. To date, joint committees exist for Atomic Energy, Defense Production, Economics, Internal Revenue Taxation, Library, Printing, and Reduction of Nonessential Federal Expenditures.

When differences of opinion arise between the two Houses, a bill is sent to a *conference committee*, where members of each House confer to iron out differences. Usually, a bill passes one House with provisions that are different or unacceptable to the other. If after discussion and compromise the bill is accepted by both Houses, it goes to the President for his signature. If it is rejected by either House, the matter in disagreement is discussed as if there had been no conference. If the conference committee does not reach an agreement, it reports that to each House. The Houses consider the parts of the bill that the conference committee failed to agree on. Practically speaking, conference committees are expected to produce a compromise bill that will need no further adjustments.

The *House Rules Committee* considers bills that some other committee has reported. Most of its work is to decide whether or not to grant special consideration for bills that otherwise might be long delayed on the various calendars of the House. When the House Rules Committee reports a special rule to the House, it is usually adopted. When it is adopted, the bill to which it refers is considered under the provisions of that rule.

After a bill has been signed into law

If a program that has been set forth in a bill needs funds that must be appropriated in addition to the fiscal budget, another bill to get those funds must be passed by Congress after the bill authorizing the program has been approved. All Congress has done at this stage is "authorize" a law, not "appropriate" funds for it. If the funding is not approved, the program cannot begin, even though a bill was passed approving the program.

Judiciary branch: the court system

Once a bill does become law, it is up to the federal courts to decide its meaning. Not only do the courts interpret Congresses's intent, but if they find that the law conflicts with the Constitution, the law is struck down.

There are two sets of courts in the United States—federal and state—and most legal matters that affect everyday life are handled by state courts. California state courts, for example, handled about 15 million cases last year. By contrast, 172,000 civil and criminal cases were begun in all federal trial courts.

Federal courts have limited jurisdiction. In general, they deal with interpretation of federal laws, treaties, or the Constitution. Their rulings have a profound effect on the course of history.

Makeup of the courts

Article III of the Constitution specifies that "the judicial power of the United States shall be vested in one Supreme Court, and in such inferior courts as the Congress may from time to time ordain and establish."

The United States and its territories are divided into eleven judicial circuits. There are now ninety-four district courts, with each state having at least one. One court of appeal is located in each circuit. Congress also has created some special courts, such as the Court of Claims, which hears claims against the federal government; the Tax Court; the Court of Customs; and the Court of Customs and Patent Appeals.

Congress has set the number of Supreme Court Justices at nine, although the court has functioned at times with as few as five and as many as ten. The Chief Justice of the United States is designated by the President when there is a vacancy in that position.

There are two main roads for a case to reach the Supreme Court—one is through the state and the other is the federal route. In the state route the following happens:
1. Defendant loses in state trial court.

2. He takes case to state appeals court.
3. State supreme court rules on case.
4. Decision can now be appealed directly to U.S. Supreme Court if a constitutional question is involved.

In the federal route the process is a three-step routine, as follows:
1. Case involving federal law is tried in a U.S. district court.
2. Loser takes case to a U.S. circuit court of appeals.
3. Court of appeals ruling can be submitted to U.S. Supreme Court for review.

Judges of the federal district courts, the appeals courts, and the Supreme Court hold lifetime jobs. They are appointed by the President with the advice and consent of the Senate and can be removed only by impeachment. Most matters that come into federal court are settled at the district court level. As a general rule, only errors of law may be appealed.

Special departments

Career federal employees, those public servants known as "bureaucrats," operate largely backstage but still wield much of the real power in government.

Staffing eleven major departments, fifty-five agencies, and 1,175 advisory boards, nearly 3 million people are ultimately responsible for executing the programs formulated by Congress and the President. No matter how beneficial a program might be, it can easily become sidetracked without the support of civil servants.

Some of the major agencies, such as the Departments of State and Treasury, have been around since colonial times and have assumed more strength and prestige with each passing decade. Others such as the Department of Transportation and the Department of Housing and Urban Development are more recent institutions. Of major interest here is the Department of Health, Education, and Welfare, formed in 1953 as a successor to the old Federal Security Agency. Given the task of administering the many Great Society programs launched in the 1960s, this department saw its payroll zoom from 87,000 employees in 1965 to about 157,000 today. The department will spend nearly $148 billion in 1977—the largest budget by far of any agency. It administers such well-known programs as Social Security, Medicare, and Medicaid. It provides financial assistance to the poor and disabled and operates many public services aimed at the economically deprived and the physically and mentally handicapped. It also conducts extensive research on the causes and treatment of diseases and establishes guidelines and aid for the operation of schools and colleges. This huge department, as well as other departments, must begin to plan its request for funding, that is, its portion of the federal fiscal budget, at least 15 months before the new fiscal year. This allows time for the President, the appropriations committees, and the whole Congress to review and approve the allotment of federal money.

FEDERAL LEGISLATION SUPPORTING NUTRITION SERVICES

The activities of the Senate Select Committee on Nutrition and Human Needs served as a catalyst for federal legislation that is concerned with the nutritional status of high-risk Americans. However, the nutritional well-being of the nation's children has been a continuing concern of the federal government. Egan[12] states that "This concern has evoked a variety of responses depending upon the interest and commitment of the leadership, the advances of science and technology, as well as the problems, pressures, priorities, and fashions of the times."

Legislation with nutritional implications began as early as 1915-1920, when the Children's Bureau, then a part of the U.S. Department of Labor, issued technical bulletins on aspects of nutrition to help health and welfare workers and teachers in their work with children and families.[13] The bureau initiated a nutritional survey of children in low-income families in the mountainous area of Kentucky. This was one of the first of many such studies on the prevalence of malnutrition.[14]

The Social Security Act of 1935 authorized grants-in-aid to the states for health services for mothers and children. Programs initiated in the area of maternal and child health introduced both preventive and curative measures in nutrition as a basic part of child health care. In the mid-1930s the Federal Surplus Commodities Corporation distributed surplus commodities to schools and employed a special representative in each state to expand the school lunch program.[15]

The National School Lunch Act of 1946 made grants-in-aid available to the states to assist them in providing an adequate supply of food and other facilities for the establishment, maintenance, operation, and expansion of the nonprofit school lunch programs.

In the 1950s there was increasing recognition that appropriate dietary treatment could prevent mental retardation by correcting inborn metabolic errors.

In the 1960s the number of nutritionists in health care programs increased as a result of the support from the Maternal and Child Health and Mental Retardation Planning Amendments of 1963. Families enrolled in maternity and child health care projects were able to receive direct nutrition services as a part of health care. In these years, too, the National Academy of Sciences studied the relationship of nutrition to pregnancy, and a health reason was recognized as a basis of need for food assistance. As a result, the Supplemental Food Program for Low Income Groups Vulnerable to Malnutrition was initiated.[16]

Other recent legislation concerned with nutrition includes the 1963 amendments to Title V of the Social Security Act, which provided for a new program of grants for maternity and infant care, especially for low-income families.

Nutrition service and dietary counseling are integral parts of these projects. In the approximately fifty-four maternity and infant care projects and in the fifty-five children and youth projects, about 400 positions have been budgeted for nutrition personnel.

There is also the Elementary and Secondary Education Act of 1965 and its 1966 amendments, which provided for financial assistance to local educational agencies for special education programs in areas having high concentrations of children from low-income families. Some of these funds can be used for supplemental health and food services.

The 1965 amendments to the Social Security Act provide for a five-year program of special project grants for comprehensive health care and services for school and preschool children, particularly in areas of low-income families. The purpose of these "Projects for Comprehensive Health Services for Children and Youth" is to increase the availability and to improve the quality of health care services, including nutrition, through screening, testing, diagnosis, and follow-up treatment. Emphasis is placed on the comprehensiveness and continuity of services. The Child Nutrition Act of 1966, authorized by the Department of Agriculture, also aided the nutrition of youngsters by broadening school feeding programs and closing gaps in these school services. However, it should be remembered that authorization of such funding does not necessarily mean that the same amount is actually appropriated by the federal budget. Special summer programs, preschool programs, and breakfast programs were some of the additional services that were initiated during the 1960s.

In the 1970s child nutrition programs were extended to residential programs and brought the benefits of food service to family day care homes and licensed nonprofit, private, residential institutions such as homes for the mentally retarded, orphanages, and temporary shelters. Congress in 1972 passed legislation that authorized the Special Supplemental Food Program for Women, Infants, and Children (WIC).

In 1975 the National School Lunch Program was available to 88% of all children enrolled in school. Other services under the Child Nutrition Programs include the Nonfood Assistance Program and the Special Milk Program.

The Department of Health, Education, and Welfare began to administer the Head Start Program, which includes the service of

NEW MENU FOR SCHOOL LUNCH

Another step was recently taken in a year-long effort to straighten out the $130 million New York City School Lunch Program as a Federal-State-City task force recommended extensive changes in the administration, delivery and quality of meals served to more than half a million youngsters.

The USDA–headed task force was organized at Congressman Richmond's request following March hearings in New York City and the release of a General Accounting office survey of New York's program, which found that 45% of the 550,000 meals served failed to meet minimal quantity standards of the Federal government.

The task force recommended a managerial reorganization of the Board of Education's Bureau of School Lunches and a redirection to the meal selection process so that parents and students can finally have a say in the types of foods served in schools. The Federal study, moreover, found that warehouse and accounting practices of the Bureau of School Lunches was costing taxpayers millions of dollars.

"We have finally developed a unique and common sense approach to New York's meal program," stated Richmond. "Local school districts will now have a greater flexibility in the types of meals served and quantity, as well as quality control procedures will be set up guaranteeing that our youngsters are not short-changed at the lunchroom counter." Most of the recommendations of the task force will be implemented in time for the September school term.

Congressman Fred Richmond: New menu for school lunches, Reports from Washington, D.C. and Brooklyn **3:**2, July, 1977.

nutritious meals and snacks, nutrition education for children and their families, as well as consultation technical assistance, and training in nutrition for Head Start staff. In fiscal year 1975 about 350,000 children were provided with nutrition services, and approximately $69 million were spent for food and labor. The program, School Health and Nutrition Services for Children from Low-Income Families, also examined ways to organize a system of comprehensive health and education services through effective coordination of existing resources. In fiscal year 1975 there were eight separate projects involving about $1.35 million and thirty elementary schools.

Other health programs that are currently

operative because of funds appropriated by Congress are Community Health Centers, Migrant Health Projects, Appalachian Health Programs, Title VII programs, National Health Service Corps projects, and Indian Health Services, among others. These are all aimed at particular population groups and contain an important nutrition component.

In addition to these which are locally specialized, other programs seek to improve nutrition regardless of age category. The Food Stamp and Food Distribution Programs fall under the general heading of Family Food Assistance and are aimed at the family unit rather than the individual. The Food Distribution Program, which gives out food products directly, is being phased out in favor of the Food Stamp Program, where money is exchanged for a higher value of food coupons.

An example of pending health legislation in President Carter's administration deals with child health assessment. This is a major expansion, and improvement in the Early Periodic Screening, Diagnosis, and Treatment Program (EPSDT) has been recommended by President Carter. The bills are S. 1392 and H.R. 6706, the Child Health Assessment Act (CHAP).

EPSDT has not been regarded as a success story. It has reached only 30% of the children eligible for Medicaid, and approximately one fifth of the children screened with medical problems do not get the required treatment. It is the purpose of CHAP to improve this performance record.

States would be encouraged to establish Child Health Advisory Committees to assist them in developing an implementation plan to carry out the requirements of this program. This might take the form of a special committee of an existing group such as the state's Medicaid advisory committee or the state's health planning and development agency.

WHERE ARE WE NOW?

For several years there has been consideration of ways to create a voice in government that will be able to speak up for consumers.

On April 16, 1977, a message was presented to the Senate from President Carter recommending measures that will help this movement:

1. Creation of an Agency for Consumer Advocacy. Its purpose will be to plead the consumers case within the government.
2. The administrator of the agency will be appointed by the President.
3. The agency should be empowered to intervene or participate in proceedings before federal agencies to assure adequate representation of consumer interests and in judicial proceeding involving Agency action.
4. The agency should have its own information-gathering authority, including, under appropriate safeguards, access to information held by other government agencies and private concerns.
5. Legislation to help consumer groups represent themselves in agency and judicial proceedings.
6. Legislation that will give citizens broader standing to initiate suits against the government in appropriate cases.
7. Legislation that will enable consumers to sue as a class to enforce their rights.

Additionally, food stamp legislation was proposed by the administration that would no longer require the purchase of food stamps. Participants would receive food stamps only for the amount now contributed by the federal government. Other proposals include regulation of eligibility standards, simplified administration, and substitution of a standard income deduction for the specific individual deductions under the existing program.

In August, 1977, President Carter announced his new welfare program. Legislation resulting from this will change pending practices related to food stamps.

At the present moment numerous bills relating to nutrition are before the House and Senate. For example, in the House of Representatives, hearings are just being conducted on H.R. 11761—the National Consumer Nutrition Information Act of 1978. Some of the major features of this bill include the establishment of USDA as the leading agency in coordinating nutrition education among federal agencies, improving coordination in nutrition education among public voluntary and private sectors, and improving methods for communicating information about food, diet, and health to the general public. However, simultaneously the Carter administration is recommending the transfer of nearly all child nutrition programs to a proposed Department of Education. Therefore, as the title of Chapter 13 indicates, "Where do we go from here?" is a very timely question.

An excellent reference for the public health nutritionist and the dietitian who plan to get involved in the legislative arena is *A Nutritionist's Guide to Washington*, which follows.

A NUTRITIONIST'S GUIDE TO WASHINGTON*

Congress

Capitol Hill Switchboard
(information)
224-3121

Senate Agriculture Committee
(farm and food programs)
322 Russell Building
224-2035

Senate Nutrition Committee
(nutrition oversight)
119 D Street N.E.
224-7326

Senate Human Resources Committee
(aging, community nutrition programs, nutrition research, food safety)
4230 Dirksen Building
224-5375

Senate Special Aging Committee
(aging oversight)
G-233 Dirksen Building
224-5364

Senate Appropriations Committee
(money bills)
1235 Dirksen Building
224-3471

House Agriculture Committee
(farm and food stamp programs)
1301 Longworth Building
225-2171

House Education and Labor Committee
(nutrition programs except food stamps)
2181 Rayburn Building
225-4527

House Aging Committee
(aging oversight)
712 H.O.B. Annex #1
225-9375

House Appropriations Committee
(money bills)
H218, Capitol
225-2771

House Commerce Health Subcommittee
(food safety)
2415 Rayburn Building
225-4952

General Accounting Office
(program evaluation)
441 G Street N.W.
275-5525

Office of Technology Assessment
(special projects)
119 D Street N.E.
224-8711

Agencies

U.S. Department of Agriculture (USDA)
Food and Nutrition Service (FNS)
(food program administration)
500 12th Street S.W.
447-8360

Agricultural Research Service (ARS)
(nutrition and consumer research)
Beltsville, Maryland
436-8221

Consumer and Food Economics Institute
(consumer research)
Hyattsville, Maryland
436-8457

Animal & Plant Health Inspection Service
(meat and poultry inspection)
14th and Independence S.W.
436-8013

---

*From Community Nutrition Institute: A nutritionist's guide to Washington **7:**29, July 28, 1977.

A NUTRITIONIST'S GUIDE TO WASHINGTON—cont'd

Agency for International Development
(world hunger)
Arlington, Virginia
235-8927

Food and Drug Administration (FDA)
(food safety)
200 C Street, S.W.
443-1544

Federal Trade Commission (FTC)
(food advertising)
9th and Constitution, N.W.
523-3830

Administration on Aging (AoA)
(elderly feeding program)
330 Independence Avenue, S.W.
245-0724

National Institutes of Health (NIH)
(nutrition research)
Bethesda, Maryland
496-4461

Office of Consumer Affairs (OCA)
(consumer issues)
300 7th Street, S.W.
755-8875

Community Services Administration (CSA)
(community food and nutrition program)
1200 19th Street, N.W.
254-5400

Private organizations

The Action Center
(student food advocacy)
1028 Connecticut Avenue, N.W.
466-3726

American Freedom from Hunger Foundation
(world hunger)
811 Vermont Avenue, N.W.
254-3487

Agribusiness Accountability Project
(agribusiness)
1000 Wisconsin Avenue, N.W.
338-6331

American Institute of Nutrition
(nutrition research)
Bethesda, Maryland
530-7050

Center for Science in the Public Interest
(food advocacy)
1757 S Street, N.W.
332-4250

Children's Foundation
(child nutrition)
1028 Connecticut Avenue, N.W.
296-4451

Community Nutrition Institute
(nutrition program and policy issues)
1910 K Street, N.W.
833-1730

Consumer Action
(consumer issues)
1625 Eye Street, N.W.
872-8660

Consumer Federation of America
(consumer issues)
1012 14th Street, N.W.
737-3732

Council on Children, Media & Merchandising
(food advertising)
466-2583

Environmental Defense Fund
(food safety)
1525 18th Street, N.W.
833-1484

Federation of American Societies for Experimental Biology
(nutrition research)
Bethesda, Md.
530-7000

Food Research and Action Center
(feeding programs)
2011 Eye Street, N.W.
452-8250

Health Research Group
(food safety)
2000 P Street, N.W.
872-0320

Interreligious Task Force
(world hunger)
110 Maryland Avenue, NE
543-2800

Institute for Local Self-Reliance
(food co-ops and urban gardens)
1717 18th Street, N.W.
232-4180

Nutrition Foundation
(research and information)
888 17th Street, N.W.
872-0778

Nutrition Today Society
(nutrition information)
Annapolis, Maryland
261-2830

Public Resource Center
(agriculture)
1747 Connecticut Avenue, N.W.
234-6485

Worldwatch Institute
(world hunger)
1776 Massachusetts Avenue, N.W.
452-1999

SUMMARY

Legislation and related public policies will determine the future of the health care system as well as the practice of the health professional. It is important that health professionals recognize the need for their advocacy in the area of health and nutrition legislation. Therefore the nutritionist should be armed with the skills and knowledge needed for successful lobbying, including awareness of existing and proposed legislation and the ability to make some compromises. The health professional should also be able to make a clear presentation of his cause, its support, and its monetary advantages. The health professional should also understand the legislative process itself, including the process of a bill through the House of Representatives and the Senate; the interaction of the three branches of government, legislature, judiciary, and executive; and how any one of these can serve as a check on the passage of a bill.

Budgetary considerations are especially vital, since a proposed program's budget must be submitted in advance of the congressional budgetary appropriation decisions, which themselves are begun one and a half years before the fiscal year to which they are applied.

Currently, legislation relating to health and nutrition is becoming more and more extensive, particularly in the areas of child nutrition programs (School Lunch Program, School Breakfast Program, Summer Feeding Program), maternal and infant feeding programs (WIC), special population programs (Appalachian and Indian Health Programs), and food assistance programs (Food Stamp Program). These are encouraging, but as yet they have not answered all the nutritional and health needs by any means.

REFERENCES

1. Grad, F. P.: Public health law manual, Washington, D.C., 1970, American Public Health Association.
2. Fischer, F. E.: The dietitian in the legislative arena, J. Am. Diet. Assoc. **64:**621, 1974.
3. Fischer, F. E.: Legislative highlights, J. Am. Diet. Assoc. **61:**50, 1972.
4. The American Dietetic Association: Position Paper on food and nutrition services in day-care centers, J. Am. Diet. Assoc. **59:**47, 1971.
5. The American Dietetic Association: Position Paper on nutrition and aging, J. Am. Diet. Assoc. **51:**623, 1972.
6. Collins, M. E., Forbes, C., Kocher, R., and Yanochik, A.: Position statement on implementation and delivery of nutritional care services in the health care system. Subpanel of Health Care System of Panel on Nutrition and Health, Senate Select Committee on Nutrition and Human Needs, Part 5, Washington, D.C., June 21, 1974, Government Printing Office.
7. Springer, N. S., and Segal, R. M.: Dietitian's attitudes toward advocacy, J. Am. Diet. Assoc. **67:**445, 1975.
8. Schlossberg, K.: What it takes to pass nutrition legislation, J. Nutr. Educ. **5:**228, 1973.
9. McGovern, G.: Statement by Senator George McGovern, Chairman, Senate Select Committee on Nutrition and Human Needs, 1976.
10. WHO Report of Conference of Directors of Schools of Public Health, WHO Technical Report Series no. 351, Geneva, 1967, World Health Organization.
11. U.S. News and World Report, The ABC's of how your government works, May 9, 1977, p. 50.
12. Egan, M. S.: Federal nutrition support programs for children, Pediatr. Clin. North Am. **24:**229, 1977.
13. Heseltine, M. M.: Nutrition as a concern of the Children's Bureau, 1912-1961, Washington, D.C., Children's Bureau, Department of Health Education and Welfare (unpublished).
14. Heseltine, M. M.: The nutritionist in public health work, J. Am. Diet. Assoc. **14:**241, 1938.
15. Food and Nutrition Service, Department of Agriculture: The National School Lunch Program: background and development, FNS-63, Washington, D.C., 1971, Government Printing Office.
16. Egan, M. C.: A supplementary feeding program—an integral aspect of health services for young children: nutrition programmes for preschool children, Zagreb, Yugoslavia, 1973, Institute of Public Health of Croatia.

GENERAL CONCEPT

Grants, a form of financial assistance from federal, voluntary, and private agencies, provide additional monies for service, training, and research for nutrition programing.

OUTCOMES

The student should be able to do the following:
- List the sources of funding from federal, voluntary, and private sectors.
- Define how extra funding can enhance service, research, or training that will improve nutritional status of population groups.
- Identify the parts of a proposal for a grant.
- List reasons why grants are denied.

Grants and grantsmanship: where the money is

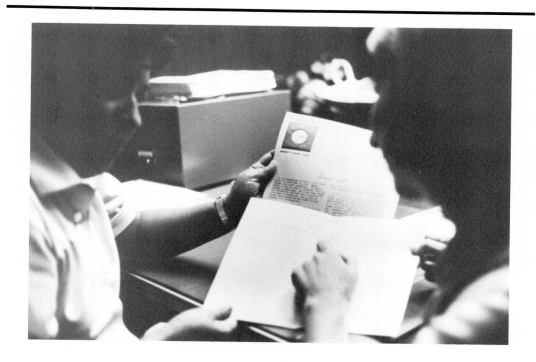

With the increasing competition for tax funds and with the uncertainties of the future role of federal grants-in-aid, financing is currently less stable than in the past. The nutritionist as a leader in agency health planning would do well to seek additional funds for service, training, and research in health programs. The financing of local and state health services has always been a critical matter in developing community health programs. In most state health agencies nutrition is included as an item in the budget funded by state legislatures as part of the total state health program. Nichaman and Collins[1] of the Center for Disease Control have reported a 1975 study of 50 states and the District of Columbia, Guam, Trust Territories of the Pacific Islands, Puerto Rico, and the Virgin Islands. This survey of nutritionists in health agencies indicated that altogether there were 496 positions budgeted (included 32 part-time positions). In addition to the 173 nutritionists in identifiable nutrition units, it was reported that there were 53 positions in health care facilities (nursing home consultant, hospital consultant, etc.), 8 in chronic disease programs, 54 in maternal and child health programs, and 125 in "other" programs all sponsored by the government.[1] However, the support for almost all health and medical research at teaching and research centers as well derives in great measure from governmental agencies, with some additional aid from organizations and private foundations. The provision of community health services in the United States today is a cooperative project, with responsibility shared by federal, state, and local units of government.

FINANCING NUTRITION SERVICES

It should be stated at the outset of this chapter that financing nutrition services is an integral part of the agency budget. Every health care program should include nutrition as an item in its budget. There may be instances such as in the case of single provider sites or in projects offering limited services in which it may not be feasible to identify a separate budget item for nutrition. However, this should be the exception and not the rule.

Salary ranges for nutritional personnel in state positions are usually determined by State Merit System Agencies. In addition, local and state dietetic associations can be helpful in providing information. The national office of The American Dietetic Association can provide information about current salary scales and prevailing wages for nutrition personnel.

A budget for nutrition services should include salaries, expenses and fringe benefits of nutrition personnel; supportive services (clerical, secretarial, etc.); space and facilities; equipment including laboratory supplies and manuals; education materials; office supplies, data processing costs, overhead and operating costs; travel costs; and expenses for staff development.

The subject of this chapter, Grants and Grantsmanship, or how to obtain funding, is concerned with additional monies from federal, voluntary, and private agencies to expand nutrition programing in the community.

From the priorities established for nutrition programing in the community, plans are designed and programs are implemented and evaluated. Baseline data are gathered, and the need for such programs is established. The quality of human life is improved by increasing the health professional's knowledge through research, improving essential services through innovation, and working toward professional training in the allied health field. Discussions regarding research, service, training, and funding mechanisms, proposal writing, and grantsmanship have long been absorbing topics of conversation among nutritionists and health providers. The main question asked is: Where are funds available for expanding one program or starting another?

With the advent of national health insurance, systems of health care, methods of prevention, and a myriad of related subjects on community health will be examined. There will be more questions than answers. Each state and local government can seek additional funds to help gather answers to these important questions. They will look to governmental agencies at federal, state, and local levels, at voluntary health organizations, and at private foundations. Through the years the system of grant awards has evolved as the most satisfactory mechanism to distribute funds available for these agencies.

GRANTS-IN-AID

Grants-in-aid represent a form of transfer of public funds for the purpose of equalizing revenue among several levels of government and among states and their contained local areas. The first purpose is to improve the quality and expand the quantity of government programs in less affluent areas and areas of special need by augmenting their revenue with legal transfers of funds from more wealthy regions.

A second justification for the increasing use of grants-in-aid is to help local government units that are more restricted as to types of revenues available for health programing. A third purpose is to provide some measure of supervision or control over the activities of the lower units of government. Related to this is a fourth purpose of grants-in-aid: the enforcement of minimum standards on the recipient of the grant. As Hanlon[2] points out, few things have been as influential in promoting the employment of qualified public health personnel as have been the conditions attached to grants by both state and federal health agencies.

BRIEF HISTORY OF GRANTS

The idea of grants-in-aid is by no means new, having been first applied in the United States for the improvement of schools in the poorer, particularly rural areas of the state. The support of constitutional law, legislation, contract law, accountancy, management, and administration related to funding has long existed. Even the first inaugural address of George Washington referred to the "promotion of science and literature" as a function of government.[3]

The grant goes back about 129 years, when the Congress of the United States gave $30,000 to Professor Samuel F. B. Morse.[4] This expenditure, authorized on March 3, 1842, by the 27th Congress, provided expense money and personal reimbursement to test for public use the feasibility of the electromagnetic telegraph system, the nucleus of which Morse had already invented. The grant to Morse was directly authorized by Congress and represents one of the first technical proposals accepted by the federal government.

Morrill Act of 1862 and Hatch Act of 1887

Congressional interest in research was manifested during the agriculturally dominated nineteenth century by the passage of the Morrill Act in 1862 and the Hatch Act in 1887. The Morrill Act entitled each state to a grant of public lands based on the total number of its members of Congress. States not containing public land were given scrip. The only condition was that not less than 90% of the gross proceeds was to be used for the establishment, endowment, and maintenance of agricultural and mechanical colleges. The Hatch Act provided $15,000 a year to each state for the establishment of agricultural experiment stations. With this act there was instituted the condition of submission of an annual financial report, to be followed eight years later by provision for a federal audit. This established a pattern that has never since been altered. These legislative enactments established land grant colleges and agricultural stations as adjuncts to these schools. The oldest continuous support of research by the federal government is thus found in the field of agriculture and nutrition.

Sheppard-Towner Act of 1921

The first federal health grants to states were instituted in 1918 for the control of venereal disease through the Public Health Service. Grants-in-aid specifically for mothers and children were provided by the Children's Bureau through the Sheppard-Towner Act of 1921, which operated through 1925. Such services and expanded public health programs and special and general grants were reinstituted in 1935 with the Social Security Act of that year.

Social Security Act of 1935

The Social Security Act of 1935 provided for federal and state cooperation in public health matters on an increased and more or less permanent basis. It provided for annual grants "to assist states, counties, health districts and other political subdivisions of states in establishing and maintaining adequate public health services."[5] Under this act, state-supported services included maternal and child health, child welfare, crippled children's care, and some grants to pay for the foster care of children. The annual appropriation was to be distributed among the states by the Surgeon General of the United States Public Health Service on the basis of three factors: population, special health problems, and financial need. The relative weight to be given these factors was left to the discretion of the Surgeon General after consultation with a conference of the state and territorial health authorities. Since the initial Social Security Act, grants have been extended to include hospitals, nursing homes, and other types of health centers, primarily through the Hospital and Construction (Hill-Burton) Act of 1946. These federal funds are matched by one third to two thirds in state and local funding.

National Cancer Institute—1937; National Institutes of Health—1944

Of further historic interest in the issuance of grants was the creation of the National Cancer Institute by Congress in 1937. This grant was used as the instrument to advance and promote research toward the solution to the mystery of cancer. In 1944, with the creation of the National Institutes of Health, Congress extended the right to use research grants to all components of the National Institutes of Health. This was followed in 1950 with the establishment of the National Science Foundation, to which Congress gave general grant authority.[6]

The term "grant" has been defined by the Director of Institutional Relations of the Division of Research Grants, National Institutes of Health, as a "conditional gift."[7] Chalkley[7] states "that there is no 'the Grant Philosophy.' It varies from agency to agency and it varies within agencies. It undergoes evolutional changes from year to year. The evolutional pressures are many; they are budgetary, they are legislative, they are bureaucratic, and they produce changes that affect the way grants are used and the purposes to which grants are put." This is important to remember as the scene in granting and funding is ever changing.

The great increase in the numbers and types of grants-in-aid programs in the health and health-related fields in the mid-1960s created serious problems of manageability. The 89th Congress alone passed acts that created 21 new health programs, 17 new educational programs, 15 new economic development programs, 12 new programs for cities, 17 new resource development programs, and 4 new manpower programs.[8] Over 170 different federal aid programs existed, financed by over 400 separate appropriations, 21 federal departments, 150 Washington bureaus, and 400 regional offices.

Comprehensive Health Planning and Public Health Service Amendments of 1966 (Public Law 89-749)

The critical situation that existed with reference to the proliferation of grants-in-aid programs without effective mechanisms for their implementation was recognized. Attempts were made at all levels of government, particularly the federal level, to coordinate efforts. A significant step was taken by the passage of Public Law 89-749, the Comprehensive Health Planning and Public Health Service Amendments of 1966, signed into law November 3, 1967. It provided for comprehensive planning for health services, health manpower, and health facilities on the state and local level. It broadened and increased the flexibility of support services in the community and provided for the interchange of federal, state, and local health personnel.

Prior to this act, grants had been given according to defined disease or health problem categories. Under the act they were given to establish and maintain adequate public health services of all kinds, based on a state plan for the planning and provision of public health services that had approval of the Surgeon General. Project grants were awarded to public or nonprofit private agencies and organizations to focus on priority health targets. The goal of this legislation was to allow for the effective utilization of all available health resources.

The passage of Public Law 89-749 resulted in changes in agency organization at the federal and state levels. An office of comprehensive health planning was established in the Public Health Service, and a major reorganization of the regional office structure of the Public Health Service became necessary. (See Table 3-1 for the location of the ten regional offices of the Department of Health, Education, and Welfare.) Applications for grants under the law passed through the appropriate regional office. Each regional health director was provided with assistance through an Advisory and Review Council, the membership of which had to be representative of wide interests, including industry, the medical profession, and universities.[9] (Public Law 89-749 is also discussed in Chapters 3 and 11.)

The National Health Planning and Resources Development Act of 1974 (Public Law 93-641)

In 1978 the United States health system is large and expensive. It employs about 4.5 million people—double the number it employed twenty-five years ago—making it one of the largest industries in the country. Spending for health care in the United States now totals in excess of $100 billion annually, or about 8% of the gross national product, and health expenditures are still rising. New developments in the health field—in financing and delivery of health care and in training—and the need for effective health resources planning led to Public Law 93-641, the National Health Planning and Resources Development Act of 1974, combining the responsibilities of Comprehensive Health Planning, Regional Medical Program, and the Health Facilities Assistance Program (Hill-Burton).

Health Systems Agencies

This act, Public Law 93-641, has established Health Systems Agencies across the country that are responsible for preparing and implementing plans designed to improve the health of the residents of its health service area; to increase the accessibility, acceptability, continuity, and quality of health services in the area; to restrain increases in the cost of providing health services; and to prevent unnecessary duplication of health resources. Under the Health Systems Agencies, funds become available for grants or contracts for health service development projects that advance the goals specified in the law. The funds may not be used for actual delivery of health services.[10] (Public Law 93-641 and Health Systems Agencies are also discussed in Chapters 3 and 11.)

GRANT VERSUS CONTRACT

A constantly repeated source of grievance in the utilization of government grants has been that "there is not a formal statement of public policy setting criteria for using the grant or the contract."[11] A constantly repeated source of confusion is the difference between the grant and the contract, since there are fundamental distinctions between grants and contracts. A grant is an award of financial or direct assistance to an eligible recipient under programs that provide for such assistance based on review and approval of an application, plan, or other document(s) setting forth a proposed activity or program. A contract is a promise or set of promises. Whereas the grant is an agreement to support research, a contract is an instrument to procure research. Grants entail ideas originated and defined by the grantee; contracts contain work requirements specified by the government.

Grant investigators do not conduct research for the governmental agency supplying the funds; rather, they explore ideas of their own choosing in health areas in which there is a high degree of public interest. Grant applications are approved and funded based on considerations of merit and relevance to the grantor organization's program objectives. Grants are supportive in character with the objective of strengthening investigators' opportunities for making valuable contributions to the governmental granting agency's mission and are made to educational and nonprofit institutions to the exclusion of commercial organizations.

Contracts, on the other hand, offer more universal competitive opportunities to all types of scientific sources and are used by the awarding agency as a means of fulfilling *its* program objectives. Because the government defines the area of work to be undertaken by contract, offerors can compete for a commonly understood requirement, and contract proposals received are evaluated with the framework of technical evaluation criteria announced to all competing sources.

Although the dividing line between grants and contracts is not always apparent, the fact remains that the Congress has used the two terms to describe essentially different transactions.[12] A grant is an award of funds, included in a written instrument executed by the head of a federal agency of a duly authorized representative. The grant is usually made for a stated purpose and contains a minimum of limiting conditions.

The grant has been distinguished from the contract in that it does not constitute the procurement of goods and services. The grant is a unilateral act. The primary concern in the grant award is the identification of the public value to be gained through the grant and the capability of the grantee to advance such a value. The grant period then follows.

In the grant system responsible investigators are asked to define their goals, analyze their previous achievements, and give evidence of the scientific value of their ideas. The ability to interest an impartial, usually unknown group of scientists in any investigative effort, large or small, ultimately determines the amount of success a scientist will enjoy in the highly competitive field of gaining financial backing.

The usual grant instrument contains a number along with the name and address of the grantee institution; the grant title is rather descriptive, summarizing the research and effort described in the proposal. It names the principal investigator who is the individual under whose direction the work is carried out. However, it should be emphasized that grants are generally made to institutions.

Almost every federal agency includes language in its regulations and literature to the effect that once a grant is made, the principal investigator, operating with the policies of the grantee institution, is in the best position to determine the means by which the research may be conducted most effectively. Accordingly, the primary responsibility for the performance under any grant is shared by the grantee institution and the principal investigator.

TYPES OF GRANTS

Grants can be classified in several ways, for example, on the basis of purpose (research, training, service, etc.) or on the basis of the method of award (formula or discretionary). A brief glossary of commonly used designations has been designed by the Public Health Service, Department of Health, Education, and Welfare, without regard to classification systems. Therefore these designations are not mutually exclusive. In the department's *Grants Policy Statement*[13] a specific grant might be described by more than one of these terms.

Biomedical research support. A grant to assist an eligible institution to maintain, develop, and advance its biomedical research capabilities. An eligible institution must have received a minimum level of PHS research project grant funds within a given period of time in order to qualify for such a grant.

Capitation. A grant awarded to an eligible institution to provide, maintain, or improve its educational program in areas such as nursing, allied health, and health-professional education. The amount of such an award is based on enrollment factors, including the number of full-time students and the potential for increased enrollments.

Conference. A grant awarded to support the costs of meetings clearly within the areas of PHS program interests.

Consortium. A grant made to one institution in support of a research project in which the program is being carried out through a cooperative arrangement between or among the grantee institution and one or more participating institutions.

Construction. A type of facilities assistance grant made to provide support for building, expanding, and modernizing health facilities. (See *Facilities assistance* below).

Consultation and education. A grant awarded to develop and coordinate the effective provision of health services and to increase public awareness of the nature of particular health problems and of the types of services available.

Continuing education. A grant, usually short term, made to provide support for additional or updated training to professionals, paraprofessionals, or nonprofessionals working in a given health field.

Demonstration. A grant, generally of limited duration, made to establish or demonstrate the feasibility of a theory or approach.

Discretionary or project. A grant made in support of an individual project in accordance with legislation that permits PHS to exercise judgment in selecting the project, the grantee, and the amount of the award.

Facilities assistance. A grant made for the acquisition, remodeling, expansion, or leasing of existing facilities, or the construction of new facilities, and for the initial equipping of such facilities.

Fellowship. An award made in behalf of an individual to support specific training that will enhance that individual's level of competence in the particular health area of concern. Under certain programs, fellowship recipients may be subject to service and payback requirements.

Financial distress. A grant awarded to an eligible institution that is in serious financial difficulty to meet operational costs required to maintain a certain level, quality, or type of health services or educational program, or that has special need for financial assistance to meet accreditation requirements.

Formula. A grant in which funds are provided to specified grantees on the basis of a specific formula, prescribed in legislation or regulations. The formula is usually based on such factors as population, per capita income, enrollment, mortality, and morbidity. In some cases, such as formula grants to States, these grants are mandatory.

Planning. A grant made to support planning, developing, designing, and establishing the means for performing research, delivering health services, or accomplishing other approved objectives.

Research. A grant made in support of investigation or experimentation aimed at the discovery and interpretation of facts, revision of accepted theories in the light of new facts, or the application of such new or revised theories.

Service. A grant made to support costs for the purpose of organizing, establishing, providing, or expanding the delivery of health services to a specified community or area.

Study and development. A grant awarded to study and develop innovative and experimental programs leading to an established health services delivery component.

Training. A grant awarded to an organization to support costs of training students, personnel, or prospective employees in research, or in the techniques or practices pertinent to the delivery of health services in the particular area of concern. Under some programs, student trainees may be subject to service and payback requirements.

SOURCES OF FUNDING

The alert administrator-nutritionist will be aware of the federal and private sources of extra monies for nutrition-related projects. Funds may be highlighted for alcoholism, drug abuse, services to mothers, infants, children, and training paraprofessionals, all of which might include a nutritional component. Or there may be a need within an

agency for gathering baseline data for a specific design for an innovative approach to examine nutritional practices.

The *Catalogue of Federal Domestic Assistance*,[14] published annually, is a comprehensive listing and description of federal programs and activities that provide assistance or benefits to the American public. It includes grants, assistance in goods, services, and properties, technical assistance, statistical and other expert information and service activities of regulatory agencies. The primary purpose of the catalogue is to aid potential beneficiaries in identifying and obtaining available assistance. It is also intended to improve coordination and communication in federal program activities among federal, state, and local governments and to coordinate programs within the federal government.

The 1976 edition of the catalogue lists 1,026 programs. Some of the new programs appearing in this edition are conservation, education, food and nutrition, health planning, health research, humanities, refugee assistance, and social services. Under "nutrition" the subject index indicates the following areas for which financial assistance is available: children, community food and nutrition, digestive diseases and nutrition research, follow through, food and nutrition in cooperative extension service, food and nutrition research, Head Start, Indians, programs for elderly, and soft tissue stomatology and nutrition research.

PUBLIC HEALTH SERVICE

The Public Health Service (PHS) is the principal health component of the Department of Health, Education, and Welfare. The basic mission of the PHS, as a whole, is to protect and advance the nation's health. According to the *Grants Policy Statement*,[13] one of the important activities that PHS carries out in pursuit of this mission is that of awarding grants in support of efforts that help PHS and the recipient institutions to achieve mutually beneficial goals.

The PHS administers a diverse array of grant programs concerned with the whole spectrum of health concerns, which are reflected in the goals of six major agencies:

The Alcohol, Drug Abuse, and Mental Health Administration. This is responsible for developing knowledge, manpower, and services to prevent mental illness, to treat and rehabilitate the mentally ill, to prevent the abuses of drugs and alcohol, and to treat and rehabilitate drug and alcohol abusers.

The Center for Disease Control. This is responsible for the national program of prevention and control of communicable and vector-borne diseases and for the control of certain other non-infectious conditions.

The Food and Drug Administration. The nation's first consumer protection agency is concerned with research and regulation in areas such as food, drugs, cosmetics, and medical devices.

The Health Resources Administration. This is responsible for health planning, research, evaluation, and development of health resources and needs, including manpower and health facilities, and the collection and dissemination of health data.

The Health Services Administration. This is responsible for the improvement of the delivery of health services to the American people.

The National Institutes of Health. This seeks to improve the nation's health by increasing the knowledge related to health and disease through the conduct and support of research, research training and biomedical communications.

These six PHS agencies and the ten PHS regional offices as shown in Table 3-1 are responsible for the award, administration, and monitoring of these grant programs under a variety of legislative authorities, governing regulations, policies, and procedures. The Health Services Administration (HSA) is the focal point for programs and health services for specific population groups of the United States and is concerned with the availability, efficiency, and quality of health care.

The Bureau of Community Health Services (BCHS) administers programs designed to provide high-quality health services primarily to those who are underserved, or unserved, by the nation's health service systems. The following are some examples of project and formula grant programs supported by BCHS:

Appalachian Health Demonstration Program (AHDP). This grant program involves a partnership between the Department of Health, Education, and Welfare and the Appalachian Regional Commission. This program authorizes support for health planning, construction, equipment, and operation of multi-county demonstration health, nutrition, and child care projects that will demonstrate the value of adequate health facilities and services to the economic development of the region.

Community Health Centers (CHC). This is a program of project grants (Community Health Center and Family Health Center Project Grants) to provide primary health care and arrange for specialty and inpatient care primarily for people living in medically underserved areas.

Comprehensive Public Health Services. This program provides for formula grants to assist states in establishing and maintaining adequate community, mental, and environmental public health services, including training of personnel for state and local public health work.

Family Planning (FP). This program provides for project grants to give families full opportunity to exercise freedom of choice to determine the number and spacing of their children through access to family planning information, educational materials, and adequate medical services.

Maternal and Child Health (MCH). This program provides for formula grants to the states to improve and extend services for reducing infant mortality, promoting the health of mothers and children, locating and providing medical, surgical, and other services and care for crippled children or those suffering from conditions that lead to crippling. In addition, it provides for a program of projects including maternity and infant care, children and youth, dental health, and intensive care of infants and special services such as pediatric pulmonary care centers, child abuse services, sudden infant death syndrome programs, and others. Also includes funds for research and training projects.

Migrant Health (MH). This program provides for project grants to improve the health status and the environment of migrant agricultural workers and seasonal farm workers and their families through the provision of comprehensive health services that are accessible to people as they migrate to work.

National Health Service Corps (NHSC). This program provides for the assignment of commissioned officers and civil service personnel of the PHS to areas of the United States to improve the delivery of health care in areas where health services are inadequate because of critical shortages of health personnel.

In the world of grants the prospective grantee, a representative of the agency known as the principal investigator, is the person who submits the proposal to the granting/funding agency. In the past it has been a customary procedure for grants to be awarded to persons well known in the field, those whose past performance made a contribution to the knowledge and practice of sound nutrition principles. Or, too often, monies were awarded to the country's top medical centers. Today, with more competitive entries, monies are being more widely dispersed. Much depends on the strength of the proposal submitted. For this reason it is essential to know the hows and whys of proposal writing.

THE PROPOSAL

A proposal writing guide is a useful tool for the grant administrator. It will not solve all the problems or provide answers to all the questions, but it is an excellent starting point and a help in creating a frame of reference. Two guides that may be useful to the person writing the proposal are those of Willner and Hendricks[6] and Crawford and Kielsmeier.[15]

The guide, *Grants Administration*,[6] evolved from instructional material prepared for a number of institutes and courses in grants and contracts given by the National Graduate University, Washington, D.C., in the early 1970s. Among the subjects presented are the rise and fall of grants, the grant instrument, role of the grants administrator, organizing the grants office, and proposal assistance.

The guide, *Proposal Writing, A Manual and Workbook*,[15] contains a text and several appendixes. The text is an overall view of proposal writing accompanied by a workbook section. The text tells what should be done; the workbook activities help develop skills

in doing. Suggested guidelines for evaluating proposals are presented in the last section and provide insight into what grant reviewers consider important.

The objective of a proposal is the award of a grant or contract that will result in a successful research, training, service, or other kind of project that will make a contribution to the improvement or advancement of society. It is most unlikely that a grant or contract would ever be awarded without a proposal. The proposal document therefore assumes a great deal of importance, magnified in recent years by the increase in competition for grant awards. Although there is no set form for proposal preparation, one method of approach will be presented. An early dialogue between the grantee and the grant administrator should precede the actual writing of the proposal.

The purpose of this early dialogue is to ensure that the author of the grant is "in tune" with the program for which the proposal is to be submitted. Although the grant writer should recruit help on the technical aspects of the proposal from peers, the grant administrator can be of considerable service by advising the seeker of funds on the probable reaction of the government review process to the proposal.

An early dialogue between the grantee and the fiscal officer within the agency is also a vital step. The purpose of this early dialogue is to alert the fiscal officer of the pending project and the application for funds. This will determine in the early stages whether such funding is acceptable within the confines of the agency's policy. Important questions can be answered at this stage also. What are the institutions indirect costs? Who will control the monies if the grant is approved? What flexibility is there in the use of funds? What are the various categories for which monies can be used?

The groups that review and evaluate project grant proposals have only the information submitted by the prospective grantee. Whereas the grant is the award, the proposal is the act of putting forward a plan or stating a scheme for consideration. Therefore

Table 12-1. Major parts of a proposal*

Topic	Function in terms of general questions answered
Introduction	
Statement of the problem	What needs to be done and why?
Review of the literature	What has been done that is relevant?
Objectives	What are the specific testable goals?
Procedure	
Design	What is the structural plan?
	What control will it afford?
Sampling	What population will be sampled?
	What size sample and how drawn?
Measurement and data	What will be measured? How?
Analysis and evaluation	How will the data from the measures be examined?
Time schedule	How much time will be needed to complete each portion of the study?
Product and use	What will be the end product of the study?
(dissemination)	What contribution can it make? How?
Personnel and facilities	Who will do the study? What is their relevant competence?
Budget	What will each part of the study cost?

*Modified from Crawford, J., and Kielsmeier, C.: Proposal writing, a manual and workbook. A Continuing Education Book, Corvallis, Ore., 1970, Oregon State University.

the project proposal should include sufficient information to enable the reviewers to determine accurately what is to be done, why it is to be done, how it is to be accomplished, the anticipated results, and the ability to carry out the project proposal submitted.

Major parts of the proposal

Reviewing groups are assisted in their evaluation when statements in the application are arranged under a uniform pattern of captions as shown in Table 12-1, which indicates the major components of the proposal.

Introduction: statement of the problem and objectives

In the introduction it is important to state the title concisely and accurately so that it clearly indicates to an unfamiliar reader the nature and intent of the project. In stating the problem, the reason why the project is being proposed should be indicated, as well as what questions are to be solved and what is the need to answer these questions or solve the problem. Information should be supplied

that will orient the reader to the setting in which the questions or problem occurs. A description of the situation, events, and characteristics in a specific setting that led to the subject of inquiry will help the reviewers with specific data and pertinent factual information that can support and justify the significance of the project. A review of work already done in the setting that relates to the question or project will establish credibility to the logic of pursuing the study further. A review of the literature, citing related work, is helpful. If the project has wider implications such as for other disciplines, it is helpful to state these. The objectives should be concise and clear. A statement of specific testable goals and how their achievement will relate to the stated questions or problem is essential (Chapter 4).

Procedure

In the procedure or methodology the plan that will help achieve the specific objectives of the study must be presented. What is the plan? How will the plan be carried out, that is, how will it be implemented and in what time schedule? How will the population be sampled?

A built-in evaluation that allows for data collection and decision making is essential and impressive. What methods and measuring devices will be used? How will the status at the beginning of the project period and progress made during the project and at the outcome of the project be determined? This outline for periodic assessment should be consistent with the project proposal and be a reasonable period for accomplishing the work to be undertaken. If evaluation tools are to be developed by project personnel as part of the project, the plans for construction of these tools should be included in the discussion of methodology (Chapter 9).

Personnel and facilities

The reviewing committee will ask who will carry out the work of the project and who will assume responsibility for its fulfillment. The program director should be the individual available and committed to undertake the work if the grant is awarded. The director should be available for an amount of time that is fully sufficient to accomplish the proposed project. It is necessary that the education and experience of the project director be appropriate or at least applicable to the problem with which the project is concerned and to the methods used to carry out the project. The application should describe the program director's educational background and prior work in the area with which the project is concerned. Other pertinent experience and information in sufficient detail to permit evaluation of anticipated direction of the plans proposed will highlight the proposal.

There are some instances when it may not be possible to have the project director under firm commitment to undertake the direction of the project at the time the proposal is submitted. In this instance, information should be included to indicate how the project director will be recruited and how successful the search will be, and the educational background and experience being sought. Specific identification of all personnel

who will be carrying out various parts of the work planned (faculty, project staff, technical assistants, consultants) will strengthen the proposal.

Other major questions that the reviewing committee will have in mind are the facilities and supporting services that will be used in carrying out the work of the project. A description of the facilities available such as special equipment, laboratory space, and communications center should be included. In addition, a list of the supporting services on hand that are pertinent to the work of the project such as technical assistance, consultation, testing services, and maintenance of equipment will add to the reviewers' understanding of the nature of the project. Are there any factors in the institutional environment that will support the project, thereby contributing to the success of the project? Are there plans to collaborate with other institutions or agencies that are not directly affiliated with the institution wherein the project is to be carried out? If so, a description of the organizational structure of that institution showing the lines of authority and the working relationships that will be used to carry out the project with other agencies is necessary. A letter of agreement signed by a responsible officer of each of the associating organizations should be included.

Budget

The reviewing committee will want to know the plans for continuing the project at the end of the grant period and how findings can be disseminated to other interested persons. The budget is all too often a source of confusion. The easiest way to get a feel for proper budget allowance is to peruse some approved budgets for projects that have already been granted by the same agency. The agency will probably include as part of the application form a rather detailed budget schedule. It is useful to construct a sample budget and review it with an experienced researcher or the fiscal officer within the institution. Omission and underestimation are the chief areas of concern to the reviewers. The typical budget consists of three categories: direct costs, indirect costs, and total costs as shown in the following outline.

A. Direct costs
  1. Personnel
    a. Research
    b. Support
    c. Secretarial/clerical
    d. Consultants
  2. Employee benefits
  3. Travel
  4. Supplies and materials
    a. Project and/or instructional materials
    b. Office supplies
    c. Books and journals
  5. Communications
  6. Services
  7. Final report
  8. Equipment and/or equipment rental
  9. Other direct costs
  10. Subtotal direct costs
B. Indirect costs
C. Total costs

Although a great deal of flexibility in the preparation of grant requests is allowed generally, almost all major sources insist on some similar information in one form or another.

Once each of the aforementioned parts of the grant proposal have been designed, it is helpful to refer to a proposal checklist (Fig. 12-1).

SHORTCOMINGS FOUND IN DISAPPROVED GRANT APPLICATIONS

Allen,[16] National Institutes of Health official, performed an extensive study as to why research grant applications are often disapproved. Based on a study section review of 605 disapproved research grant applications during the period of April through May, 1959, a breakdown of the shortcomings occurred as follows: the problem 58% (Class I); the approach 73% (Class II); personnel 55% (Class III); other 16% (Class IV). Table 12-2 enumerates these shortcomings in detail.

Although a great deal of flexibility in the preparation of grant requests is allowed generally, almost all major sources insist on the presentation of similar information in one

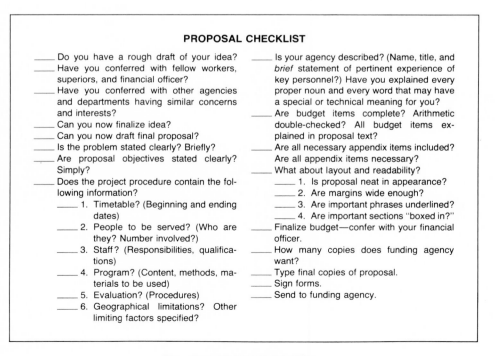

PROPOSAL CHECKLIST

_____ Do you have a rough draft of your idea?
_____ Have you conferred with fellow workers, superiors, and financial officer?
_____ Have you conferred with other agencies and departments having similar concerns and interests?
_____ Can you now finalize idea?
_____ Can you now draft final proposal?
_____ Is the problem stated clearly? Briefly?
_____ Are proposal objectives stated clearly? Simply?
_____ Does the project procedure contain the following information?
  _____ 1. Timetable? (Beginning and ending dates)
  _____ 2. People to be served? (Who are they? Number involved?)
  _____ 3. Staff? (Responsibilities, qualifications)
  _____ 4. Program? (Content, methods, materials to be used)
  _____ 5. Evaluation? (Procedures)
  _____ 6. Geographical limitations? Other limiting factors specified?

_____ Is your agency described? (Name, title, and _brief_ statement of pertinent experience of key personnel?) Have you explained every proper noun and every word that may have a special or technical meaning for you?
_____ Are budget items complete? Arithmetic double-checked? All budget items explained in proposal text?
_____ Are all necessary appendix items included? Are all appendix items necessary?
_____ What about layout and readability?
  _____ 1. Is proposal neat in appearance?
  _____ 2. Are margins wide enough?
  _____ 3. Are important phrases underlined?
  _____ 4. Are important sections "boxed in?"
_____ Finalize budget—confer with your financial officer.
_____ How many copies does funding agency want?
_____ Type final copies of proposal.
_____ Sign forms.
_____ Send to funding agency.

Fig. 12-1. Proposal checklist.

Table 12-2. Shortcomings found in study-section review of 605 disapproved research grant applications, April-May, 1959*

No.	Shortcoming	%
Class I: Problem (58%)		
1.	The problem is of insufficient importance or is unlikely to produce any new or useful information.	33.1
2.	The proposed research is based on a hypothesis that rests on insufficient evidence, is doubtful or is unsound.	8.9
3.	The problem is more complex than the investigator appears to realize.	8.1
4.	The problem has only local significance, or is one of production, or control, or otherwise fails to fall sufficiently clearly within the general field of health-related research.	4.8
5.	The problem is scientifically premature and warrants, at most, only a pilot study.	3.1
6.	The research as proposed is over-involved, with too many elements under simultaneous investigation.	3.0
7.	The description of the nature of the research and of its significance leaves the proposal nebulous and diffuse and without clear research aim.	2.6
Class II: Approach (73%)		
8.	The proposed tests, or methods, or scientific procedures are unsuited to the stated objective.	34.7
9.	The description of the approach is too nebulous, diffuse, and lacking in clarity to permit adequate evaluation.	28.8
10.	The over-all design of the study has not been carefully thought out.	14.7
11.	The statistical aspects of the approach have not been given sufficient consideration.	8.1
12.	The approach lacks scientific imagination.	7.4
13.	Controls are either inadequately conceived or inadequately described.	6.8
14.	The material the investigator proposed to use is unsuited to the objectives of the study or is difficult to obtain.	3.8
15.	The number of observations is unsuitable.	2.5
16.	The equipment contemplated is outmoded or otherwise unsuitable.	1.0
Class III: Man (55%)		
17.	The investigator does not have adequate experience or training or both, for this research.	32.6
18.	The investigator appears to be unfamiliar with recent pertinent literature or methods, or both.	13.7
19.	The investigator's previously published work in this field does not inspire confidence.	12.6
20.	The investigator proposed to rely too heavily on insufficiently experienced associates.	5.0
21.	The investigator is spreading himself too thin; he will be more productive if he concentrates on fewer projects.	3.8
22.	The investigator needs more liaison with colleagues in this field, or in collateral fields.	1.7
Class IV: Other (16%)		
23.	The requirements for equipment or personnel, or both, are unrealistic.	10.1
24.	It appears that other responsibilities would prevent devotion of sufficient time and attention to this research.	3.0
25.	The institutional setting is unfavorable.	2.33
26.	Research grants to the investigator, now in force, are adequate in scope and amount to cover the proposed research.	1.5

*From Allen, E. M.: Why the research grant applications disapproved? Science **132**:1533, Nov. 25, 1960. Copyright 1960 by the American Association for the Advancement of Science.

form or another. The reviewer should be convinced as to the scientific merit of the study and the competence of the investigator. Remember, it is in the formulation and offering of the specific proposal plan that the conscience and imagination of the reviewer of the grant are captured.

GRANTS APPEAL PROCEDURE

A grantee institution may seek a review with respect to an adverse determination. The Secretary of Health, Education, and Welfare has established a Departmental Grant Appeals Board for the purpose of reviewing and providing hearings on postaward

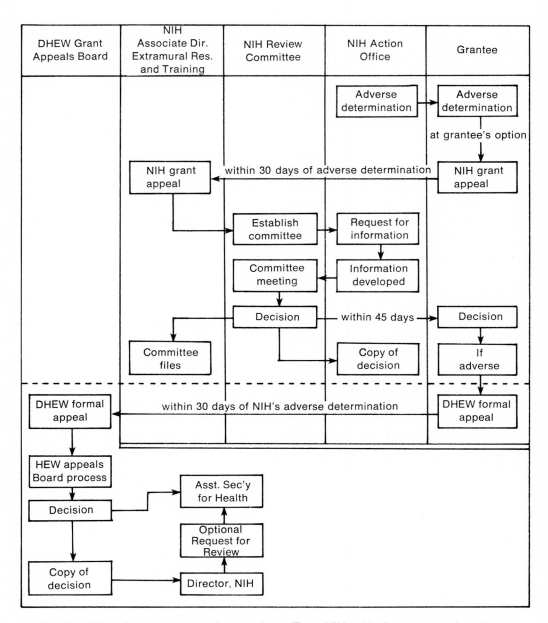

Fig. 12-2. Flow chart grant appeals procedure. (From NIH guide for grants and contracts, Vol. 3, Bethesda, Md., Nov. 13, 1974, U.S. Department of Health, Education, and Welfare.)

disputes that may arise in the administration of Department of Health, Education, and Welfare grants. A flow chart (Fig. 12-2) outlines the procedure that is followed for a grant appeal.[17] Although the request for review need not follow any prescribed form, it must contain a full statement of the grantee's position with respect to the disputed matter and the facts and reasons in support of the position.

SUMMARY

Grant monies have helped to build clinics and medical schools and trained men and women to staff them, have supported medical research, and have underwritten methods of delivering better health care in urban ghettos and Appalachian hills. Grant monies have helped to fund the nutrition component of health services and allowed for innovative method of delivery of service and training of health workers.

Society has called on the government to become increasingly involved in improving health care, whereas government, traditionally, has looked to the private sector, the health professionals, for help in developing and operating the kinds of programs that the public wants and needs.

This partnership of public and private initiative has been strengthened, its work immeasurably advanced, by the many grant programs administered by the Public Health Service since 1918 and carried out by its grantee partners. Today these programs distribute more than $3 billion annually to help finance thousands of projects in all parts of the United States.

The Public Health Service is assigned the task of protecting and advancing the nation's health, and thus it is involved, directly or indirectly, in almost everything that happens in the United States health care system, which in total is a $100-billion enterprise.

There are six Public Health Service agencies covering all aspects of health research, service training, and dissemination of information, and ten regional offices.

When submitting a grant proposal to a government agency, it is well to keep in mind the difference between a grant and a contract. Contracts entail work requirements that are specified by the government; grants, on the other hand, do research and work on ideas that were originated and defined outside the government. Thus it is of major importance to present a clear and detailed proposal to the proper government agency. The government publications, *The Catalogue of Federal Domestic Assistance*, which lists programs and subject areas that offer financial assistance, and the *Grants Policy Statement*, should both be consulted.

The major parts of a grant proposal should include an introduction or statement of the project and its objectives, the procedure or methodology to be followed, how and when the operation will be evaluated, the projected time length of the operation, the personnel and their qualifications, the facilities already available, and a detailed and realistic budget. Should the grant proposal be rejected, the grantee may request an appeal through a specified procedure.

Too often grants are written to comply with existing funds. For example, an announcement that monies are available for community hypertension screening may lead to a flurry of activity to design such a program for the sole purpose of obtaining funds. However, hypertension may not be the priority for the specific community. The nutritionist should assume a leadership role in promoting legislation that will produce funding for health issues that are basic to community needs. Chapter 11 discusses the legislative process as it pertains to nutrition programs.

REFERENCES

1. Nichaman, M. Z., and Collins, G. E.: Nutrition programs in state health agencies, Nutr. Rev. **32:** 65, 1974.
2. Hanlon, J. J.: Public health administration and practice, ed. 6, St. Louis, 1974, The C. V. Mosby Co., p. 151.
3. Bledsoe, E. P., and Ravitz, H. I.: The evolution of research and development as a procurement function of the federal government, Federal Bar J. **17:** 189, July-Sept., 1957.
4. U.S. Congress Report of the Select Committee on Government Research of the House of Representatives, 88th Congress, 2nd session, July 31, 1964, p. 3.
5. Smolensky, J., and Haar, F. B.: Principles of community health, Philadelphia, 1972, W. B. Saunders Co., p. 175.
6. Willner, W., and Hendricks, P. B., Jr.: Grants administration, Washington, D. C., 1972, National Graduate University.
7. Chalkley, D. T.: The grant philosophy, Federal Grants Management Proceedings, Bethesda, Md., 1970, National Graduate University, p. 3.
8. Reston, J.: Johnson's administrative monstrosity, The New York Times, Nov. 26, 1966.
9. Cavanaugh, J., and McHisock, J.: Comprehensive Health Planning and Public Health Service Act of 1966 (P.L. 89-749), Health, Education and Welfare Indicators, Jan., 1967.
10. Public Health Service Health Planning and Resources Development Act of Washington, D.C., 1974, HEW publication no. (HRA) 76-14015, Government Printing Office.
11. Grossbaum, J. J.: Choosing between research project grants and contracts in mission agencies, Nat. Contract Management J. **5:**40, Spring, 1971.
12. Willcox, A. W., General Counsel, U.S. Department of Health, Education, and Welfare: Letter to M. Wesker, Assistant Solicitor, U.S. Department of Interior, Dec. 20, 1968.
13. Public Health Service: Grants policy statement, Washington, D.C., Oct. 1, 1976, HEW publication no. (OS) 77-50,000, pp. 6-7.
14. Catalogue of federal domestic assistance, Washington, D.C., 1976, Executive Office of the President, Office of Management and Budget.
15. Crawford, J., and Kielsmeier, C.: Proposal writing, a manual and workbook. A Continuing Education Book, Corvallis, Ore., 1970, Oregon State University.
16. Allen, E. M.: Why are research grant applications disapproved? Science **132:**1533, Nov. 25, 1960.
17. NIH guide for grants and contracts, HEW publication, Nov. 13, 1974, Washington, D.C., Government Printing Office.

SUGGESTED READINGS
U.S. Department of Health, Education, and Welfare, Washington, D.C., Government Printing Office

NIH guide for grants and contracts. Published at irregular intervals to provide policy, program, and administrative information to individuals and organizations who need to be kept informed of requirements and changes in grants and contracts activities administered by The National Institutes of Health.

Office of Education support for research and related activities (free on request). This 22-page manual provides summary information on patterns of support and application procedures through the U.S. Office of Education. It is a helpful reference guide for anyone involved in education research.

Programs and services ($2.00). This is a useful and comprehensive guide to federal programs administered through the Department of Health, Education, and Welfare. It is highly recommended as a valuable reference source.

Public Health Service: Profiles of grant programs, HEW publication no. (OS) 75-50,002, Oct., 1974.

Public Health Service: Grants policy statement, HEW publication no. (OS) 77-50,000, Oct. 1, 1976.

Review and approval procedures Public Health Service research grant and award programs, Bethesda, Md., 1965, National Institutes of Health Division of Research Grants.

Other publications

Church, D. M.: Seeking foundation funds, New York, 1956, New York Health and Welfare Services, National Public Relations Council.

College and University Reporter (Topical Law Reports), Commercial Clearinghouse, Inc., 420 Lexington Ave., New York ($55 annual subscription includes weekly bulletin on recent developments in Washington, D.C., in legislation relating to education and research). This is an expensive reference source, but the services provided to the subscriber are well worth the investment. Two large loose-leaf books are included, containing detailed and completely up-to-date information on all major developments in the field of education. The volumes are revised each week when the company (CC) mails supplementary loose-leaf pages to all subscribers. Included, too, are weekly bulletins dealing with recent developments in Washington, D.C., and a copy of each law or pending law in both the House and Senate pertaining to education. This is a must for a larger research organization.

Elliott, R., and Michak, H. B.: Raising funds from foundations, Nurs. Outlook **20**:108, Feb., 1972.

Federal grants reporter: basic reference guide, Washington, D.C., 1976, ($85.00). This is a resource volume that pulls together all circulars, regulations guidelines, executive orders, court decisions and statutes affecting grant management. It is designed for the front-line grant administrator, coordinator, lawyer, or finance officer who needs comprehensive information efficiently organized in a single reference work. It consists of a *Basic Reference Guide*, which collects and analyzes executive, agency, and judicial decisions affecting all federal grant recipients, and individual chapters, which probe the makeup and set forth the requirements for twenty-one major federal grant-making agencies. These individual agency chapters devote a separate chapter to each of the twenty-one major federal grant-making agencies. Each individual chapter is indexed and crossreferenced to the *Basic Reference Guide*. The chapters, available at an additional $10.00, contain specific guidelines, issuances, and regulations for each agency's own grant programs; a list of all grant programs administered by the agency; grantee hearing rights; and formal and informal dispute resolution procedures. The chapter most helpful for the nutritionist is the special chapter on Public Health Service (HEW grants from PHS, NIH, and NIMH for health planning, services and construction, maternal and child health; drug abuse, mental health, alcohol research and training). Others might be Agriculture Department (school lunch, soil conservation, Farmers Home Administration); Community Action Program (CAP); Education (HEW educational grants including adult, bilingual, handicapped, follow-through, Indian, right-to-read, research and development grants); Human Development (HEW grants for Head Start, aging, youth development, delinquency, R & D grants); Interior Department (Indian programs, outdoor recreation, fisheries and wildlife); Labor Department (employment, training and manpower programs); National Science Foundation; Social and Rehabilitation Service (HEW grants including public assistance and social services such as child welfare, work incentive, rehabilitation, developmental disabilities).

Fish, M., editor: National organizations of the U.S., ed. 7, Detroit, 1972, Yale Research Co., Vol. 1.

Grant Data Quarterly, Academic Media, Inc., 10835 Santa Monica Blvd., Los Angeles, Calif. 90025. (single subscription $35.00; 10% on two or more). The first four issues (1967) present detailed information on government support programs, business and professional organization support programs, and foundation support programs. This quarterly would be valuable as a reference source for college libraries or progressive departments contemplating a substantial volume of research and development activities.

Guide to support programs for education, ed. 2, St. Paul, 1967, Education Service Press, Visual Products, 3M Company ($12.00). This is a worthwhile investment for the novice. It discusses federal laws aiding education and aid from business and foundation sources, and it provides helpful hints on how and where to obtain support for research, development, or training programs.

Krathwol, D. R.: How to prepare a research proposal, Syracuse ($1.00). 1966, Syracuse University Bookstore.

Larocque, G. M.: Consumerism, federal grants and you: the consumer of services and the inexperienced —and not so inexperienced—grant applicant, Exposition Press, Inc., 900 So. Oyster Bay Rd., Hicksville, N.Y. 11801 (8.75). In concise, readable style, this book offers expert technical assistance and tells absolutely all you need to know about the world of federal grants including special techniques for preparing written grant proposals, method of accounting, understanding government reports, negotiating budgets and contracts, conducting reviews and audits, defining objectives, evaluating projects, and much more.

Lewis, M. Q., editor: The foundation directory, ed. 4, New York, 1971, Columbia University Press.

Rowland, H. S.: New York Times guide to federal aid for cities and towns, New York, 1971, Quadrangle/ The New York Times Book Co.

The Grantsmanship Center, 1015 West Olympic Blvd., Los Angeles, Calif. 90015 ($10.00 annually).

Willner, W., and Hendricks, P. B., Jr.: Grants administration, Washington, D.C., 1972. National Graduate University. This book evolved from instructional materials prepared for a number of institutes and courses on grants and contracts given by the National Graduate University in the early 1970s. It was prepared to offer assistance to college and university administrators in diverse field of grants and contracts with federal agencies, but it is equally useful for state, county, and city governmental agencies as well as with other nonprofit institutions and foundations. The frame of reference is applicable to hospitals, community health centers, model cities, and nonprofit research, training, and social action entities of all kinds, sizes, shapes, and varieties, both financially dependent on and financially independent of the federal government.

GENERAL CONCEPTS

There is a horizon on which nutritionists can plot their future course involving the commitment of the health professional, the government, the medical insurance industry, and the people in the community.

OUTCOMES

The student should be able to do the following:
- Characterize the role of nutrition and community-level services in health care today.
- Identify what is meant by "wellness" as opposed to "absence of disease."
- Identify the areas of nutrition research that require further study.
- Point out the implications of a national health insurance plan.

The outlook for nutrition services: where do we go from here?

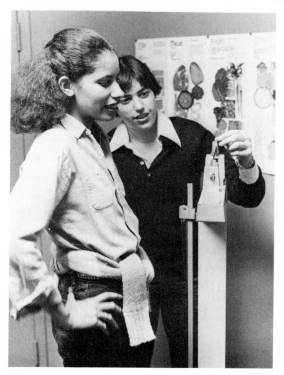

Photograph by Gary O. Goldsmith, M.D.

VIEWPOINT OF THE AUTHORS

In the preceding chapters the subjects and issues discussed should be considered by the student and the practitioner when planning and providing nutrition services as a component of health care in community programs. These subjects and issues, including a national nutrition policy, the role of the public health nutritionist, the role of the community, the art and essentials of program planning, budgeting, and legislation, have been examined from our viewpoint, and we are both practicing public health nutritionists

and teachers. The approach has been to present a step-by-step method for the planning, implementation, and evaluation of community nutrition programs.

We have attempted to show how to take a broad view of the subject of community nutrition, although the models here hardly present the only answer or do they cover every aspect of the material. Rather, the models, examples, and procedures should be considered stimuli for exploring other theories and challenging creativity in the development of other methods of practical application.

343

AN AFTERWORD ABOUT COMMUNITY MEDICINE*

Community medicine, then, provides a way whereby health professionals can keep their activities in context; that is it provides a horizon upon which they can plot their own course on some relatively fixed points of reference . . . Community medicine then gives its practitioners a series of reference points for raising new questions and perhaps for challenging old answers. To its proponents it is an ever-changing, dynamic discipline, borrowing and synthesizing concepts and procedures from a variety of sources. To its detractors it sometimes appears ill-defined and uncertain, and often confusing. To its poets and philosophers it is "a star to every wandering bark, whose worth's unknown, although its height be taken."

*The authors relate this to an afterword about community nutrition.

Robert L. Kane, editor: The challenges of community medicine, New York, 1974, Springer Publishing Co., Inc. Reprinted by permission. Copyright © 1974 by Springer Publishing Co., Inc., New York.

NUTRITION IN THE COMMUNITY

We have defined community nutrition as that discipline which deals with the identification and solution of health problems related to nutrition in communities or particular population groups. When focusing on the community, the common denominator should be the entire population rather than only those who present themselves for care.

We believe that the current changes in the health care delivery system have emphasized the values of services at the community or neighborhood level. In the future many of the services that are now offered in hospitals and physicians' offices are more likely to be based in the community, where it is hoped that they will be more accessible and acceptable to the resident population. The trend is for students and practitioners to become more community oriented, to share more responsibility in the planning, implementation, and evaluation of community health care services.

Our primary unit of concern, the community, is the most realistic place for the practitioner and the student to obtain the information and experience necessary to guide decision making and future professional performance. Everyone in the community—consumer, practitioner, and student, health care agency, and others—needs to become involved in identifying and ordering the problems. The community is made up of individuals who wield considerable political and social power. Consumers can be a potent force in health planning.

Health decision making on a community level consists of the following four phases: (1) assessment, containing the elements of data collection, analysis of data, and statement of conclusions; (2) planning, with the elements of setting priorities, defining objectives, and selecting the appropriate solutions; (3) implementation, the action; and (4) evaluation, measuring and judging actions. Operationally, these four steps are continuous and at times occur simultaneously. It is not unreasonable to implement a plan to meet an immediate goal while assessment continues to enable long-range planning. Planning and the resulting intervention imply concern with a change process. The process of planned change involves a change agent who is concerned and knowledgeable about possible change and a client. They will work together to apply their combined efforts in solving a problem. The evaluation process is ongoing to provide continuous feedback for reassessment and reordering of priorities based on new data.

To accomplish all this, there are methods and sources for getting information. Specific tools are required for community diagnosis, which draws on such diverse fields as sociology, political science, economics, biostatistics, epidemiology, and health service research (the application of the epidemiologic technique to analyzing the effects of medical care on health). The tools for nutritional assessment—dietary, biochemical, clinical, and anthropometric—have been used in the various stages of the individual life cycle, as well as in the composite picture of the community.

The mathematical science of biostatistics, once the boring manipulation of complex mathematical procedures, has been freed by

WHO IS RESPONSIBLE FOR HEALTH?

Most individuals do not worry about their health until they lose it. . . .The individual must realize that perpetuating the present system of high-cost, after-the-fact medicine will only result in higher costs and greater frustration. The next major advances in the health of the American people will be determined by what the individual is willing to do for himself and for society at large. If he is willing to follow reasonable rules for healthy living, he can extend his life and enhance his own and the nation's productivity. If he is willing to reassert his authority with his children, he can provide for their optimal mental and physical development. If he participates fully in private and public efforts to reduce the hazards of the environment, he can reduce the causes of premature death and disability. If he is unwilling to do these things, he should stop complaining about the rising costs of medical care and the disproportionate share of the gross national product that is consumed by health care. He can either remain the problem or become the solution to it; beneficent government cannot.

John H. Knowles: Responsibility for health, Science **198:** 1103, Dec., 1977. Copyright 1977 by the American Association for the Advancement of Science.

---

the computer to expand into fruitful areas such as medical diagnosis, simulation models of health situations, and rapid processing of large volumes of data.

WELLNESS: BEYOND GOOD HEALTH

Often there seems to be confusion among the concepts of "health" and "medicine" and "health care" and "medical care"—words that are often used loosely and interchangeably. Medicine and medical care are appropriate when referring to sickness, although health is more than the absence of sickness. Health is a positive state of well-being—a feeling of being on top of one's form or possessing a high quality of life.

The prevention of disease is only a part of the maintenance of good health. Too often prevention has been viewed by both the individual and institutions as merely that which can be done to forestall disease. Thus the disease model pervades everyone's thinking about good health. As Mico and Ross[1] state, "Practically all that is done in health care now for prevention-diagnosis-treatment-rehabili-

tation purposes is done from within the context of disease-oriented programs and organizations." Health professionals, especially, should be acquainted not only with what individuals can do to avoid being sick but, more importantly, with what they can do in a positive way to remain healthy or to achieve even better health.

What is health?

The World Health Organization[2] has stated that *"Health* is a state of complete physical, emotional, and social well-being, and is not merely the absence of disease and infirmity." However, others such as Dubos[3] and Dunn[4] consider that this definition is utopian and unrealistic. Instead Dunn prefers to define high-level wellness as follows:

High-level wellness for the individual is defined as an integrated method of functioning which is oriented toward maximizing the potential of which the individual is capable. It requires that the individual maintain a continuum of balance and purposeful directions within the environment where he is functioning.

This allows for the particular individual, his environment, and the opportunity for change, presumably, to improve.

Furthermore, Kirk and associates[5] remind us that although wellness is an individual personal responsibility, the tasks it requires of the individual are mostly determined by the larger social system. If society does not enhance or support the completion of wellness tasks, it is difficult for individuals to maintain the proper motivation to develop a complete sense of well-being.[5] Unfortunately, as yet, there are no statistics, no index or cluster of factors, no baseline data that can be used to measure or to assess an individual's health.[6]

What really contributes to health wellness? Or as Jourard[7] asks, "What ways of behaving in the world will promote health?" He states that the most obvious answers relate to diet, rest, and exercise. That person who attempts to keep fit, who finds his life challenging and satisfying, and who resists infections and illness better is labeled "a phys-

THE WELLNESS PROCESS

Good health is only a part of what individuals can experience; they also can experience "wellness." Wellness can only be experienced by individuals, however, if they actively pattern their behavior and lifestyle to suit their circumstances. Wellness is not a static state of being. Rather it is a continually evolving and changing process in which individuals may participate; it is, as much as possible, an integration of all aspects of their physical, mental, social, and environmental well-being . . . One might assume from the emphasis given to health by the mass media that good health is highly valued in our society, but the lack of healthful behavior on the part of many people leads us to question this assumption.

John G. Bruhn, F. David Cordova, James A. Williams, and *Raymond G. Fuentes, Jr.:* The wellness process, J. Commun. Health **2**:209-221, Fall, 1977.

ical-health-promoting personality" by Jourard. On the other hand, that person who does not pay attention to eating, sleeping, and exercise routine and who has a lack of satisfaction in interpersonal relationships, problems with self-image and self-identity, lack of emotional spontaneity, and an overdeveloped sense of duty is labeled an "illness yielding personality." He notes that, in reality, periods of illness may be periods of respite from a dispiriting way of life for some people.[7]

What about life-style?

Recently, there has been much concern and discussion about life-styles. It is now apparent that the health status and general well-being of a given population are determined by a complex ecologic network of forces that operate within a community. These forces include the environment, genetic endowment, habits, and the availability of health care services. The environment itself includes the economic, social psychological, and cultural factors that influence not only matters of disease control, health attitudes, and behavior but also the provision, organization, and utilization of health services.[8] Health reflects the quality of life, and therefore it is an indicator of the total community profile.

The community nutritionist must now view the health and social problems of an individual or a family within the context of how all these forces affect the community.

It is apparent that many health professions have failed dismally in changing behavior. Many variable conditions, such as obesity, exercise, diet, and cigarette smoking are risk factors in disease, and it is vital that health professionals identify the distribution, extent, and nature of their client's health knowledge, attitudes, and behavior. The community nutritionist is in a position to have grass roots experience and knowledge that should be shared for effective program planning.

A look at successful programs demonstrates that often prevention can be cost effective, particularly in situations of individual primary prevention (adoption of a healthful life-style) and selective screening and appropriate early therapy. We believe that a significant reduction in sedentary living and overnutrition, alcoholism, hypertension, and excessive cigarette smoking would save more lives in the age range of 40 to 64 years than the best current medical practice. The significantly lower incidence of disease among Mormons and Seventh-Day Adventists, and their lower mortalities, are indications of the preventive effects of healthful life-styles.[9]

As health care professionals, we support continued improvements in clinical medicine and fundamental research, of course. The issue is one of priorities and resources, since it is obvious that cost-effective selective screening and risk-factor reduction can lower morbidity, mortality, and medical costs, thus leading to an increase in total real national output. If a national, comprehensive preventive program is to be implemented and succeed, it must have the enthusiastic support of *all health professions* to which the public has entrusted its well-being, especially the medical profession; the support of the *government*, which alone has the resources to create a national approach and to provide the necessary incentives; the support of the *medical insurance industry*, which must cooperate with the government in this effort; and the support of the *individual*, who must accept a greater responsibility for his or her own well-being and exert the required self-discipline in the modification of life-style habits.

PERSONAL COMMITMENT

It is a paradox that health professionals, in their efforts to improve people's health-related practices, seem to expect more from the ordinary consumer than they do of themselves. It is mistakenly assumed that if people know what is most healthful, they will do it. As Milio[10] has reminded us, too often there is a lack of commitment by the professionals toward the very goals that they are attempting to establish for others:

If *knowing* what is health-generating were directly related to *doing*, then surely we in the health field would be among the most robust in the nation, slim, agile, nonsmoking, temperate eaters of complementary protein, low fat and cholesterol, low-sucrose, and nonrefined carbohydrate foods, avoiders of drugging levels of alcohol and other artificial mood-changers, evenly paced in our daily patterns.

Rather, the mere realization that a health need exists is not enough, but it is the translation of need to demand that provides the stimulus. There are variable influences that have great impact as determinants of the conversion of need to demand: sociocultural (education level, attitudes, values toward health), economic (income level, methods available for financing), and spatial (location and type of facilities required). The health care delivery system is one in which economic motivations are at least equally as strong as the service motivation. As Bruhn and co-workers[11] state, "In any case, an individual's economic resources determine how well he uses the system and how much health care is available to him. In health care, dollars are destiny. There is no such incentive as yet in our society for individuals to become well."

Above all else, our commitment must be to

THE AMERICAN DIETETIC ASSOCIATION POSITION PAPER ON CONTINUING EDUCATION*

The "Goals of the Lifetime Education of the Dietitian"[1] serve as a basis for the on-going continuing education and development throughout the lifetime of each dietitian. The American Dietetic Association defines continuing education as that which follows the basic preparation for the profession of dietetics and recognizes that this is a life-long process.

The objectives of continuing education are:

(a) To enhance the knowledge of the individual member, thereby improving her competency.

(b) To enable the individual member to contribute to the advancement of the profession of dietetics.

The consumer of dietetic services has the right to expect excellence of dietetic practice. The dietitian recognizes that continuing education is an essential element of professional competence. Each dietitian has the responsibility to evaluate her own educational needs and to initiate a plan for self-development. The individual accepts the responsibility for determining the value of an educational activity in terms of her own needs.

The American Dietetic Association recognizes its responsibility for setting and maintaining standards for dietetic education. National, affiliated, and district associations assume responsibility for sponsoring and informing members of continuing education opportunities.

The American Dietetic Association shares in the responsibility for the continuing education of its members. Primarily, self-development is the member's commitment to the realization of her professional goals. Continuing education is the intellectual stimulation to open new vistas related to job enrichment and the prevention of professional obsolescence. It is an extension of the dietitian's field of knowledge which may prepare her for assuming greater professional responsibilities. The dietitian benefits not only herself, but is better able to serve those who are recipients of her services. In turn, this contributes to the strength of the profession.

*Approved by the Executive Board on November 30, 1973, as Position Paper No. 0000L.

Reference

1. Comm. on goals of education for dietetics, Dietetic Internship Council, The Amer. Dietetic Assoc.: Goals of the lifetime education of the dietitian. J. Am. Dietet. A. **54**:91, 1969.

   Position paper on continuing education, J. Am. Diet. Assoc. **64**:289, 1974.

ourselves as professionals to design an on-going, continuing education and development program to guide us throughout our careers. The objectives of continuing education are (1) to enhance the knowledge ourselves, thereby improving our competency, and (2) to enable us to contribute to the advancement of our profession. *The American Dietetic Association Position Paper on Continuing Education* recognizes that this is a lifelong process.

GOVERNMENT COMMITMENT

Earlier chapters referred to the Senate's involvement in national nutrition policy. New allies in the effort to define individual nutritional needs have been the Subcommittee on Domestic and International Scientific Planning, Analysis and Cooperation (DISPAC) of the House Science and Technology Committee. Hearings held in the summer of 1977 examined subjects such as the nature and extent of malnutrition and nutritional status in the United States, nutrition surveillance and monitoring within the United States and efforts outside the United States, and nutrition research priorities and accomplishments in the United States and elsewhere.[12]

Esther Peterson,[13] Special Assistant to the President for Consumer Affairs, made the following preface to her testimony at the subcommittee on DISPAC:

The nutrition of people is not only affected by what scientists know or what doctors tell them, or even by what they, themselves, understand. It is affected by decisions in the area of agricultural policy, in economic and tax policy, in export and import policy, as well as by decisions in almost every other area of activity with which the government is concerned. Nutrition is a complex subject which involves decisions of food production, transportation, processing, marketing, consumer choice, income, and education, as well as food availability and palatability.

I am reminded almost sadly that one of the reasons why I resigned from the food advisory panel of the Office of Technology Assessment is that it seemed unable to break away from the preoccupation with agricultural production which has domi-

nated government concern in the food policy area . . . All of that, of course is changing and changing rapidly.

At this same Hearing, Wilbur J. Cohen[14] and his colleagues from University of Michigan, where he is currently Dean and Professor of Public Welfare Administration, School of Education, and who was formerly the Secretary of Health, Education, and Welfare, commented on the need for government commitment to the prevention of disease through expanded nutrition research, knowledge, and dissemination of information: "I only wish I knew in 1968 what I know now, so that I could have unleashed the full power of the Department of Health, Education, and Welfare in strengthening this aspect of disease prevention on behalf of the American people."

Cohen was heartened with the recent activity of the Nutrition Coordinating Committee in the National Institutes of Health, the special concern for nutrition in the National Institute of Child Health and Human Development, and the approval by the present Secretary of Health, Education, and Welfare of a policy statement on the "Health Aspects of Nutrition" in March, 1975.[15] He nevertheless believed that nutrition policy and research could be strengthened by congressional action and he called on Congress to enact legislation specifically authorizing and directing the Secretary of Health, Education, and Welfare to be responsible for developing and implementing nutritional research projects and policies.

Congressman Fred Richmond[16] is calling on the government to make a more organized effort to coordinate nutrition education activities. He has blatantly stated that consumers are deprived of reliable nutrition education.

We are spending more than $70 million a year on a patchwork of more than 30 uncoordinated and unfocused programs administered by 11 different agencies which are going blithely about their business in splendid isolation from each other and the contemporary world in which we live.

We are, of course, living in the age of electronic media. Instant replay brings us from one corner of the globe to the other. Yet when we want answers to our questions from the Federal government, we must wait six weeks or more to receive a pamphlet from the Government Printing Office.

Today, we are doing something unique in the history of this Committee. Instead of having producers, technocrats and marketers tell us what is good for the consumer, we are going to hear consumers and their representatives tell us directly of their concerns, demands and needs.

Be assured that this Subcommittee shall deliver your message next week to the Government policy-makers whom Congress has mandated to inform and counsel the public. This Subcommittee takes its jurisdiction very seriously. Our charge is to protect the interests of the consumer in matters pertaining to food and nutrition. You have the right to receive answers to your questions when you want them, where you want them and how you want them. We promise you who have come to participate in our hearings that your words will guide us.

National Consumer Health Information and Health Promotion Act (Public Law 94-317)

The National Consumer Health Information and Health Promotion Act, Public Law 94-317, signed by President Carter, June 23, 1976, requires health education in delivery systems and sets up mechanisms for nationwide development, testing, and dissemination of methods to promote health-generating behavior. It requires the Secretary of Health, Education, and Welfare to develop national goals and strategies for preventive health services and to explore innovative health promotion concepts, and it also provides for technical assistance in these areas. There is also a section devoted to assistance particularly for research programs, including cost and effectiveness assessment, and community programs, including developing models for planning, operation, and evaluation of community programs.

The Child Nutrition Act of 1977

In a major compromise the House and Senate have passed the Child Nutrition Bill under which states would receive an automatic entitlement of 50 cents for each schoolchild, with no state receiving less than $75,000 a year, for nutrition education in fis-

cal years 1978 and 1979. In fiscal year 1980 the entitlement would be subject to the regular congressional appropriations process.

Research

According to a statement from The American Dietetic Association made late in 1976, there are major gaps in knowledge regarding human nutrition, and in the areas where dietary studies do exist, they do not provide readily useful data for the community level. Certain issues require much more research, for example, the availability of iron and other nutrients to the human body and their utilization, the relationship between nutrition and degenerative diseases such as cancer and diabetes, the effect of diet on recovery from illness, the interrelationships between nutrients in mixed diets as opposed to usage of isolated nutrients, the effects of fad diets, the long-term effect of a vegetarian diet, and the complete analysis of all foods.

There is also a need to arrive at nutritional standards for the aging and also for other population groups aside from the most typically "normal," such as handicapped or hypermetabolic individuals for instance. In addition, the standards that have been developed by various programs and studies should be coordinated and considered in terms of cost effectiveness.

Another important area for research occurs with the need to bring together knowledge and standards and the nutritional activities of the food production industry, which actually supplies most food to the consumer.

Furthermore, there is a need for research into the health services system itself. As Lewis[17] points out, health services research is evaluative research that studies all or part of the health care system, including the workings of the various subsystems, the follow-up after initial contact with the patient, the utilization of goods and facilities, and the costs.

According to a report prepared by the Subcommittee on Domestic Marketing, Consumer Relations and Nutrition, entitled *The Role of the Federal Government in Nutrition Education*,[18] there is great justification for health services research. This report lists and describes thirty different nutrition education programs administered by various government agencies, but it indicates no single federal policy or coordination among these programs or does it indicate how much they cost and the number of people served. Certainly, integration and coordination of such programs would eliminate waste and help them perform with increased impact.[18]

PROFESSIONAL COMMITMENTS: ASTPHND AND AGFPHN

Specific recommendations that will influence future planning for public health nutrition were made at The National Public Health Nutrition Workshop held in Chicago in May, 1977. This was a joint venture of the members of the Association of State and Territorial Public Health Nutrition Directors (ASTPHND) and the Association of Graduate Faculties of Schools of Public Health Nutrition (AGFPHN). Top priority was given to national nutrition standards, health planning, payment mechanisms for nutrition services, surveillance, and cost effectiveness and staffing patterns.

National nutrition standards

It was recommended that there should be a nationally coordinated effort in the development and implementation of nutrition standards. The standards for ambulatory care should be written to include process and outcome criteria, and they should be adapted to promote optimal nutritional care in local circumstances.

Health planning

ASTPHND should give its assistance to the federal health planning agency and participate in the community planning process as well through local agencies such as Health Systems Agency (HSA). As standards and other data become available, they should be included in HSA plans. A document entitled "Community Nutrition in Preventive Health Care Programs" was prepared for the National Health Planning Information Center to address priority number eight of the Health

Planning Legislation, which states, "the promotion of activities for the prevention of disease includes studies of nutritional and environmental factors affecting health and the provision of preventive health care services." This document covers the state of the art in nutrition services with a review of 230 papers.[19]

Payment mechanisms

It was recommended that nutrition service be recognized by insurance companies as a reimbursable service and that dietitians and nutritionists be included as health care providers in all pending legislation.

Surveillance

All data gleaned from nutrition surveillance systems, both public and private, should be pooled in a national system so that progress of programs can be measured and local nutrition situations can be compared with national standards. Also, nutrition data should be included in all health screening activities.

Cost effectiveness and staffing patterns

Nutritionists should develop cost-effectiveness data on nutrition as a component of prevention, early diagnosis, and treatment. There should also be a prescribed staffing ratio, with the following as a proposed standard:

Ratio for general population
   1 Public health nutritionist/50,000 population
   5 Supportive personnel/50,000 population
   ½ Clerical position/1 nutritionist
Ratio for ambulatory care programs for a target population
   1 Public health nutritionist/1,000 client population
   2 Supportive personnel/1,000 client population
   ½ Clerical position/1 nutritionist

POPULATION

The issues of population, especially an increasing population in terms of actual numbers, and adequate nutrition for all the world's peoples are closely connected. It is clear that the increase in population and the increase in material consumption per capita must reach limits in a finite world. In addition to educating populations about the necessity of fertility control, which in itself requires great cultural and social adjustments, it is certain that there must be economic adjustments as well. However, before such fundamental and massive environmental changes can become a reality, it is vital that family planning programs be a part of any comprehensive health care system.

NATIONAL HEALTH INSURANCE

No doubt, if this book had been written a year or so later, further comments pertinent to the practical application of a national health insurance plan would be available. Nevertheless, when that day comes, the guidelines discussed herein will be ready to be included in the ensuing programs.

Prior to the establishment of a national health insurance system, specific changes must first be made in the health care delivery system. Briefly, it appears necessary that (1) planning, rate setting, reimbursement, and regulation be firmly linked and coordinated; (2) a system of regionalization be planned for and established; (3) consumers be encouraged to use "lower levels" of care when appropriate; (4) bold new experiments in health care delivery be tried and tested; and (5) prevention of disease, as far as possible, through massive health education be a "must." Without such ground rules any system of national health insurance will become a financial disaster, similar to the Medicaid experience.

When national health insurance becomes a reality, disease prevention will be even more important than it is now because prevention of illness may be the most effective way to control the enormous and mounting costs of delivering personal health services. Thus the need for sound and efficient systems of delivering community preventive services will be intensified rather than obviated by the passage of a national health insurance plan.

The passage of a national health insurance plan in the near future seems certain. How-

ever, many erroneously believe that national health insurance will answer the needs of disease prevention by providing health care to all. This position ignores the difference between personal preventive health services delivered to an individual and community preventive health services. It also ignores the fact that whereas some plans cover some personal preventive health services, none of the current national health insurance proposals covers community preventive health services.

The health insurance plan recommended to the President by the Department of Health, Education, and Welfare[20] will be consistent with the following basic principles that have already been set forth by President Carter:

1. The inclusion of preventive health care services, particularly for children
2. Equality in our health care system, and thus a universal and mandatory health insurance program
3. Management efficiency
4. Quality assurance mechanisms
5. Citizen/consumer participation in the administration of national health insurance and community participation in decisions about health care services
6. The need for a phased national health insurance plan and coordination with the administration's welfare reform plan

Community preventive health services include those directed at unmet environmental needs, public health laboratories, disease control and prevention, family planning, migrant health, health education, nutrition, maternal and child health, and dental health. To deliver these services, the supportive activities of outreach and community management are necessary. Such services may be delivered by state and local health departments, through the know-how of personnel specifically trained in the areas of nutrition and preventive care on a community level.[21]

The 1970s have already brought some comprehensive planning (Chapter 4) and allied health legislation that will foster providing the means for meeting preventive care manpower needs. Thus nutritionists now have greater visibility, more services of nutritional care outside the hospital have been brought about, and new levels of care and emphasis on the quality of care are apparent. As nutritionists work with community health planning agencies, it becomes more and more likely that an effective, preventive and comprehensive health care system can become a reality.

SUMMARY

Once again, the need for including a nutrition component in any community health care system is emphasized. There is a trend showing that practitioners and students are becoming more involved in the planning, implementation, and evaluation of community health care services. Concomitant with this is the idea that wellness or health is not simply the absence of sickness but is a positive state of well-being and a high quality of life and that people can be educated to conduct their lives in a physically health-promoting manner. Certainly this requires effort and commitment from both the professional and the government and the need for them to work together. Mutual cooperation would involve sharing of data, coordinated research programs, and a national nutrition policy. Ideally, the outcome would be a national health insurance system that includes comprehensive health care on the community level, and thus ensures a healthier society.

REFERENCES

1. Mico, P. R., and Ross, H. S.: Health education and behavioral science, ed. 1, Oakland, Calif., 1975, California Third Party Associates.
2. Interim Commission: Constitution of the World Health Organization, WHO Chron. 1, Geneva, 1947.
3. Dubos, R.: Man adapting, New Haven, Conn., 1965, Yale University Press.
4. Dunn, H.: High-level wellness, Arlington, Va., 1961, R. W. Beatty, Ltd.
5. Kirk, R. Hl., Mayshark, C., and Horsby, R. P.: Personal health in ecologic perspective, St. Louis, 1972, The C. V. Mosby Co.
6. Lerner, M.: Conceptualization of health and social well-being. In Berg, R. L., editor: Health status indexes, Chicago, 1973, Hospital Research and Educational Trust.
7. Jourard, S. M.: Healthy personality: an approach from the viewpoint of humanistic psychology, New York, 1974, The Macmillan Co.
8. Blum, H. L., et al: Health planning 1969—Notes on comprehensive planning for health, San Francisco, 1969, Western Regional Office, American Public Health Association.
9. Fuchs, V.: Who shall live, New York, 1974, Basic Books, Inc., Publishers.
10. Milio, N.: A framework for prevention: changing health-damaging to health-generating life patterns, Am. J. Public Health 65:435, 1976.
11. Bruhn, J. G., Cordova, F. D., Williams, J. A., and Fuentes, R. G., Jr.: The wellness process, J. Commun. Health 2:209, 1977.
12. Scheurer, J. H.: Presentation at Hearings of U.S. Congress, Domestic and International Scientific Planning, Analysis and Cooperation Subcommittee, U.S. House of Representatives, Washington, D.C., Aug. 3, 1977.
13. Peterson, E.: Testimony at Hearings of U.S. Congress, Domestic and International Scientific Planning, Analysis and Cooperation Subcommittee, Committee on Science and Technology, Nutrition Oversight Review, Washington, D.C., Aug. 3, 1977.
14. Cohen, W.: Testimony at Hearings of U.S. Congress, Domestic and International Scientific Planning, Analysis and Cooperation Subcommittee, Committee on Science and Technology, Nutrition Oversight Review, Washington, D.C., Aug. 3, 1977.
15. Public Health Service: Forward plan for health, FY 1978-82, Bethesda, Md., Aug., 1976, U.S. Department of Health, Education, and Welfare.
16. Richmond, F.: Press release, Sept. 27, 1977.
17. Lewis, C. E.: Health services research: asking the painful questions. In Kane, R. L., editor: The challenges of community medicine, New York, 1974, Springer Publishing Co., Inc.
18. U.S. House of Representatives, Committee on Agriculture: The role of the federal government in nutrition education. A study prepared by Congres-

sional Research Services, Library of Congress for Subcommittee on Domestic Marketing, Consumer Relation and Nutrition, Washington, D.C., March, 1977, Government Printing Office.

19. Owen, A. Y.: Community nutrition in preventive health care programs, National Health Planning Information Center, June, 1978, Government Printing Office.

20. U.S. Department of Health, Education, and Welfare: National Health Insurance: statement of issues, Washington, D.C., 1977, Government Printing Office.

21. Public Health Service, Center for Disease Control: Funding community preventive health services under national health insurance, Bethesda, Md., April 18, 1975, U.S. Department of Health, Education, and Welfare.

Common abbreviations

AHA	American Hospital Association	**MBO**	Management By Objectives
BCHS	Bureau of Community Health Services	**MCHS**	Maternal and Child Health Service
		MCE	Medical Care Evaluation
BHI	Bureau of Health Insurance	**NAS/NRC**	National Academy of Science/National Research Council
BQA	Bureau of Quality Assurance		
CDC	Center For Disease Control	**NHI**	National Health Insurance
CIHP	Coalition of Independent Health Professions	**NIH**	National Institutes of Health
		NSF	National Science Foundation
DHEW	Department of Health, Education, and Welfare	**OLTCSE**	Office of Long-Term Care Standards Enforcement
DLTC	Division of Long-Term Care	**OPSR**	Office of Professional Standards Review
DPSC	Division of Provider Standards and Certification		
		PEP	Performance Evaluation Procedure
DQ&S	Division of Quality and Standards	**PSRO**	Professional Standards Review Organization
FAO	Food and Agriculture Organization of United Nations		
		PHS	Project Head Start
FDA	Food and Drug Administration	**PHS**	Public Health Service
HANES	Health and Nutrition Examination Survey	**QAP**	Quality Assurance Program
		RDA	Recommended Dietary Allowances
HMO	Health Maintenance Organization	**SNF**	Skilled Nursing Facility
HRF	Health-Related Facility	**SRS**	Social and Rehabilitation Service
HRA	Health Resources Administration	**SSA**	Social Security Administration
HSA	Health Service Administration Health Systems Agency	**TAP**	Trustee, Administrator, Physician
		UHDDS	Uniform Hospital Discharge Data Set
ICNND	Interdepartmental Committee on Nutrition for National Defense		
		USDA	United States Department of Agriculture
ICF	Intermediate Care Facility		
IHS	Indian Health Service	**USDHEW**	United States Department of Health, Education and Welfare
IUNS	International Union of Nutritional Science		
		UR	Utilization Review
JCAH	Joint Commission on Accreditation of Hospitals	**WHO**	World Health Organization

Glossary

abstract sheet A sheet prepared by the medical record practitioner from the list of criteria for the purpose of recording data (for each criterion) abstracted from patient records.

abstracting or chart review The process of collecting data from the patient records.

action planning An element of program planning that addresses itself to presenting the steps involved in achieving program objectives and subobjectives.

action plans or work statements or methods States the means by which objectives are to be achieved.

activity The performance of a function by an organization unit toward the achievement of a stated objective.

actual level of performance A percentage discovered through a review of charts that describes the actual pattern of care for each criterion.

administration The planning, facilitation, execution, evaluation, and control of services.

admission review certification A form of concurrent health care review in which an assessment is made of the medical necessity of a patient's admission to a hospital.

ambulatory health care center A public or private organizational unit (free standing or institution based) that provides, directly or through contractual arrangements, health care services to meet the needs of noninstitutionalized or non-homebound patients.

American Dietetic Association, The A professional organization responsible for establishing educational and supervised clinical experience requirements and standards of practice in the profession of dietetics.

anthropometric assessment Measurement of the physical dimensions and gross composition of the body at different age levels and degrees of nutrition.

attending physician The primary physician for a patient while he is in a health care facility.

audit topic A subject selected for investigation of possible health care problems for a particular group of patients. (See *objective/focus.*)

balanced diet Oversimplified term that implies ideal proportions of all proteins, minerals, fats, and carbohydrates for "optimum" nutrition. Since no one "diet" can be quantitatively "balanced" for "optimum" needs of all individuals, the term "balanced diet" should be used only in properly informative statements where its meaning is plainly evident and free of misleading implications.

baseline or benchmark The recorded status of the situation before action is taken to effect change, to which subsequent action or accomplishment can be referred; normative data of health care delivery in a PSRO area prior to PSRO implementation.

brainstorming A technique to be used with groups for eliciting verbally a maximum number of ideas on a particular topic with no evaluation or comments allowed on any of the generated ideas.

budget (as defined by USPHS grant) The financial expenditure plan approved by PHS to carry out the purposes of the grant-supported project.

The budget comprises both the federal share and any nonfederal share of such plan and any subsequent authorized rebudgeting of funds (see *prior approval*); except that for those programs which do not involve federal approval of the nonfederal share of costs, such as research grants, the term "budget" means the financial expenditure plan approved by PHS, including funds only. Any expenditures charged to an approved budget consisting of federal and nonfederal shares are deemed to be borne by the grant in the same proportion as the percentage of federal/nonfederal participation in the overall budget.

budget period The interval of time (usually 12 months) into which the grant project period is divided for budgetary and reporting purposes.

community assessment Practical method of obtaining an overview of nutritional status of a given community.

community nutrition Academic discipline that deals with identification and solution of health problems with nutritional implications in communities or human population groups.

community and public health nutritionist Primarily an educator or communicator who functions as a member of the health team in assessing nutritional needs of individuals and groups in the community; plans, organizes, coordinates, and evaluates the nutritional component of health care services; works in public or private health agencies, industry, or extension services and provides information through various media to the general public and to other health professionals in public health nutrition; has unique expertise in the area of health care administration; is responsible for program planning that identifies nutritional problems in the population, implements corrective action, and evaluates program results through changes in the nutritional status of the community. This position requires graduate training in public health in addition to the core knowledge and experience in the science and practice of nutrition. An advanced degree is also required for the extension specialist.

concurrent review Review of patient services that is performed while the patient is hospitalized.

conditional PSROs A PSRO that is designated by DHEW to implement a satisfactory formal plan for review of designated health care services and is in the process of developing and expanding its review activities and capacity to qualify as a PSRO.

constraints Limitations on cost that may have to be accepted or limits imposed on planning.

consumer (of health care) An individual who is either a patient or a potential patient and whose primary source of income is not based on the delivery of health care or health care products.

cost-benefit analysis Process that is based on the assumption that a specific problem can be identified; that the cost effectiveness of its consequence is within a permissible range of accuracy; that it can be controlled at some predetermined level by a new program; and that the cost of the new program can also be measured.

cost effectiveness Variation of the original cost-benefit analysis model. Its purpose is to find the best way or alternative, at the least cost, for obtaining a desired objective. Cost effectiveness includes analyses of both monetary and nonmonetary data.

criteria Predetermined elements against which aspects of the quality of a medical service may be compared. They are developed by professionals relying on professional expertise and on the professional literature.

outcome criteria Used to evaluate optimal quality of health care by measurement of the results of treatment in terms of health status of the individual or a target population or group.

process criteria Used to evaluate optimal quality of health care by measurement or management or specific elements of care provided in the course of treatment.

cross-sectional data Data collected over a short interval describing given parameters in groups of various ages.

data display form A form for display of the abstract data for a set of criteria, usually including the criteria (as ratified), expected levels of performance, actual levels of performance, and for each criterion, a ratio of the number of charts meeting the criterion to the number of charts audited.

deficiency diseases Disorders or disease conditions with characteristic clinical signs caused by a dietary deficiency of nutrients; they can be cured or prevented by supplying the nutrients that are lacking.

Delbecq technique A group technique for eliciting ideas from every participant. It can be divided into the following steps:

1. Individuals silently record all ideas.
2. "Round robin," where each participant states

one of his ideas, which is recorded on flip chart. Continue around room until all participants have all of their ideas recorded. No evaluation is allowed during this process.

3. Period of discussion of each recorded idea.
4. Participants rank ideas in order of priority.

demographic data Quantitative data on characteristics of human population such as size, growth, density, distribution, and vital statistics.

demonstration area An area or region selected for the purpose of demonstrating methods (such as agricultural food production or food processing) or the effectiveness of following some procedure such as a particular nutrition program.

determinants of change Factors that can be identified by study and research as being responsible for change in the attitudes, beliefs, or behavior of individuals or groups, especially with regard to the acceptance of new food products and new methods for food preparation.

diet counseling Providing individualized professional guidance to assist a person in adjusting his daily food consumption to meet his health needs. This process actually involves three components: interviewing, counseling, and consulting. Success depends on one's ability to explain the nutrition plan in simplest language, considering the patient's background, socioeconomic needs, and personal preference.

dietary history A detailed account of the kind, estimated amount, and preparation methods of the usual daily food intake and variations for an individual, obtained in an interview by a professional worker. It should include socioeconomic factors.

dietary study (survey) Method of determining or evaluating the dietary intake of an individual, group, or population at large. The adequacy of a given diet is determined by qualitative comparison with the basic food groups or by quantitative comparison with the recommended dietary standard of a particular country. A dietary study is used to detect adequacy or inadequacy of diets to give valuable information concerning food habits, menu preparation, and food procurement, availability, and distribution.

dietary study methodology Methods of obtaining dietary information include the following:

Individuals

1. Estimation by recall, with the client or client's parent recalling food intake of previous 24 hours or longer.
2. Food intake record, which is a listing of all foods eaten (including between-meal intakes)

for varying lengths of time, usually 3 to 7 days.

3. Dietary history taken by recall or repeated food records or both to discover the usual food pattern over relatively long periods of time.
4. Weighed food intake of the client, or the client himself.

Groups

1. Food account or running reports of food purchased or produced for household use.
2. Food list or recall of estimated amounts of various foods consumed during the previous days, usually the past 7 days.
3. Food record or weighed inventory of foods at the beginning and end of the study, with or without records of kitchen and plate wastes.

dietetics A profession concerned with the science and art of human nutritional care, an essential component of health science. It includes the extending and imparting of knowledge concerning foods that will provide nutrients sufficient to health and during disease throughout the life cycle and the management of group feeding.

dietetic practice Performance of activities in fulfilling a professional position in nutritional care.

dietitian The professional dietitian has earned a baccalaureate degree and has met basic academic and experience requirements for eligibility to write the qualifying examination for professional registration in dietetics. The registration program is maintained by The American Dietetic Association as a service to both the profession and the public. Three defined subdivisions in dietetics, based on employment areas, are administrative, clinical, and community.

administrative dietitian One who manages an institutional food service program and must be capable of utilizing effectively the human and facilitating resources of a food service system to provide nutritionally adequate, quality food and to influence, directly or indirectly, the behavior of individuals to achieve appropriate nutrient intake. Although all hospital and health care facility dietitians are concerned to some degree with therapeutic diets, the administrative dietitian's role is primarily that of managing food production and service. Department heads in large institutions administer dietetic and nutrition services as well as educational programs.

clinical dietitian A specialist in the area of therapeutic dietetics, who may function in a hospital, in ambulatory care services, or as a consultant; assesses nutritional needs and status of patients, develops and implements nutritional care plans, and evaluates the results; may serve as part of a clinical research team or in epidemiologic studies requiring the collection and interpretation of dietary intake data.

consultant dietitian One who has followed a prescribed academic program resulting in a baccalaureate degree from an accredited college or university and has satisfactorily completed an approved dietetic internship or qualifying experience; advises and assists public and private establishments, such as child care centers, hospitals, nursing homes, and schools in food service management and nutritional problems in group feeding; plans, organizes, and conducts such activities as in-service training courses, conferences, and institutes for food service managers, food handlers, and other workers; develops and evaluates informational materials; studies food service practices and facilities and makes recommendations for improvement; confers with architects and equipment personnel in planning for building or remodeling food service units.

dietitian in a community setting One who provides consultation to individuals, groups, or organizations serving food in the community setting. This position requires the same bachelor's level of training as the other two subdefinitions of dietitian.

therapeutic dietitian One who has followed a prescribed academic program resulting in a baccalaureate degree from an accredited college or university and has satisfactorily completed an approved dietetic internship or qualifying experience; plans and directs preparation and service of modified diets prescribed by the physician; consults medical, nursing, and social service staffs concerning problems affecting patients' food habits and needs; formulates menus for therapeutic diets based on indicated physiologic and ethnic needs of patients and integrates them with basic institutional menus; establishes and maintains standards of palatability and appearance of patient meals; counsels patients and their families on the requirements and importance of their modified diets and on how to plan and prepare the food; may engage in research; may teach nutrition and diet therapy to dietetic, medical, dental, and nursing students.

direct assistance A grant under which goods or services are furnished in lieu of cash. It generally involves the detail of federal personnel or the provision of supplies, such as vaccines. Prerequisite to the use of direct assistance is authorization by statute or regulation and pre-establishment of agreements between PHS and the grantee.

double-blind technique A method that eliminates much of the conscious or unconscious bias of both subject and investigator by keeping them unaware of who is getting what specific treatment. Classically, this involves the use of the look-alike placebo in intervention studies.

draft criteria Criteria developed by an audit committee or audit task force that have *not* been ratified and are subject to change by those whose practice will be audited.

effectiveness A measure of the actual accomplishment of a program compared with the amount intended or planned, which may be less than total eradication or prevention. The effectiveness of a prophylactic measure is the percentage of cases expected in a population that are prevented by the measure.

efficiency A measure of the cost in resources necessary to accomplish the program's objectives or the ratio between an output (net attainment of program objectives) and an input (program resources expended).

episodes of care A specified period of time during which health services are rendered to a patient.

evaluation The process of determining the value or amount of success in achieving a predetermined objective. It includes at least the following steps: formulation of the objective, identification of the proper criteria to be used in measuring success, determination and explanation of the degree of success, and recommendations for further program activity.

expected level of performance A percentage developed for a criterion that indicates the minimum accepted level.

family composition The number of persons in the family group, including the age, sex, and kinship of the group.

family eating patterns The order of serving food to family members, who eats with the men of the family, and when and with whom the children and women eat.

family food distribution The way in which food is

distributed within the family, particularly what kind and amount of food is given the father or men in the family and what foods are given to the women and children.

food checklist A list of foods that an individual may be requested to check in some way, for those foods he usually or regularly eats. It also may be arranged to check for likes and dislikes or other specific reactions to a given list of foods.

Food and Nutrition Board, NAS/NRC This board, established in 1940 under the Division of Biology and Agriculture of the National Academy of Sciences/National Research Council serves as an advisory body in the field of food and preparation. Its earliest activity was the preparation of Recommended Dietary Allowances (RDAs), which are revised periodically.

food patterns The kinds of foods customarily used by people in a given area, region, or ethnic group and the way those foods are prepared and served.

food science and technology The food scientist utilizes the disciplines of biology and chemistry to understand the nature of food, its composition and properties, and the chemical reactions that take place therein. The food technologist is concerned with the application of the laws and processes of biology, physics, chemistry, and engineering in the preparation, preservation, and analysis of food products that, in the interest of public health, are of high nutritional quality, are safe, and can be stored for reasonable periods of time to allow for maximum distribution. Qualifications vary depending on the place of employment and responsibilities involved. High-level positions in industry usually require training beyond the bachelor's degree. Academic positions either in teaching or research or a combination of the two almost always require a Ph.D. Food scientists and technologists often come into the field through related areas such as microbiology, chemistry, physics, or engineering.

format to complete objectives

Format: To / action verb / desired result / time frame / resources required

Example: To reduce the prevalence of anemia in 1- to 2-year-olds by 30% in one year using the nutrition staff.

function An area of responsibility whose discharge is required to meet program objectives.

administrative function Involves the planning, evaluation, advice, facilitation, and coordination of health effort; modifies and controls the operating functions.

operating function Contributes directly toward the achievement of the objective.

goal Statement of broad direction, general purpose, or interest. It may be somewhat unreachable, and it is often not quantifiable.

government (local) A unit of government below the state level, including specifically a county, municipality, city, town, township, school district, council of governments, sponsor group, representative organization, and other regional or interstate government entity, or any agency or instrumentality of a local government, exclusive of institutions of higher education and hospitals. This term also includes federally recognized Indian tribal governments.

government (state) Any governing body of the several states of the United States, the District of Columbia, the Commonwealth of Puerto Rico, any territory or possession of the United States, or any agency or instrumentality of a state, exclusive of state institutions of higher education and hospitals.

grant An award of financial or direct assistance to an eligible recipient under programs that provide for such assistance based on review and approval of an application, plan, or other document(s) setting forth a proposed activity or program.

grantee The institution, public or private corporation, organization, agency, or other legally accountable entity that receives a grant and assumes legal and financial responsibility and accountability both for the awarded funds and for the performance of the grant-supported activity. In certain cases a grantee may be an individual.

grants management officer The individual designated to serve as the PHS official responsible for the business management aspects of a particular grant project(s); serves as the counterpart to the business officer of the grantee institution and is the focal point for matters such as interpretations of grant policies and provisions; works closely with the program or project officer who is responsible for the scientific, technical, and programatic aspects of the grant project. (See *program/project officer.*)

grant-supported activities/project Those activities specified or described in a grant application or other document that are approved by PHS funding, whether or not such funding constitutes all or only a portion of the financial support necessary to carry out such activities.

guideline A list of indications for future action.

health A state of complete physical, mental, and social well-being and not merely the absence of disease or infirmity (World Health Organization).

health care Elements concerning the health of an individual including environment, nutrition, patient care, etc.

health care consumer See *consumer (of health care).*

health (medical) care evaluation A program of an organized health care staff designed to measure the quality of care in a health care institution. Health (medical) care evaluation is concerned with two dimensions of quality:

    health care (medical) audit Retrospective examination of clinical application of health care knowledge as revealed by medical record.

    utilization review Examination of efficiency of institutional use and appropriateness of admissions, services ordered and provided, length of stay, and discharge practices on a prospective and concurrent basis.

health care practitioners (other than physicians) Those health professionals who (1) do not hold a Doctor of Medicine or Doctor of Osteopathy Degree; (2) are qualified by education, experience, and/or licensure to practice their profession; and (3) are involved in the delivery of direct patient care or services in hospitals and other institutional or noninstitutional settings (also referred to as nonphysician health care practitioners).

health care team A group of health care professionals who provide coordinated services to achieve optimal health care of the client.

health maintenance Preventive, diagnostic, curative, and restorative health services available to a client, group, or community.

Health Maintenance Organization (HMO) An organized system of health care that accepts the responsibility to provide or otherwise assure the delivery of an agreed-on set of comprehensive health maintenance and treatment services for a voluntarily enrolled group of persons in a geographic area and is reimbursed through a pre-negotiated and fixed periodic payment made by or on behalf of each person or family unit enrolled in the plan. The HMO provides comprehensive care with major emphasis on prevention, care continuity, and maximum health service at a reasonable cost. The American Dietetic Association has proposed that nutritional care be a basic service of HMO.

Health and Nutrition Examination Survey (HANES) The National Center for Health Statistics is conducting nutritional status surveys of the United States' population on a two-year cycle. The sample consists of persons from 1 through 74 years of age who are not institutionalized. There is an oversampling of groups that are susceptible to nutritional difficulties such as poor children of preschool age, women of childbearing age, and the aged. The survey includes household interviews, questionnaires, physical measurements, physical examinations, tests and procedures, and biochemical determinations on blood and urine samples.

Health Systems Agency (HSA) Authorized in P.L. 93-641, the HSA is responsible for health planning and development throughout the country in health service areas designated by the governor of each state. These agencies are responsible for preparing and implementing plans for the development of health services, manpower and facilities, and for the prevention of unnecessary duplication of health resources or of other inefficiencies in the health care delivery system.

immediate outcomes The status as measured by specific criteria at the end of treatment in a particular level of care.

implementation A phase in the planning process that makes a plan operational and in which definite action is taken to commit resources for the purpose of achieving desired results.

implicit method of assessment A method of review in which practitioners read an abstract of each case and judge whether the care provided was necessary and appropriate based on their own knowledge, skills, and experiences.

incidence The number of *new* cases during a period of time. (See *prevalence.*)

infant An individual in the age period of 29 days through 12 months.

infant feeding practices Methods of feeding (breast or bottle fed), the kind and amount of supplements given, weaning age, method and kind of foods given at weaning, and similar information.

in-kind contributions They represent the value of noncash contributions provided by the grantee or third parties. In-kind contributions may consist of charges for real property and nonexpendable personal property and the value of goods and services directly benefiting and specifically identifiable to the grant-supported activity.

institutions for health care For the purpose of the

PSRO program these comprise short-term general hospitals, tuberculosis hospitals, mental health hospitals, skilled nursing facilities, and intermediate care facilities.

Interdepartmental Committee on Nutrition for National Defense (ICNND) A group established to assess, assist, and learn about the food and nutrition situation in countries to which the United States is giving military support. Local specialists in each country assist personnel from the United States in defining the major nutritional problems.

intermediate outcomes The status as measured by specific criteria at intermediate points during the course of treatment in a particular level of care. Such measurements may be used as indicators of anticipated immediate outcomes.

International Council of Scientific Unions An organization that sponsors international congresses of nutrition every three years. It consists of sixteen unions, one of which is the International Union for Nutritional Sciences.

International Dietetic Association An organization whose aim is to raise the level of the dietetics profession in member countries.

International Union for Nutritional Sciences (IUNS) One of sixteen unions of the International Council of Scientific Unions. Its aim is to provide a means for international cooperation in the study of basic and applied nutrition. Information is exchanged at international congresses.

length of stay The number of days a patient remains in a specific institution, from the day of admission to the day of discharge.

licensed to practice Authorized under law to engage in the unrestricted practice of a specific profession, e.g., medicine, osteopathy, nursing.

life-style An individual's mode of living as affected by physiologic, psychosocial, environmental, economic, and religious influences.

local government (See *government* [*local*].)

longitudinal data Data derived from measurements in the same person periodically over a long period of time.

longitudinal studies Continuous or repeated experimental observations and measurements carried on for many years with the same group of human subjects or through one or more generations of animals.

maintenance of effort A requirement contained in certain legislation, regulations, or administrative policies stating that a grantee must maintain a specified level of financial effort in a specific area to receive federal grant funds and that the federal grant funds may be used only to supplement, not supplant, the level of grantee funds.

malnutrition A state of poor health with symptoms that can be identified clinically as due to inadequate intake of one or more essential nutrients over a sustained period.

Management by Objectives (MBO) A management tool by which a definition of work objectives for each department, division and employee within an organization is established. Its basic philosophy is that employers and employees work together to (1) set specific measurable objectives, (2) make dated action plans for their implementation, and (3) periodically review the results of these objectives and plans together. All activities must be related to overall organizational goals.

    milestones (as related to MBO) Specific events that will be tracked during the periodic review. There are two types of milestones:

        cumulative milestones Represent gradual progress toward the objective throughout the year and are chartered on a quarterly basis.

        discrete milestones Represent completion of major pieces of work that will occur once during the year and specify an anticipated completion date.

management team Individuals who, through coordinated effort, apply the principles and practices of management to an organization's operation.

marasmus A condition occurring mostly in infants (3 to 18 months of age) as a result of gross deficiency of calories over a period of time and an accompanying lack of protein and other nutrients. It is frequently accompanied by diarrhea and characterized by low body weight, loss of subcutaneous fat, and wasting of muscle tissue. (Some cases of marasmus show edema and are best described as kwashiorkor rather than marasmic kwashiorkor.)

matching A study technique for neutralizing confounding variables. It matches each individual exposed with an unexposed individual who is identical with respect to all confounding factors.

meal patterns The kind and amounts of food eaten at the various meals of the day.

Medicaid (Title XIX) The program under federal

law that provides payments for medical care services to recipients of categorical public assistance. This program is administered by the individual states, which in turn receive matching federal funds to support it.

medical care That portion of care under the control of the physician.

medical care evaluation studies A form of retrospective health care review in which in-depth assessments of the quality and/or nature of the utilization of health care services are made, sometimes stated as "patient care process."

Medicare (Title XVIII) An amendment to the Social Security Act, which provides a federal health insurance program to persons over 65 years of age.

memorandum of understanding An agreement between a PSRO and Medicare intermediaries, Medicaid state agencies, state and maternal and child health and crippled children's agencies or institutions that specifies the review and monitoring roles of each of the contractors.

morbidity ratio A ratio of the sick/well in a given area; expressed in terms of population, usually 100,000.

mortality (death rate) A measure of the frequency of death for a specified period of time, usually a year, in relation to the total population.

National Academy of Sciences/National Research Council (NAS/NRC) Government group that established the Food and Nutrition Board, which is concerned with nutrition policy and the development of materials for use by professionals. It also advises national and international groups about nutrition.

National Center for Health Statistics Federal agency established specifically to collect and disseminate data on health in the United States; designs and maintains national data collection systems, conducts research in statistical and survey methodology, and cooperates with other agencies in the United States and in foreign countries in activities to increase the availability and usefulness of health data.

National Institutes of Health (NIH) Research unit of the Public Health Service in the DHEW. It is engaged in clinical research of diseases of public health importance, such as allergic, dental, mental, and metabolic diseases.

National Nutrition Consortium An organization in which all of the major professional societies in food, nutrition, and dietetics participate, representing more than 50,000 scientists, clini-

cians, and educators who have a background and training in nutrition and can speak with authority on sound nutrition practices. These organizations are The American Dietetic Association, American Institute of Nutrition, American Society for Clinical Nutrition, Institute of Food Technologists, Society for Nutrition Education, American Academy of Pediatrics, and The Food and Nutrition Board.

National Nutrition Survey In 1967 Congress requested that the DHEW survey malnutrition and related health programs in the United States. Kentucky, Louisiana, South Carolina, Texas, West Virginia, California, Massachusetts, Michigan, New York, and Washington were surveyed. From 1968 to 1970, data were collected regarding general demographic, dietary intake, clinical and anthropometric, dental, and biochemical considerations.

national poverty line The income level in cash, or cash equivalent, determined as the amount below which poverty exists.

National Professional Standards Review Council A group of eleven physicians appointed by the Secretary of DHEW that arranges for collection and distribution of information to PSROs and makes recommendations to the Secretary of DHEW and Congress for improvement of the PSRO program.

National Science Foundation (NSF) A foundation established in 1950 for the purpose of improving scientific research and education in the United States. Grants are awarded to universities and other nonprofit institutions to support research. The foundation also maintains a register of scientific personnel.

need That state or condition in the community which shows a lack of essential public health protection and well-being.

neonate An individual in the age period from birth through 28 days.

norms (medical care appraisal norms) Numerical or statistical measures of usual, observed performance.

nutrition Nutrition is the science of food, the nutrients and other substances therein, their action, interaction, and balance in relation to health and disease, and the processes by which the organism ingests, digests, absorbs, transports, utilizes, and excretes food substances. In addition, nutrition must be concerned with social, economic, cultural, and psychological implications of food and eating. Furthermore, it includes an evaluation of nutritional status and effect on the individual's health of an inadequacy or imbalance of nutrients consumed. For this diverse field of study a number of subspecialties have evolved that require varying competences and depth of knowledge in the biologic, medical, chemical, and social sciences.

nutrition education specialist A person who coordinates and facilitates the many varied aspects of a school nutrition education program, integrating it with the school health and food service programs as well as the health education and general educational curriculum, interprets the school nutrition program to parents and the community and utilize community resources within the program.

nutrition educator One with knowledge of the basic principles of applied nutrition and competence in educational skills and techniques; works in formal educational settings such as schools and colleges and in informal educational programs such as continuing education, extensions, adult education, and health intervention programs. Academic preparation requires a degree in either nutrition or education with sufficient supporting work in the other field to provide competence to function effectively as a professional. An advanced degree is desirable for more responsible positions.

Nutrition Foundation, Inc. A public nonprofit institution that was established in 1941 for "the advancement of nutrition knowledge and its effective application in improving the health and welfare of mankind." It is supported by food and allied industries. The foundation publishes *Nutrition Reviews*, monographs, and pamphlets for lay persons. It also sponsors conferences on nutrition.

nutrition history An informative and comprehensive description of laboratory and clinical findings as well as dietary history of an individual. (See *dietary history; nutritional status.*)

nutrition interdisciplinary ("**interface**") **areas** Emerging as distinct subspecialties in nutrition are interface areas, requiring varying degrees of expertise in sociology, economics, anthropology, or other social sciences. Such areas are nutritional anthropology, nutrition policy planning, and the components of dietary services in public health and health care institutions. Qualifications cannot be precisely defined at this point because the fields are relatively new and are still in the process of developing. Clearly, however, the expertise required likely could not be acquired at the undergraduate

level, and advanced training, probably at the Ph.D. level, would be most desirable.

nutrition, public health The theory and practice of nutrition as a science through organized community effort, with the family as the smallest unit under study. The overall aim of public health nutrition is to improve or maintain good health through proper nutrition. Various agencies, governmental or nongovernmental, are concerned with nutrition work at local, national, or international levels.

nutrition scientist A trained nutritionist who has undergone advanced study leading to an advanced degree in nutrition or in allied science, has attained the competencies required for a degree in nutrition, and in addition, has developed competence in research techniques and methodologies as applied to nutrition such that the individual is capable of independent research in nutrition.

nutritional care The application of the science and art of human nutrition in helping people select and obtain food for the primary purpose of nourishing their bodies in health or disease throughout the life cycle. This participation may be in single or combined functions; in food service systems management to groups; in extending knowledge of food and nutrition principles; in teaching these principles for application according to particular situations; and in dietary counseling.

nutritional status State of the body resulting from the consumption and utilization of nutrients. Clinical observations, biochemical analyses, anthropometric measurements, and dietary studies are used to determine this state.

nutritional status assessment An evaluation of one's nutritional state is accomplished by one or more of the following methods:
1. Dietary survey (to detect a faulty diet, i.e., primary factor)
2. Medical and clinical examination (to detect conditioning factors)
3. Biochemical tests (to detect tissue levels)
4. Anthropometric tests (to detect anatomic changes)

These methods are used in nutrition surveys. Other sources of information helpful in appraising the nutritional status of groups of individuals or populations are vital and health statistics, food balance sheets, and other pertinent data compiled by government agencies, hospitals, clinics, insurance companies, etc.

nutritional survey Study of the nutritional status

of a population group in a given area of operation. The population may be homogeneous (e.g., teen-aged girls or diabetics) or heterogeneous (e.g., hospital patients). Thus the survey may be slanted with respect to various factors such as age, sex, race, or socioeconomic, geographic, physiologic, or pathologic condition, depending on the aims of the study. In general the main objectives of the nutrition survey are to determine the extent of malnutrition and ascertain feeding problems, to provide ways and means of correcting or preventing nutritional problems, and to help in nutrition education, economic planning, and other programs for the improvement of the health status of the population or group.

nutritionist One who has followed a prescribed academic program and received a master's degree in public health nutrition from an accredited college or university; organizes, plans, and conducts programs concerning nutrition to assist in promotion of health and control of disease; instructs auxiliary medical personnel and allied professional workers on food values and utilization of foods by human body; advises health and other agencies on nutritional phases of their food programs; conducts in-service courses pertaining to nutrition in clinics and similar institutions; interprets and evaluates food and nutrient information designed for public acceptance and use; studies and analyzes scientific discoveries in nutrition for adaptation and application to various dietary problems; may be employed by voluntary or public health agency.

   clinical nutritionist A specialist in some branch of medicine (internal medicine, pediatrics, obstetrics, etc.) as well as in nutrition who is concerned with nutritional care of patients as well as overall medical supervision. The principles of nutrition that are of concern to the medical student and physician include the metabolism of foods; the quantitative and qualitative requirements of nutrients for growth, development, and maintenance of health, and their alterations by environment, disease, surgery, injuries, drugs, or antimetabolites; nutritional symbioses of humans and microorganisms; the influences of certain nutrients on normal or abnormal metabolism; the delayed effects of early nutrition that may modify genetic, prenatal or postnatal influences toward disease; and the composition and biologic effects of foods, including beneficial and harmful effects. The clinical nutritionist is concerned with the use of nutritional measures for the maintenance of health, the management of disease and trauma, and the prevention of disease. The clinical nutritionist may act as consultant to those nutritionists not medically trained but involved in health care services that require graduate nutrition training. Advanced training, such as a Ph.D., a residency, or postgraduate training is required beyond the Doctor of Medicine degree.

   experimental nutritionist One who conducts research related to nutrient metabolism and requirements of humans, experimental and domestic animals, and nutrition problems related to modern life-styles and technology; generally works in academic or research institutions, most often combining teaching and research in the academic field. An advanced degree, preferably a Ph.D., is essential for the experimental nutritionist, and the fields of study may emphasize physiology or biochemistry as well as nutrition per se. In any case, a strong background in basic biologic and chemical sciences is mandatory.

   public health nutritionist One who has followed a prescribed academic program and received a master's degree in public health nutrition from an accredited college or university; in a public health agency, interprets and applies scientific knowledge of nutrition to planning, organizing, and carrying out or directing programs for the promotion of positive health, the prevention of chronic and debilitating diseases, and the treatment and rehabilitation of individuals; consults with administrators and medical and paramedical personnel on current scientific findings in food and nutrition and their application to agency programs; conducts or participates in preservice and in-service education of professional staff of own and related agencies; may design, conduct, or participate in dietary and nutrition studies and other studies with a nutrition component; prepares and evaluates technical and popular educational material; cooperates with other agencies in the formulation and coordination of nutrition programs involving professional or lay groups; should have postgraduate education in nutrition as it relates to public health and qualifying experience for the responsibilities entailed.

   teaching nutritionist One who has followed a

prescribed academic program and received a master's degree in public health nutrition from an accredited college or university. Plans, organizes, and conducts education programs in nutrition for the preparation of professional workers as well as for the public; develops curricula, course outlines, visual aids, pamphlets, and other materials used in teaching. The nutritionist in the college teaches the basic science and application of science of food and nutrition and often engages in research. The nutritionist in the extension service advises agency administrators and county home economists and participates with the agent in training lay leaders. In business the nutritionist gives technical advice and guidance in preparing and conducting consumer education programs; should have postgraduate education in nutrition as it relates to public health, research, and teaching and qualifying experience.

objective A defined end result of specific public health activity, to be achieved in a finite period of time. Objectives are stated as definite aims or goals of action, which should be quantitatively measurable and capable of being reflected in standards performance. Objectives can be long range, intermediate, and short range. (See *format to complete objectives.*)

subobjectives Set forth the generally shorter term, more detailed program accomplishments that will be necessary for attainment of the objectives. Subobjectives represent the means by which a program is to be carried out.

objective/focus A narrower aspect of an audit topic chosen for focused attention in evaluating patient care for possible health care problems and planning remedial actions to solve those problems. (See *audit topic.*)

Office of Professional Standards Review A department in DHEW administering provisions of Public Law 92-603 relative to Professional Standards Review.

operation A specific task or series of tasks that, when completed, advances work to the next operation.

outcomes

immediate outcomes The status as measured by specific criteria at the end of treatment in a particular level of care.

intermediate outcomes The status as measured by specific criteria at intermediate points during the course of treatment in a particular level of care. Such measurements may be used as indicators of anticipated immediate outcomes.

outcome criteria Criteria used to evaluate optimal quality of health care by measurement of the results of treatment in terms of health status of the individual or a target population or group.

parameters of patient population Those items which narrow the scope of the patient population who will be audited, e.g., age, sex, type of surgical procedure.

patient care Everything done for the patient by the physician and other health care personnel.

patient care audit The team approach of health care professionals for the improvement of patient care using predetermined, objective criteria developed by professionals for the purpose of identifying areas requiring improvement through educational programs or through procedural or technical changes. It is a continuous process with the capability for describing trends in the quality of patient care.

patient sample That patient population to which the criteria for care set for an audit topic objective will be applied.

peer review The formal assessment by health care practitioners of the quality and efficiency of services ordered or provided by other members of their profession.

performance gap The difference between the desired level of performance and the actual level of performance.

physician coordinator The physician designated by the PSRO or hospital responsible for making health care review determinations when the review process indicates the need for such consultation.

physician professional activities Direct patient care and related clinical activities, administrative duties in a medical facility or other related institution, and/or medical or osteopathic teaching or research activities.

plan An orderly construction of the major objectives and the steps needed for their achievement. It includes (1) formulation of objectives, (2) assessment of resources available to realize these objectives, and (3) preparation of a work program to achieve the objectives.

planning A process for determining a future course of action, the purpose of which is to bring about a certain condition or goal. This process involves a series of recurring phases, beginning with goal formulation and proceeding to the development of alternative plans for goal achievement, plan implementation, plan evaluation, and plan updating.

policy The controlling principles of an organization that determine the boundaries of action in the selection of objectives and in the promulgation of the work of the organization.

preadmission certification Review of the medical necessity of admission to a hospital prior to the admission.

preliminary draft criteria Those elements of care selected as critical for measuring care by the group whose task it is to prepare draft criteria for an audit topic.

preschool child An individual in the age period of 1 through 5 years.

prevalence The number of persons with a given condition in a population during a specified time. (See *incidence*.) Prevalence = Incidence × Duration.

> **period prevalence** Prevalence over a specified period of time.

> **point prevalence** Prevalence at one point in time.

prevention The avoidance of a disease and/or its morbid consequences.

> **primary prevention** The actual prevention of a disease from occurring.

> **secondary prevention** Detection and early action taken to minimize the ramifications of the disease.

> **tertiary prevention** Often called clinical medicine, i.e., treatment and the prevention of complications.

> **rehabilitation** Prevention only to the extent that it may discourage the development of sequelae that lead to further deterioration after the arrest of a disease process.

primary care A type of medical care delivery characterized by a coordinated approach to patient care encompassing the following functions:

1. It includes "first-contact" care, serving as the patient's point of entry into the health care system.
2. It assumes the responsibility for outreach and follow-up for both the patient and the community.
3. It is comprehensive, including knowledge of all major disciplines.
4. It assumes continuing responsibility for the patient, both in health and in sickness.
5. It assumes the role of coordinating the care for all the patient's health problems.
6. It is personal care in the broadest sense.

prior approval Written permission provided by an authorized official in advance of an act that would result in either (1) the obligation or expenditure of funds or (2) the performance or modification of an activity under the grant-supported project, where such approval is required. Prior approval must be obtained from the designated Grants Management Officer for the grant involved, except that certain grantee institutions may approve some rebudgeting actions under an institutional prior approval system. Documentation of the approved budget on the Notice of Grant Award constitutes prior approval for the performance of activities and the expenditure of funds for specific purposes and items described in the grant application unless otherwise restricted by the Notice of Grant Award.

probability scale An ordered list of mutually exclusive and collectively exhaustive categories, with systematic assignment of intervals, including a meaningful absolute reference point, but with the scale altered to reflect not only the relationship of each value to a reference point but of the distribution of all values to a standard theoretic distribution.

problem analysis The procedure used to analyze performance gaps discovered during an audit to determine whether or not a problem exists, its most probable cause(s), and who is responsible.

procedure The prescribed sequence of defined activities required to meet a program objective within the framework of the organization and in line with definite policies.

process criteria Criteria used to evaluate optimal quality of health care by measurement of management or specific elements of care provided in the course of treatment.

profession A career requiring specialized knowledge and intensive preparation, including instruction in skills and methods, and in scientific, historic, or scholarly principles underlying such skills and methods, maintaining by force of organization or concerted opinion high standards of achievement and conduct, and committing its members to continued study and to a kind of work that has for its prime purpose the rendering of a public service (*Webster's Third International Dictionary*).

Professional Activity Survey–Medical Audit Program (PAS–MAP) An automated data reporting system that supplies information about hospital activities and diagnoses.

professional education A prescribed program of study and experience to develop competence in the practice of a profession, social understanding, ethical behavior, and scholarly concern.

professional person A person who, in the practice of his occupation, exhibits a service orientation, perceives the needs of the individual or collective clients that are relevant to his competence, and attends to these needs by competent performance. The professional person proceeds by his own judgment and authority and thus enjoys autonomy restrained by responsibility.

Professional Standards Review Organizations (PSROs) Empowered by federal law (Public Law 92-603) to monitor health care services paid for wholly or partially under Titles V, XVIII, and XIX of the Social Security Act.

profile A presentation of patterns of health care information during a defined period of time.

profile analysis A form of health care review that examines patterns of practice to identify problem areas in the delivery of health care and to evaluate the effects of peer review.

program The prescribed sequence of defined activities required to meet a program objective within the framework of the organization and in line with definite policies.

Program Director/Project Director/Principal Investigator A qualified individual designated by the grantee and, where required, approved by PHS to direct the project or program being supported by the grant. This individual is responsible to grantee institution officials for the proper management and conduct of the project or program. The grantee institution is, in turn, legally and financially responsible and accountable to PHS for performance of the grant-supported activity.

program evaluation That part of the manager's job which calls for measuring outcomes and assessing relative and absolute worth of specific undertakings.

program planning The process of determining the organization's plan of action to be performed within a specified time interval. It includes the delineation of the program content, objectives, procedures, criteria for evaluation, timetable of activities, and coordination with related activities.

Program/Project Officer The PHS official who is responsible for the technical, scientific, and programmatic aspects of a grant project; is involved in many day-to-day contacts with project staff on the grantee institution and works closely with the Grants Management Officer in the administration of grants.

project The activity required to achieve a subob-

jective. Projects are the means by which a program is carried out.

project costs Those costs, direct and indirect, incurred to carry out an approved grant-supported project. Only project costs incurred during the budget period indicated on the Notice of Grant Award are allowable unless specific approval to include other costs is given by PHS.

Project Head Start Program started in 1965 by the Office of Economic Opportunity to help disadvantaged preschool children from poverty areas attain their potential in growth and physical and mental development before entering school. Nutrition is an important part of this project. Meals and snacks are provided at the Head Start centers. In addition, meal planning and preparation classes are held for the parents of these children.

project period The total time for which support of a project has been approved, including any extensions thereof.

prospective study A study planned to observe events that have not yet occurred. (See *retrospective study.*)

PSRO Manual A manual issued by the Bureau of Quality Assurance (BQA) that reflects the legislative intent as well as the interpretation made by the BQA.

PSRO member A physician who meets PSRO membership requirements and has voluntarily signed a written statement indicating a desire to be a PSRO member and a willingness to abide by the by-laws and to participate in the review functions of the PSRO.

Public Law 89-749 The Comprehensive Health Planning and Public Health Service Amendments (1966).

Public Law 92-603 The Social Security Act Amendments of 1972 (H.R.I.) passed by the 92nd Congress and signed into law by the President on October 30, 1972. PSROs were established by section 249F(b) of this law and added as sections 1151-1170 of the Social Security Act of 1935.

Public Law 93-641 The National Health Planning and Resources Development Act (1974).

Public Law 94-317 National Consumer Health Information and Health Promotion Act (1977).

public representative An individual who may be a health care consumer or provider, who has distinguished himself by objective scholarship and/or leadership in the health field or a related field and is not identified with a single interest point of view.

quality assurance programs Programs organized

and administered by practitioners designed to certify continuously optimal quality and cost effectiveness of care provided within an institution or set of institutions. It is implied that, in these programs, health care (patient care) evaluation will be followed by appropriate corrective action whenever suboptimal care is identified. Change is effected through feedback of the results of evaluation to the entire professional staff and by educational programs with a positive incentive rather than by punitive programs with a negative incentive.

ratification The process of submitting a set of criteria to those whose practice will be audited for acceptance, rejection, and/or modification until at least some criteria are accepted unanimously.

ratified criteria Those critical indicators of care pertaining to a particular audit topic objective which have been ratified (approved) by the whole group whose delivery of health care is being audited.

re-audit The procedure that follows remedial action of applying criteria a second time to a new sample of charts to determine if the remedial action was effective in correcting a problem.

recall A method used in dietary surveys where the client is asked to recall everything he has eaten for the past 24 hours or other specific period; the reliability of this procedure is highly variable.

Recommended Dietary Allowances (R.D.A.) The amounts of various nutrients recommended by the Food and Nutrition Board of the National Research Council as normally desirable objectives toward which to aim in planning practical dietaries in the United States; sufficiently higher than the minimal requirements of persons in normal health. Allowances are related to body size and are stated for the reference men and women at moderate physical activity; for pregnancy and lactation; and for children and adolescent boys and girls of various age groups.

reference man Standard originally used by the FAO Committee on Caloric Requirements and now adopted by the Food and Nutrition Board in the recommended dietary allowances. He is described as a man, 22 years old, weighing 70 kg, living in a moderate climate with a mean temperature of 20° C, wearing light clothing, and engaged in light physical activity. His estimated caloric allowance is 2700 kcal. This baseline can be used to adjust calorie allowances of individuals in different circumstances.

reference woman She is 22 years old, weighs 58 kg, lives in a moderate climate with a mean temperature of 20° C, wears light clothing, and is engaged in light physical activity. Her estimated caloric allowance is 2000 kcal.

reliability The reproducibility of a result, i.e., how closely a second go-around would yield the same answer.

remedial action The action taken to correct a deficiency discovered by an audit.

retrospective study A study that deals with persons who have already developed the condition and examines the record for the characteristic; often called the case-control study. (See *prospective study.*)

review coordinator A person—paraprofessional, nurse, medical records analyst, etc.—who, with or without automated equipment, performs many essential functions related to particular types of review.

RUMBA Acronym representing desirable characteristics of criteria:
Relevant
Understandable
Measurable
Behavioral
Achievable

science and art Science as systematized knowledge derived from exact observations or experimentation and evaluation carried on to identify facts, phenomena, laws, and proximate causes; art as skill in performance acquired by study, observation, and experience.

screening A process in which norms, criteria, and standards are used to process large numbers of items, activities, or transactions to identify a smaller sample for study in detail.

secondary care Care provided by medical specialists, community hospitals, and other such providers who generally do not have first contact with patients.

selection The method for obtaining a population for study; generally used with the negative connotation of obtaining an unrepresentative group from a population.

sensitivity (of a predictor or a screening test) The proportion of true cases correctly identified. Sensitivity = True positives ÷ (True positives + False negatives).

skilled nursing facility A specially qualified facility that has the staff and equipment to provide skilled nursing care or rehabilitation services in addition to other health services.

skinfold thickness Measurement, with calibrated calipers, of thickness of a fold of skin at a selected body site. These measurements indicate subcutaneous fat and the state of nutriture. Commonly selected sites for measurement, particularly in nutrition surveys, are the upper arms or triceps, subscapular region (just below the shoulder blade), and upper abdomen.

specific rate A rate for a segment of the population, selected by age, race, sex, or other characteristic.

specificity (of a predictor or a screening test) The percentage of healthy persons (true noncases) correctly assessed by a negative report as healthy. Specificity = True negatives ÷ (True negatives + False positives).

standards Professionally developed statements for the level of performance for health care.

standard of performance The prescribed amount and quality of accomplishment, an accepted yardstick with which performance can be measured. A standard of performance may be based on cost, the output of effort, or the public health effect of this effort.

standard or unit of measurement A known quantitative element or component of an operation that is recognized as a completed step process or action.

starvation Complete or partial deprivation of food for varying lengths of time; the resulting condition may be classified as mild, moderate, severe, or extreme.

state advisory groups A group formed of representatives of hospitals and other health care institutions as well as nonphysician health care practitioners who advise and assist statewide councils or, in states with no council, each PSRO with particular regard to nonphysician input and participation.

state government (See *government [state]*.)

Statewide Professional Standards Review Council A group of physicians and public representatives formed in states that have three or more PSROs to coordinate activities of PSROs within that state, disseminate information to PSROs within that state, and review PSRO performance.

Statewide PSRO support centers Centers awarded contracts by DHEW to furnish educational, organizational, administrative, and professional assistance to applicants or designated planning, conditional, or operational PSROs within a state.

stipend A payment made to an individual under a fellowship or training grant in accordance with preestablished levels. Such payments are intended to provide for the individual's living expenses during the period of training.

surveillance The process of gathering routine data for the purpose of identifying and responding to problems. As contrasted to survey, implies continuity, a frequent and continuous "watching over."

techniques The specific skills required for the performance of a specific operation or function.

terms and conditions All legal requirements imposed on a grant by the federal government, whether by statute, regulations, the grant award document itself, or other documents.

tertiary care Services are provided by highly specialized providers (e.g., neurologists, neurosurgeons, thoracic surgeons, intensive care units). Such services frequently require highly sophisticated technologic and support facilities. The development of these services has largely been a function of diagnostic and therapeutic advances attained through basic and clinical biomedical research.

threshold for action The point at which, looking at a specific group of patients, one would become anxious about the quality of care they are receiving and would be willing to mobilize resources to take major action for change.

Title V, Social Security Act This title authorizes health programs for mothers and children, including maternity care, well child services, crippled children's service, training, and research. It is a federally supported, state operated program in which the state funds match or exceed the federal funds.

Title XVIII, Social Security Act This title, known as Medicare, authorizes the Social Security health insurance program. It is federally operated with funds contributed through the Social Security tax system.

Title XIX, Social Security Act This title authorizes a program of a wide range of benefits to needy persons. Among its provisions are a medical assistance program known as Medicaid for the indigent, aged, dependent children, and blind and permanently disabled persons. Other medically needy persons can be included. It is a state operated program, supported largely by federal funds.

tools of nutritional assessment Tools of individuals and population groups follow.

1. Biochemical measurements of nutrients in body fluids and tissues
2. Clinical examination including assessment of growth by utilizing body measurements
3. Collection of dietary information

Uniform Hospital Discharge Data Set (UHDDS) A discharge set based on the work done by the Uniform Abstract Subcommittee of the United States National Committee on Vital and Health Statistics, the Uniform Hospital Discharge Data Demonstration, and the work group on Uniform Hospitalization Data for DHEW programs. It is the minimum basic data anticipated to be used for judgments about elements of quality of care, such as patient management, planning and providing services, and claims processing.

undernutrition Inadequate intake of one or more nutrients and/or of calories. (The converse term "overnutrition" is not a recommended term.)

United States Department of Agriculture (USDA) Department of the federal government consisting of a Human Nutrition Research Division, experiment stations, and extension services, all of which are concerned with nutrition. These divisions carry out research and program services such as the Food Stamp Program and publish data on the nutritive value of common foods and information on the eating patterns of persons residing in the United States.

United States Department of Health, Education, and Welfare (HEW) Department of the federal government that has several agencies that deal with nutrition, such as the Maternal and Child Health Service, the Office of Education, the Food and Drug Administration, and the National Institutes of Health and its Public Health Services agency.

validity The degree to which the data actually assess the phenomenon of interest; the extent to which a situation as observed reflects the "true" situation, or the situation as evaluated by other criteria that are thought to reflect the true situation accurately.

veto Of Latin derivation, meaning "I forbid." The President is authorized by the Constitution to refuse his assent to any measure presented by Congress for his approval. In such case he returns the measure to the House in which it orig-inated, at the same time indicating his objections—the so-called veto message. The veto goes to the entire measure; the President is not authorized, as are the governors of some states, to veto separate items in a bill.

pocket veto By the Constitution the President is allowed 10 days (exclusive of Sundays) from the date of receiving a bill within which to give it his approval; if, within 10 days, Congress adjourns and so prevents the return of a bill to which the President objects, that bill does not become law. In many cases, where bills have been sent to him toward the close of a session, the President has taken advantage of this provision and has held until after adjournment measures of which he disapproved but which for some reason he did not wish to return with his objections to Congress for their further action. This action is the so-called pocket veto.

White House Conference on Food, Nutrition and Health As a result of the concern for hunger and malnutrition in the United States, a conference was held in December, 1969, in Washington, D.C. Its objectives were to advise the President and to create a national nutrition policy. The areas discussed at the conference included methods for continual evaluation of (1) the nutritional status of the American people; (2) nutritional needs of vulnerable groups such as children, pregnant and lactating women, adolescents, and the aged; (3) foods to meet the nutritional needs of the people; (4) nutrition education; and (5) the role of voluntary groups in improving the nutritional state of the people of the United States.

World Health Organization (WHO) International organization that aims to eliminate all kinds of diseases. In the field of nutrition, WHO has been involved in developing and testing new protein-rich foods; combating protein-calorie malnutrition, nutritional anemias, vitamin A deficiency, endemic goiter, and rickets; assessing nutritional status; determining nutritional requirements; and developing coordinated applied nutrition programs and training personnel for them. WHO was created in 1948 and is composed of about ninety member countries with headquarters in Geneva, Switzerland.

Recommended bookshelf for the community nutritionist*

BASIC NUTRITION BOOKS

Alfin-Slater, R., and Aftergood, L.: Nutrition for today, Dubuque, Iowa, 1973, William C. Brown Co., Publishers, 64 pp. (softcover, $1.25). Additives, calories, carbohydrates, fats, malnutrition, minerals, proteins, vitamins are included.

Arlin, M. T.: The science of nutrition, ed. 2, New York, 1977, The Macmillan Co., 462 pp. ($10.95). A physiologic approach to nutrition is emphasized; chapters on food supply and safety are included.

Bogert, L. J., Briggs, G. M., and Calloway, D. H.: Nutrition and physical fitness, ed. 9, (rev. ed. 1978), Philadelphia, 1973, W. B. Saunders Co. ($11.50). A comprehensive basic nutrition text; chapters on food habits and beliefs and food processing are included.

Clydesdale, F. M., and Francis, F. J.: Food, nutrition and you, Englewood Cliffs, N.J., 1977, Prentice-Hall, Inc., 248 pp. (hardcover, $9.95; softcover, $4.95). Basic nutrition and our food supply are examined along with additives, food fads, processing techniques, nutritive content, and regulations.

Deutsch, R. M.: Realities of nutrition, Palo Alto, Calif., 1976, Bull Publishing Co., 405 pp. ($9.95). A popularized approach exposes facts and fallacies and discusses the basis of present nutrition knowledge.

Guthrie, H. A.: Introductory nutrition, ed. 3, St.

Louis, 1975, The C. V. Mosby Co. ($13.95). The comprehensive coverage of basic nutrition also includes a discussion of contemporary concerns. (Edition 4, 1979, in preparation.)

Lamb, M. W., and Harden, M. L.: The meaning of human nutrition, Elmsford, N.Y., 1973, Pergamon Press, 284 pp. (softcover, $11.50). College texts, consumer aspects, diets, energy balance, nutrient functions, nutrient sources, nutritional status, programed instruction are included.

Mayer, J.: A diet for living, New York, 1975, David McKay Co., Inc., 293 pp. (hardcover, $8.95; softcover from Book Department, CO 36, Consumers Union, Orangeburg, N.Y. 10962, $4.50.) Numerous consumer questions about basic nutrition, weight problems, "healthy" foods, and buying and preparing foods are answered.

McNutt, K., and McNutt, D.: Nutrition and food choices, Palo Alto, Calif., 1978, Science Research Associates, Inc., 506 pp. ($12.95). Highlights the latest in nutritional research; emphasizes the relationship of nutrition and current life-styles; relates nutrition to the varying needs of individuals at different stages of their lives; explains technical processes in simple terms without sacrificing depth; stresses the relationship between diet and the prevention of illness.

McWilliams, M.: Nutrition for the growing years, ed. 2, New York, 1975, John Wiley & Sons, Inc., 452 pp. ($10.95). Basic nutrition and physical and mental development from conception through maturity and the special nutritional requirements of pregnancy, lactation, and the growing years are covered.

*Modified from Society for Nutrition: Nutrition information sources for the whole family, Berkeley, Calif., Jan., 1978, National Nutrition Education Clearing House.

Runyan, T. J.: Nutrition for today, New York, 1976, Harper & Row, Publishers, 472 pp. ($11.95). Health, nutrition, and contemporary issues are stressed.

Stare, F., and McWilliams, M.: Living nutrition, ed. 2, New York, 1977, John Wiley & Sons, Inc., 497 pp. ($12.95). Sociopsychological aspects of nutrition are explored along with basic information.

Whitney, E., and Hamilton, M.: Understanding nutrition, St. Paul, 1977, West Publishing Co., 607 pp. ($14.95). Understanding is stressed through explorations of contemporary issues related to the basic concepts of nutrition.

NUTRITION AND DIET THERAPY BOOKS

Robinson, C. H.: Basic nutrition and diet therapy, ed. 3, New York, 1975, The Macmillan Co., 369 pp. ($5.25).

Robinson, C., and Lawler, M.: Normal and therapeutic nutrition, ed. 17, New York, 1977, The Macmillan Co., 739 pp. ($12.95).

Mitchell, H. S., Rynbergen, H. J., Anderson, L., and Dibble, M. V.: Nutrition in health and disease, ed. 16, Philadelphia, 1976, J. B. Lippincott Co., 652 pp. ($14.50).

Williams, S. R.: Mowry's basic nutrition and diet therapy, ed. 5, St. Louis, 1975, The C. V. Mosby Co., 215 pp. (softcover, $5.95).

Williams, S. R.: Nutrition and diet therapy, ed. 3, St. Louis, 1977, The C. V. Mosby Co., 723 pp. ($12.75).

ADVANCED AND SPECIALIZED BOOKS

Fomon, S. J.: Infant nutrition, ed. 2, Philadelphia, 1974, W. B. Saunders, Co., 575 pp. ($22.50). This comprehensive review of the literature and history of infant feeding includes data on food patterns, nutrient intake and retention, growth, gastrointestinal function, methods of measurement and determinations, nutritional problems, and status determinations.

Gifft, H. H., Washbon, M. B., and Harrison, G. G.: Nutrition, behavior and change, Englewood Cliffs, N.J., Prentice-Hall, Inc., 1972, 392 pp. ($9.95). Factors that influence food habits and food consumption patterns and the results of those patterns are explored.

Goodhart, R. S., and Shils, M. F.: Modern nutrition in health and disease: dietotherapy, ed. 5, Philadelphia, 1973, Lea & Febiger, 1153 pp. ($35.00). Each chapter of this advanced text on nutrition and dietotherapy is written by a leading authority and includes an extensive bibliography.

Hafen, B. Q., editor: Overweight and obesity: causes, fallacies, treatment, Provo, 1975, Brigham Young University Press, 410 pp. (softcover, $6.95). Seventy-five previously published essays and research papers on the etiology and treatment of obesity comprise this basic reference.

Lowenberg, M. E., Todhunter, E. N., Wilson, E. D., Savage, J. R., and Lubawski, J. L.: Food and man, ed. 2, New York, 1974, John Wiley & Sons, Inc. ($11.50). This book traces the importance of food in man's history.

Mason, M., Wenberg, B. G., and Welsch, P. K.: The dynamics of clinical dietetics, New York, 1977, John Wiley & Sons, 137 pp. ($11.95). Text designed to prepare dietetic professionals for careers in clinical dietetics. Teaches skills necessary for nutritional counseling and educating the patient concerning foods that meet his nutritional needs.

McLaren, D. S., editor: Nutrition in the community: a text for public health workers, New York, 1976, John Wiley & Sons, 391 pp. ($28.50). This multi-author collection of papers discusses community nutrition problems, e.g., the diagnosis, nature, complexity, or intervention needed for solutions.

Nutrition Reviews' Present knowledge in nutrition, ed. 4, Washington, D.C., 1976, The Nutrition Foundation, Inc., 624 pp. (softcover, $6.95). A collection of reviews written by leading authorities that discusses recent advances in specialized interest areas. Excellent bibliographies complete each chapter.

Pike, R., and Brown, M.: Nutrition: an integrated approach, ed. 2, New York, 1975, John Wiley & Sons, Inc., 1082 pp. ($18.95). This advanced nutrition text offers a more detailed biochemical and physiologic background.

Rockstein, M., and Sussman, M. L., editors: Nutrition, longevity and aging, New York, 1976, Academic Press Inc., 284 pp. ($15.50). This collection of papers reviews studies of physical and biochemical changes that occur with aging and the role of nutrition.

Schneider, H. A., Anderson, C. E., and Coursin, D. B.: Nutritional support of medical practice, New York, 1977, Harper & Row, Publishers, 555 pp. ($25.00). A core of information on basic nutrition and diet therapy is presented in addition to nutrition information as it relates to specific medical specialties.

Serban, G., editor: Nutrition and mental functions, New York, 1975, Plenum Publishing Corp., 281 pp. ($22.50). The structural, biochemical, and behavioral effects of malnutrition in various experimental animals, the antecedents and sequelae of malnutrition in children, and the presumed relation between vitamin nutrition and illness are the three major areas of presentation in this collection of papers.

Thiele, V. F.: Clinical nutrition, St. Louis, 1976, The C. V. Mosby Co., 225 pp. (softcover, $6.95). Past and current diet therapy practices as well as useful basic data are included in this reference manual.

Winick, M.: Malnutrition and brain development, New York, 1976, Oxford University Press, 169 pp. ($9.95). A review of the most important animal and human studies that give evidence of the consequences of malnutrition to brain development are discussed.

OTHER BOOKS OF INTEREST

Abelson, P. H., editor: Food: politics, economics, nutrition and research, Washington, D.C., 1975, American Association for the Advancement of Science, (hardcover, $12.95; softcover, $4.95). World food supply, trends in agricultural practices, climatic trends, energy and water usage, and plant research are some of the topics discussed in this collection of articles by various authors on current food problems.

Deutsch, R. M.: The new nuts among the berries, Palo Alto, Calif., 1977, Bull Publishing Co., 359 pp. (hardcover, $9.95; softcover, $4.95). New and old dietary fads and their promoters and followers are documented.

Food and agriculture, a Scientific American book, San Francisco, 1976, W. H. Freeman & Co., Publishers, 154 pp. (hardcover, $9; softcover, $4.95). Food problems, human requirements, sources of food, agricultural systems, resources available, and agriculture in the developing countries are a few of the topics covered by well-known scientists.

Galton, L.: The truth about fiber in your food, New York, 1976, Crown Publishers, Inc., 246 pp. ($8.95). This book details the scientific thinking that has led to the belief by some that lack of fiber may be responsible for many present health problems. Tables of the crude fiber content in foods are given.

Lappe, F. M.: Diet for a small planet, Westminster, Md., 1975, Ballantine Books, 411 pp. ($1.95). Alternatives to eating animal protein are discussed, and useful information is given on complementing plant proteins to assure a balanced essential amino acid intake. This is a good reference for the vegetarian.

Lappe, F. M., and Collins, J.: Food first—beyond the myth of scarcity, Boston, 1977, Houghton Mifflin Co., 466 pp. ($10.95). The causes of hunger throughout the developing countries are discussed, and land reform is the major solution offered.

National Nutrition Consortium, Inc., with Deutsch, R. M.: Nutrition labeling: how it can work for you, Nutrition Labeling, P.O. Box 4110, Kankakee, Ill., 60901, 1975, 134 pp. (softcover, $2.00). A guide to learning and understanding the science and the law of nutrition labeling is written in a popular style.

Robertson, L., Flinders, C., and Godfrey, B.: Laurel's kitchen: a handbook for vegetarian cookery and nutrition, Petaluma, Calif., 1976, Nilgiri Press, 508 pp. ($12.95). Nutrition basics, the nutrient content of foods, recipes, and menus for the vegetarian are discussed.

DICTIONARIES

Dorland's medical dictionary, Philadelphia, latest edition, W. B. Saunders Co.

Webster's new world dictionary of the American language, New York, latest edition, World Publishing Co.

JOURNALS
Recommended nutrition journals

American Journal of Clinical Nutrition, published monthly by the American Society for Clinical Nutrition, Inc., 9650 Rockville Pike, Bethesda, Md. 20014 ($30.00 annually).

Ecology of Food and Nutrition, published quarterly by Gordon and Breach Science Publishers, 1 Park Ave., New York, N.Y. 10016 ($38.00 annually).

Journal of the American Dietetic Association, published monthly by The American Dietetic Association, 430 North Michigan Ave., Chicago, Ill. 60611 ($24.00 annually).

Journal of Nutrition, published monthly by the American Institute of Nutrition, 9650 Rockville Pike, Bethesda, Md. 20014 ($38.00 annually).

Journal of Nutrition Education, published quarterly by the Society of Nutrition Education, 2140 Shattuck Ave., Suite 1110, Berkeley, Calif. 94704 ($12.00 annually).

Nutrition Abstracts and Reviews, published quarterly by the Commonwealth Agricultural Bureau, Farnham Royal, Slough, SL2 3BN, England (prices vary; current volume, $143.00).

Nutrition Reviews, published monthly by The Nutrition Foundation, Inc., 489 Fifth Ave., New York, N.Y. 10017 ($12.00 annually).

Nutrition Today, published bimonthly by Nutrition Today Society, Director of Circulation, Box 1829, Annapolis, Md. 21404 ($3.00 per copy).

Proceedings of the Nutrition Society, published three times a year by the Cambridge University Press for The Nutrition Society (U.K.), 32 East 57th St., New York, N.Y. 10022 (American Branch) ($30.00 annually).

Other journals

American Journal of Obstetrics and Gynecology, published semimonthly by The C. V. Mosby Co., 11830 Westline Industrial Dr., St. Louis, Mo. 63141 ($30.00 annually).

American Journal of Public Health, published monthly by The American Public Health Association, Inc., 1015 Eighteenth St., N.W., Washington, D.C. 20036 ($30.00 annually).

Clinical Pediatrics, published monthly by J. B. Lippincott Co., East Washington Square, Philadelphia, Pa. 19105 ($18.50 annually).

Federation Proceedings, published monthly by the Federation of American Societies for Experimental Biology (American Institute of Nutrition), 9650 Rockville Pike, Bethesda, Md. 20014 ($40.00 annually).

Food Technology, published monthly by the Institute of Food Technologists, Suite 2120, 221 N. LaSalle St., Chicago, Ill. 60601 ($30.00 annually).

Geriatrics, published monthly by Lancet Publications, Inc., 4015 W. 65th St., Minneapolis, Minn. 55435 ($15.00 annually).

Home Economics Research Journal, published quarterly by the American Home Economics Association, 2010 Massachusetts Ave., N.W., Washington, D.C. 20036 ($15.00 annually).

Journal of The American Dental Association, published monthly by the American Dental Association, 211 E. Chicago Ave., Chicago, Ill. 60611 ($15.00 annually).

Journal of The American Medical Association, published weekly by The American Medical Association, 535 N. Dearborn St., Chicago, Ill. 60610 ($30.00 annually).

Journal of Home Economics, published bimonthly by the American Home Economics Association, 2010 Massachusetts Ave., N.W., Washington, D.C. 20036 ($13.00 annually).

Journal of Pediatrics, published monthly by The C. V. Mosby Co., 11830 Westline Industrial Dr., St. Louis, Mo. 63141 ($22.50 annually).

Journal of School Health, published ten times a year by The American School Health Association, P.O. Box 708, Kent, Ohio 44240 ($25.00 annually).

Lancet, published weekly by Little, Brown & Co., Inc., 34 Beacon St., Boston, Mass. 02106 ($30.00 annually).

New England Journal of Medicine, published weekly by the Massachusetts Medical Society, 10 Shattuck, Boston, Mass. 02115 ($22.00 annually).

Pediatrics, published monthly by The American Academy of Pediatrics, P.O. Box 1034, Evanston, Ill. 60204 ($21.00 annually).

School Foodservice Journal, published ten times a year by the American School Food Service Association, 4101 East Iliff Ave., Denver, Colo. 80222 ($20.00 annually).

School Foodservice Research Review, published twice a year by American School Food Service Association, 4104 East Iliff Ave., Denver, Colo. 80222 ($5.00 annually).

Science, published weekly by the American Association for the Advancement of Science, 1515 Massachusetts Ave., N.W., Washington, D.C. 20005 ($50.00 annually).

PERIODICALS

CNI Weekly Report, published weekly by the Community Nutrition Institute, 1910 K St., N.W., Washington, D.C. 20006 ($25.00 annually).

Nutrition Action, published monthly by the Center for Science in the Public Interest, 1755 S St., N.W., Washington, D.C. 20009 ($10.00 annually).

Nutrition and the M.D., published monthly, P.O. Box 4128, North Hollywood, Calif. 91607 ($26.00 annually).

PAMPHLETS—BASIC REFERENCES

Nutritive value of American foods in common units, Washington, D.C. 1975, Agriculture Handbook no. 456, Government Printing Office ($5.15).

Handbook of food preparation, ed. 7, Washington, D.C., 1975, American Home Economics Association ($4.00).

Recommended dietary allowances, ed. 8, Washington, D.C., 1974, National Academy of Sciences ($2.50).

PROFESSIONAL ASSOCIATIONS

National Academy of Sciences, 2101 Constitution Ave., Washington, D.C. 20418.

The American Dental Association, 211 E. Chicago Ave., Chicago, Ill. 60611.

The American Dietetic Association, 430 N. Michigan Ave., Chicago, Ill. 60611.

The American Home Economics Association, 2010 Massachusetts Ave., N.W., Washington, D.C. 20036.

The American Institute of Nutrition, 9650 Rockville Pike, Bethesda, Md. 20014.

The American Medical Association, 535 N. Dearborn St., Chicago, Ill. 60610.

The American Public Health Association, 1015 Eighteenth St., N.W., Washington, D.C. 20036.

The American School Food Service Association, 4101 East Iliff Ave., Denver, Colo. 80222.

The Society for Nutrition Education, 2140 Shattuck Ave., Suite 1110, Berkeley, Calif. 94704.

VOLUNTARY HEALTH ORGANIZATIONS

The American Diabetes Association, 18 E. 48th St., New York, N.Y. 10020.

The American Heart Association, 7320 Greenville Ave., Dallas, Texas 75231.

The National Foundation/March of Dimes, Box 2000, White Plains, N.Y. 10605.

Index

Boldface page numbers indicate main discussions; italics, illustrations; t, tables; n, footnotes.